RACE, PLACE, AND MEDICINE

RACE, PLACE, AND MEDICINE

The Idea of the Tropics in Nineteenth-Century

Brazilian Medicine

Julyan G. Peard

Duke University Press   Durham and London   1999

© 1999 Duke University Press

All rights reserved

Printed in the United States of America on acid-free paper ∞

Typeset in Carter & Cone Galliard by Tseng Information Systems, Inc.

Library of Congress Cataloging-in-Publication Data appear

on the last printed page of this book.

For Lalo and Maxine

CONTENTS

ACKNOWLEDGMENTS

In researching and writing this book I have become indebted to many people. Kátia M. de Queirós Mattoso first told me about the Bahian doctors when she was a visiting professor at Columbia University many years ago. In Salvador, Maria José Rabello de Freitas, then Director of the Memorial da Medicina, and historian Consuelo Pondé de Sena were particularly helpful in locating sources and directing me to various archives in the city. I also used sources from the collections at the National Library of Medicine at Bethesda, the Health Sciences Library at Columbia, the National Academy of Medicine, New York, and the Paul and Lydia Kalmanovitz Library at the University of California at San Francisco. I would like to thank the librarians at all these institutions for their invaluable help.

My research was funded in part by a fellowship from the American Council of Learned Societies in 1996, a Travel to Collections grant and a summer stipend from the National Endowment for the Humanities in 1992 and 1995, a San Francisco State University Affirmative Action Award in 1992, and a Sabbatical Grant in 1998. I am deeply grateful to all these institutions. Parts of chapters 1, 2, and 3 appeared as "Tropical Medicine in Nineteenth-Century Brazil: The Case of the 'Escola Tropicalista Bahiana,' 1860–1890," in *Warm Climates and Western Medicine: The Emergence of Tropical Medicine, 1500–1900,* ed. David Arnold (Amsterdam: Rodopi, 1996) 108–32; and "Tropical Disorders and the Forging of a Brazilian Medical Identity, 1860–1890," *Hispanic American Historical Review* 77 (1997): 1–44.

I would especially like to thank Nancy Leys Stepan, who always provided intellectual support and strong encouragement; Herbert Klein, who kept on prodding me to get the project finished; Marcos Cueto, who was always willing to help me with sources and contacts; and Günter Risse, who generously asked me to join the Thursday sessions of the History of Medicine Seminar at the University of California at San Francisco. I would also like to thank the anonymous reviewers who read the manuscript closely and made many useful suggestions and the meticulous editors at Duke University Press. Responsibility for the final contents is of course mine.

INTRODUCTION

In what terms were the nineteenth-century elites of the new Latin American nations, like Brazil, to define their relationship with the Europeans? When Europeans talked of "we" as opposed to "they," where were Latin Americans to situate themselves? How could Latin Americans resist European racial and cultural notions of inferiority? This book explores the development of early tropical medicine in Brazil as an attempt to grapple with such questions. It considers the history of a group of nineteenth-century doctors in Brazil, known as the Escola Tropicalista Bahiana, who, in attempting to adapt Western medicine to more fully engage with the problems of their tropical country, sought novel answers to the age-old question of whether the diseases of warm climates were distinct from those of temperate Europe. In their search, they used the tools of Western medicine to confront European ideas about the fatalism of the tropics and its people, and to argue in favor of Brazilian expertise.[1]

The Escola Tropicalista Bahiana, an informal school formed by about thirty Brazilian and a handful of foreign physicians, made new discoveries in parasitology, contributed to ongoing debates on beriberi, leprosy, and parasitological disorders, and helped reformulate the then accepted pattern of Brazilian nosology, questioning whether Europeans really knew more about Brazilian health problems than they themselves did. The Tropicalistas practiced in Salvador da Bahia, one of two cities in nineteenth-century Brazil with state-funded medical schools. As a medical center, Bahia was second to that of the capital city, Rio de Janeiro, where more doctors were trained, the medical school was more generously funded, and the government honored its doctors more highly. In spite of this, the Bahian Tropicalistas founded the most successful privately financed medical journal in nineteenth-century Latin America, a prestigious publication widely quoted in the European medical press and a trendsetter for later Brazilian medical journals seeking to highlight Brazil's distinctive medical contribution.

One of the most significant aspects of the Escola Tropicalista Bahiana was that it started in the 1860s before the bacteriological revolution and the great push in European colonial expansion, and several decades before the institutionalization of tropical medicine by European powers.[2] I use this early attempt to take Brazilian preoccupations as a starting point—an attempt that differed significantly from the tropical medicine developed into a specialization by European colonial powers and imported into Brazil at the turn of the century—to frame the idea of illness in the tropics. In looking at this neglected episode in Latin American history, I draw on insights and theoretical orientations advanced in the last twenty years by historians of medicine and culture.

A central theoretical orientation informing my work comes from the new history of medicine that views medicine as a site of complex social interactions rather than one of universal biological truths. What especially interests me is the problem of European medical authority within nineteenth-century Latin America; that is, what happens when knowledge produced in a particular social milieu is transferred to a different set of social conditions? Just as the new scholarship has made it clear that disease and medicine are never wholly biological, so historians of medicine and of science have become increasingly aware that the transfer of Western science involves far more than simply transplanting and importing ideas. The specific social and cultural framework within which Western ideas are received and modified are crucial determining forces on the final outcome of those ideas, and the historian must grapple with all of these factors in seeking to understand how scientific ideas are recast in new social environments. This is a key research problem in the agenda of the new Latin American history of medicine and public health.[3]

Once we question the transparency of medical truth, how medical authority is constituted has to be explained. Given the long cultural relationship between nineteenth-century Latin America and Europe, it was inevitable that Western medicine, particularly that of France, would dominate the region.[4] However, the shaping of that authority was neither automatic nor devoid of historical interest. To dismiss Latin American physicians as passive imitators of European medical science and, indeed, of science in general is to gloss over the nuanced shifts in the history of Western medical authority in Latin America, and to ignore the ways in which Latin Americans tried to assert their own authority and challenge European cultural hegemony. In the first half of the nineteenth century, imitation was a strategy that many Latin Americans adopted for resolving anxieties central to the new nations. The outer replication of European social, cultural, and political institutions was a sign of continuity with Latin America's own colonial past and a way of demonstrating the Latin American proximity to the Europeans in the pageant of civilization. It was also an admission, born of cultural insecurity, that there was only one path to civilization and that the Europeans led the way. But after midcentury, some individuals, like the Tropicalistas, dared to question such assumptions. Their call for originality should be understood as an attempt to claim that there could be more than one path to knowledge, and that Latin Americans must make their own original contributions. It did not matter that the idea of "originality" was itself imported from the European repertoire; what was important was that the idea provided an inspiration to reframe European cultural authority. Like Europeans, the Tropicalistas believed in science, but they looked to science produced in the tropics, about the tropics, to help them confront what they saw as the distinctive problems of the torrid zone. At stake were competing constructs of the idea of the nation, of the caliber of the people, of the possibilities for improvement, and of where the boundaries within the nation should be set.

The difficulty for the Tropicalistas, as for many other scientists and intellectuals in nineteenth-century Latin America, was that although they resisted aspects of European cultural authority that harped on Brazilian, and Latin American, inferiority, they wanted to gain the mantle of legitimacy that they believed only European science, as the leader in universal science, could bestow on them. I argue that this tension was central to the Tropicalistas' medical theories and research, and that the ways in which they used their medical facts and the manner in which they selected, adapted, and rejected aspects of European science were born not of ignorance of European advances in medicine, nor of incompetence, but were closely related to the peculiar ideological, political, and cultural requirements of their society. Thus, although the Tropicalistas' medical science had much to do with nineteenth-century medical knowledge, it was also informed by the fact that the doctors, who were actors in a slave nation and citizens of a country where most residents were of African descent, were anxious to project and believe in an image of progress and civilization in the tropics. That is, this book is about an aspect in the transference of nineteenth-century medical ideas, ideas that, when modified for the Latin American context, served to underwrite Brazilian definitions of national identity.[5]

The recent literature on the rise of tropical medicine has been crucial to my study of the Tropicalistas.[6] My work contributes to the many-sided prism emerging as a truer image of early tropical medicine than the initial model of a medicine created by Europeans and transported outward to rule empires. The idea of tropical medicine stems from the recognition that, as Patrick Manson, the father of tropical medicine, put it, "a number of diseases are peculiar to, if not confined to, warm climates."[7] Beyond the idea of the relationship of place and disease, however, tropical medicine is often blurred and for more than a century has been the site of competing and conflicting definitions that range from viewing tropical medicine as primarily concerned with geographically specific disorders to seeing it as more related to the diseases of poverty and underdevelopment.[8] Historically, there is also the problem of where to place illnesses like malaria, cholera, and leprosy, once prominent in temperate climates but today associated with tropical regions. I focus on a region of the world hardly studied in this new context and concentrate on the early stage of tropical medicine when nineteenth-century doctors, moving beyond a concern with naval medicine and the nutritional problems of long sea voyages, began to probe the notion that there might be something special about tropical pathology.[9] In the last two decades, historians of medicine have noted how the rise of tropical medicine as an important specialty within Western medicine occurred around the turn of the nineteenth century, when ancient notions about the relevance of geography and climate to disease were, in a sense, reinvigorated by discoveries in bacteriology and the rapid advances in parasitology. During these years, doctor-scientists came to understand that the tropics provided the environment necessary for the complex propagation—often via vectors such as insects—of microorganisms, leading to specific disorders upon entry into a human host.[10]

Originally, in the telling of this history, traditional historians reconstructed a more or less unbroken chain of ideas and discoveries leading to the unraveling of the causes of numerous illnesses. The heroic protagonist in the story was Western science; its disciples, the committed doctor-scientists, a few of whom risked everything by spending long stints investigating in the tropics.[11] More recently, historians of medicine, arguing that the significance and visibility of disease in any society is always interwoven with cultural strands into historically specific textures, have turned away from such internally coherent and triumphant accounts of medical conquest to explore, instead, the social and political contexts of medical knowledge and practice.[12] In the case of tropical medicine, they have moved beyond explaining its rise purely in terms of the germ theory of disease. Rather, they have analyzed it within the setting of European empire and colonialism and have pointed to the 1890s—the decade of the great scramble for "a place in the sun"—as, not coincidentally, the decade leading to the founding of the first tropical schools of medicine in Europe. They have traced the ways in which the rise of tropical medicine furthered the purposes of the colonial powers by helping to promote the health of white administrator and native worker, by reinforcing the image of the white man as a wielder of superior knowledge, and by providing a "scientific" justification for policies of population segregation.[13] Others have asked whether the much trumpeted miracle of Western medicine was not put to work more on diseases created by colonialism than on native endemic illness.[14] Lately, historians have noted the stresses in the hegemonic depiction of tropical medicine as a "tool of empire." For example, they have looked at the ways in which indigenous people actively participated in shaping Western tropical medicine in their localities, and at the ideological conflicts among colonial administrators, providing a rather more "messy" and less formidable view of colonial tropical medicine.[15] Aside from their diverse emphases and perspectives, all of these accounts agree that the successful incorporation of tropical medicine as a new specialty within the bastion of traditional Western medicine had as much to do with considerations of political and social power as with questions of biological discovery.

My book adds to this more complicated idea of tropical medicine by inserting Brazil into the history of the emergence of tropical medicine and arguing that the Tropicalistas were part of a generation that attempted to frame a distinct tropical medicine for national reasons—not, like the leading European powers, for reasons of colonial expansion—and that in contrast to the model of tropical medicine developed by the European colonial powers that tended to perpetuate stereotypes of passive and unhealthy natives of the tropics, they forged their own definition of tropical medicine. For Brazilian doctors the production of a national medicine was a way of contesting European medicine's social construction of tropical disorders, which was largely detrimental to the notion of Brazil as a healthy country.

European analyses of the disorders of tropical climates in the nineteenth century assumed the climates had negative consequences for the dwellers of those regions. The effects of hot climates were believed to be so powerful that they not only left doctors practicing in the tropics bereft of real agency but dimmed the hopes of the new Latin American elites for the transformation of their countries into progressive, healthy, and civilized nations. It was around this problematic that the Escola Tropicalista Bahiana organized itself. At the heart of its model stood a malleable notion about the possibility of human melioration and a belief about the relation between social conditions and illness.

My history of the Escola Tropicalista Bahiana has also drawn on the interdisciplinary work of cultural historians, anthropologists, and literary critics who have focused on colonial and postcolonial discourse and viewed nations as "socially engineered" artifacts of modernity.[16] Within the history of European imperial expansion there now exists an impressive body of work analyzing European representations of the exotic "other," representations that, it is argued, became constituent elements in systems of knowledge fundamental to European imperial domination. The case of Latin America has been less studied in this way, although it offers a fascinating counterpoint to existing studies of European colonialism.[17] The new nations of Latin America were forging the contours of their nationhood in the image of Europe at precisely the time when the leading European powers were expanding their imperialistic quest. Within the context of these two broad, and sometimes clashing, processes, Latin Americans had to reformulate their relationship to Europe. I refer here not to an economic relationship—which has been much studied—but to a cultural rethinking. The Latin American elites saw themselves as European, yet they were not *of* Europe; they defined themselves as white, and yet their ranks included mulatto and mestizo; they lived in the tropics, which Europeans held to be a degenerating place, especially for whites, yet they believed their destiny was more than one of decay.[18] Would Europeans accept the Latin Americans as their equals? European narratives about countries like Brazil seemed to answer in negative terms.

In trying to situate themselves vis-à-vis Europeans, the Brazilian elites, like other Latin American elites, were forced to look inward, defining and identifying social groups and making decisions about the role of those groups within the nations being constructed. How could the racially heterogeneous Latin Americans, the hybridized and often ignorant and superstitious descendants of Indians, African slaves, and Europeans, be molded into a homogeneously modern nation that could be seen as the equal of a European nation? One of the most interesting aspects of the Latin American case, and where it can most contribute to the existing literature of colonial discourse, concerns the way in which Latin Americans substituted the Europeans' sharp cleavages between the civilized and the primitive by blurring and shifting boundaries.[19] The idea of "whitening," for example, both in its biological and cultural forms, is a particularly Latin American, and Brazilian, solution to the problem. The history of the Escola Tropicalista Bahiana, which used its medical theory to suggest ways in which Brazilians could be remolded for a modern nation, is one example of the negotiation of such boundaries.

For Brazil, a further and related problem was the question of slavery, which lasted until 1888. The institution sailed through Brazil's assertion of independence from Portugal in 1822 virtually unscathed.[20] Here, as in the rest of the new Latin American nations forged by a *mazombo* upper class, popular nationalism was a force largely absent in the nineteenth century.[21] Unsurprisingly, the Latin American elites did not consider incorporating a majority of the population as citizens within the new nations in an attempt to redress the colonial legacies of poverty and backwardness. But, while many of the Spanish American nations passed laws to abolish slavery either immediately or gradually, Brazil retained the institution as the centerpiece of its economy.[22] In the second half of the century, slavery became the burning issue confronting the Brazilian intelligentsia. At a time of growing acceptance within Brazil of positivism and social Darwinism—with their categories of evolution and a hierarchy of nations—Brazilians had to face the fact that in the European mind, slavery was one of the measures of their backwardness. Although slavery was not abolished until 1888, the most prescient Brazilians recognized the crisis of the institution as early as 1850, when the Atlantic slave trade was outlawed in Brazil. The crisis was further underscored by events in the United States; until the American Civil War resulted in the abolition of slavery, Brazil had clung to the United States as a model illustrating the possibility of modern progress *and* slavery.[23] For those members of the intelligentsia who looked beyond the immediate political problems posed by slavery to long-term questions about the nation, the continued existence of slavery exacerbated the worry about the mixed racial character of the Brazilian people. Brazil's near defeat in the Paraguayan War (1865–70), a war fought against a smaller, poorer nation, confirmed their worst fears that the Brazilian people were unfit, which did not bode well for the transformation of Brazil into a modern nation in the tropics. The final decades of the century witnessed an urgent debate among the Brazilian upper class concerning the improvement of Brazil's racial stock and the modernization of society.[24]

The debate was directed to two audiences: one external to Brazil; the other, internal. For Europeans, the Brazilian intelligentsia attempted to redefine the idea of Brazil, shedding it of exoticisms and inevitable backwardness. For Brazilians, the intelligentsia tried to weld together in a European ideal of nation an area of varied ethnic groups and racial mixtures, of huge class differences, with divisive local traditions of dispersed, unconnected geographical regions and economies more closely linked to the European than to each others. What unifying tale of national identity could be told?

The ruling groups took what they saw as the typical nation-building steps of the era. They counted populations, they clarified and protected frontiers, they set up state schools, they built railroads, they sponsored national literature, they funded scientific journals, they set up a national army, they trained a national bureaucracy, they discussed in often heated tones which institutions should be abolished or drastically reformed. But underlying the business of nation building remained the negative definition of Brazil as a country whose place and race situated it, in many ways, closer to the "barbarous" than the civilized nations. Doctors played a central role in the process of "debarbarizing" Brazil.[25] They argued that the doctor's task was to help count, measure, and cleanse populations, to weld fragmented groups into the fold of the civilized nation by entering all houses to cure and to counsel in prevention, to improve the health and vigor of the young by, for example, extending the realm of modern obstetrics.

The Tropicalistas approved of all these enlarged roles for Brazilian doctors and went one step further by demanding that the physician in Brazil study the importance of the effects of a hot climate in order to understand illness in that country. The Brazilian doctor, they believed, should make the disorders of warm climates his specialization and, in doing so, use the tools of the emerging laboratory medicine. Central to his task was to show that illness in Brazil was not the result of some ill-defined, ubiquitous tropical miasma, but that it could be scientifically traced to specific causes and combated through sanitation, social reforms, and a scientific approach to medicine. Above all, physicians like the Tropicalistas believed they could show the world that the barriers to health in Brazil were no more formidable than in any other country or region of the world, including Western Europe, and that there was nothing in the tropical climate that led inevitably and irreversibly to physical, mental, or moral decay. Thus, unlike European doctors who often saw the diseases of the tropics as medical facts that underscored the inherent differences of the natives of temperate zones and the natives of the tropics, the Tropicalistas maintained that neither climate nor race was in itself a barrier to progress—obstacles, perhaps, but not obstacles that human science and wise government could not overcome.

The Tropicalistas were of central importance in constructing the idea of a progressive Brazilian nation because they could make recommendations for improving the health of all classes of Brazilians and, more crucially, because they provided conceptual tools with which the national intelligentsia could resist derogatory labels of difference and inferiority produced by European scientific and medical discourse. When they argued that understanding the disorders of Brazil was really no different from understanding the disorders of temperate Europe, they appealed to those members of the Brazilian elite struggling to assert that although Brazilians were racially mixed and natives of the tropics, this merely made them different from Europeans, neither better nor worse. By the end of the century some Brazilian doctors, extrapolating from Tropicalista arguments and echoing themes raised by other intellectuals, especially literary critics, went so far as to assert that through hybridization and acclimatization, Brazilians had evolved as the "race" best adapted to live and work in the tropics, the one that offered the best promise of an advanced tropical civilization.[26]

Another key problem for nineteenth-century nation builders in Latin America was the articulation of central and regional authority, each crucial but essentially antagonistic parts of the nation. In Latin American history, this articulation has usually been viewed through political and economic processes. The story of the Tropicalistas provides a nuanced and as yet almost wholly unexplored medical perspective for understanding this articulation, particularly that of a provincial city, Salvador, with the imperial center, Rio de Janeiro. For example, when the Tropicalistas selected and used their European sources differently from the way in which the medical leaders in Rio de Janeiro did, criticizing older French models of environmentalism and praising instead the new German medical sciences, they were subtly critiquing the Brazilian status quo in medicine. Thus, armed with their microscopes and home laboratories, experimenting with animals, networking with other similarly geographically isolated doctor-scientists working in warm climates, the Tropicalistas confronted the Rio de Janeiro community where the French hygiene movement of the early nineteenth century and naked-eye pathological anatomy still centrally informed medical practice. The Bahian doctors' effrontery can be fully grasped only within the context of both old and new medical knowledge and the political confrontation of regions, rivals, and constituencies within the Brazilian nation. In this sense, the Tropicalistas provide a fascinating new layer to the history of the turbulence of ideas in the final decades of the Brazilian Empire, and to the intricate intertwining of politics, culture, and knowledge during the period. Above all, they represented a new conception of "Brazilianized" medicine that challenged the medical establishment's idea of what Brazilian medicine should be. In addition, their story shows how, in this instance, the flow of ideas was from the northeast to the south, placing my work within a recent trend in Brazilian historiography that has begun to redress the balance of historical scholarship between the south and northeast regions of Brazil and to question histories that subsume change in the northeast within the transformations of southern Brazil.

Within Latin American historiography more broadly, my book contributes to the small but fast-growing body of literature on the history of medicine in Latin America, recently reinvigorated by historians bringing to the field lessons learned and questions raised by the debates in the history of medicine and culture in the United States and Europe. This burgeoning field has been called the "new" history of medicine and public health in Latin America because, like its counterparts in the United States and Europe, it is no longer dominated by older physicians writing about heroes in their field but, rather, by social and cultural historians. Indeed, the history of medicine, which used to be a sideline in Latin American history, is now becoming one of the most innovative ways of looking at old problems in new ways. Questions about race, gender, the relationship between state and individual rights, the transference of scientific ideas, popular movements, resistance, and the forging of national identities, to mention but a few, are all research areas that have been significantly enriched by historians using the methodologies and insights of the new history of medicine. My work fits squarely within this expanding area of investigation in Latin American history.[27]

Finally, my work is part of a shift in Latin American history away from the focus on issues of development and economic domination within a world capitalist system.²⁸ This important scholarship has led to the rich vein in Latin American scholarship concerning such broad questions as the ways in which the structures of European and Latin American markets and labor forces were interlocked.²⁹ This has meant that the dominant trend in historical methodology in Latin America has been materialist, to the detriment of cultural and ideological concerns. The balance is now being redressed.³⁰ This book, like the new medical history in Latin America, is an attempt to explore new directions in Latin American history.

Chapter 1 provides the historical context within which to understand the impact and novelty of the Tropicalistas. Formal medical teaching in Brazil, and thus the establishment of Brazilian medical communities, began after 1808, when the Portuguese Crown set up medical schools in Rio de Janeiro and Salvador da Bahia. In the first half of the nineteenth century, medical ideas and practice in Brazil were marked by conformity and replication of Western medicine, particularly French. Essentially, medicine in Brazil was Western medicine transported to a warm region; there was little distinctive about it. Neither in Rio de Janeiro nor in Bahia was there any encouragement of innovation; conformity won promotions, not challenge. In the 1860s, the Tropicalistas emerged in Salvador da Bahia in opposition to the medical status quo in Brazil, making new discoveries about the hookworm, filaria, ainhum, beriberi, and dracunculiasis. I give an account of the school's main founding figures and of the group's early development, showing how its members, although without an official framework from which to operate, managed to carve out an institutional base from where they negotiated a new way of thinking about sickness in tropical Brazil. To the extent that they did so, I argue, they can be considered an early example, albeit a short-lived one, of successful nineteenth-century science in Latin America.

Chapter 2 looks in detail at the Tropicalistas' main discoveries, discoveries the physicians "appropriated," building up international renown, and which led them into confrontations with the Brazilian medical establishment. I examine these confrontations as the result not so much of differing interpretations of scientific facts but of the challenges that the new knowledge and its styles and techniques presented to those constituencies built on an older form of knowledge. Ultimately, the Tropicalistas' international recognition led the medical communities in both Rio de Janeiro and Bahia to a more or less grudging recognition of the upstart group. For Bahia, in particular, it soon became evident that the Tropicalistas' search to produce a medical science relevant to the special circumstances of Brazil, and especially of the northern regions of the country, was very much in line with a rising Brazilian nationalism that stressed regionalism over imperial centralism and looked for a national identity that would move Brazil away from a deferential imitation of Europe.

In chapter 3, I focus on a central strand in the Tropicalistas' medical theory and practice, namely, the resistance to European and North American stereotypes about Brazilian inferiority. In their rejection of racial and climatological determinism, the Tropicalistas were moving toward an assumption that would later underpin the rise of tropical medicine: that is, nothing inherent in tropical climates or peoples led inevitably to physical and moral degeneration. There were increased dangers, certainly, but if scientifically understood, these could be reduced and even reversed. I contrast this position to that held by one of their younger colleagues, Raimundo Nina Rodrigues, who moved beyond the Tropicalistas to embrace a "hard" form of racial determinism.

Chapter 4 focuses on the relationship between the Tropicalistas, women patients, and female midwives. A part of the European condemnation of the tropics as deleterious was the idea that it was unfit for European breeding. This was another aspect of the tropics as inherently degenerating that the Tropicalistas strove to thwart by moving into the field of women's disorders, a field long the preserve of untrained midwives. Their interest in entering the territory of women's health can also be viewed as an attempt to weaken old colonial hierarchies, such as the "unhealthy" patriarchal family, and replace them with more modern, urban-centered, "bourgeois" institutions. This shift involved new ideas about the family, the positioning of women in society, their ideal roles, and how women should participate in the production of good citizens. It also involved wresting the control of women's health away from the traditional midwife and healer, which the Tropicalistas were not fully successful in doing.

In chapter 5, I examine how by the 1880s the Tropicalistas, who had initially been outsiders, became part of the mainstream, finding accommodation and identification with the Bahian medical establishment and—limited—recognition from Rio de Janeiro. I argue that although the Tropicalistas often depicted themselves as scientists "above" politics, they were always an inherently political group. If in the early years the role of outside critics promised them the greater rewards, later, during the struggles for regional autonomy, the role of inside political players proved the most effective means of advancing their own professional, and political, interests. To illustrate their shift, I trace the evolution of the relationship between the Tropicalistas and the medical school in Bahia, their participation in some of the great political debates of the Empire, and how their early, more creative period in the production of new medical knowledge ended.

CHAPTER ONE

The Escola Tropicalista Bahiana:
A Creative Response in Adversity

When in 1865 in Salvador da Bahia some fourteen doctors started meeting regularly to discuss their local cases and original research, they initiated one of the few significant episodes of successful science in nineteenth-century Brazil and, indeed, in Latin America. The men met every two weeks at each others' houses and, after a long day's work, talked late into the night about unusual cases they had come across, medical articles that had caught their attention, the advances of parasitology and microscopy, and how it could all be applied to Brazil. They dreamed of producing original research that would "clarify and develop the study of Brazilian medicine." This seemingly innocuous intention jolted the Brazilian medical establishment in which medical ideas and practice were marked by conformity and replication of Western European medicine, particularly French. The group, known retrospectively as the Escola Tropicalista Bahiana, proposed to develop a distinctive medicine of the tropics that although attuned to the newest European advances, adapted those advances to the particular concerns of Brazil, especially the Northeast. The regional specification was important because from its very inception the school challenged Rio de Janeiro's medical hegemony. One of the group's early problems was that, having no official framework within Salvador from which to operate, they had to carve out their own institutional base. They did this by using the main charity hospital as their "teaching" base, creating an influential medical journal, and, following the lead of three foreign founders with little insertion in the established patronage network, they struck out in new and original ways.

The Evolution of a Medical Community in Salvador

From its inception, medical education in Brazil was characterized by its adherence to French medical models, centralization, and the importance of patronage connections for advancement. Medical teaching in Brazil began in 1808 when the Portuguese Crown, fleeing Napoleon I, moved from Lisbon to Brazil.[1] The arrival of King João VI in Brazil in 1808, accompanied by some fifteen thousand persons, under the protection of a squadron from the English fleet, inaugurated a period of fundamental change in Brazilian history. During his stay in Brazil, King João VI ushered in a number of momentous economic and social reforms as part of his attempt to upgrade the status of Brazil from peripheral colony to center of the Brazilian Empire. For example, all Brazilian ports were opened to foreign trade, thus undoing almost three centuries of mercantilist policy; prohibitions on manufacturing enterprises in Brazil were revoked; a Royal Committee of Commerce, Agriculture, Factories, and Navigation was appointed to encourage the expansion of these activities in Brazil; and the Bank of Brazil was established in Rio de Janeiro with branches in São Paulo and Salvador.

Equally important were the cultural changes introduced largely because the king recognized that, given the uncertainty of the outcome of events in Europe, the ruling elite would have to be trained on Brazilian soil rather than on Portuguese, as had been the custom. Thus printing presses became legal for the first time in Brazil and papers such as the *Gazeta do Rio de Janeiro* (1808) and the *Idade d'Ouro do Brasil* (1811) commenced publication. The first public library was established in 1810 in Rio de Janeiro with sixty thousand volumes. Realizing it needed to produce locally trained military and naval officers, engineers, and other experts, the government created a Naval Academy in 1808 and a Royal Military Academy in 1810, and organized courses in economics, agriculture, and industry in Salvador and Rio de Janeiro. The government quickly recognized, too, the need for schools of medicine to train Brazilians as doctors. The high death rate among soldiers in Brazilian hospitals had long been a source of denunciation by colonial authorities and some voices had long clamored for the creation of local medical schools. Now, these voices were joined by those of king and court who wanted to see health care practices in their newly adoptive country conform more closely to those in Portugal. In 1808, at the instigation of the surgeon-general, José Correia Picanço, João VI set up two chairs in the instruction of surgery and anatomy, and later two more in obstetrics and pharmacy in Salvador and in Rio de Janeiro.[2]

The teaching took place in the most precarious of conditions, at the military hospitals in the two cities. At the end of four years a candidate could petition the surgeon-general for certification and on satisfying the requirements was recommended to receive a degree from the University of Coimbra in Portugal. By 1815 the Crown had upgraded the medical chairs in Rio de Janeiro and Salvador to medical-surgical colleges with a longer five-year curriculum, and more demanding entry requirements. In an attempt to replicate the European medical practice, the Crown aimed to create a sharp separation between the "empiricism" of barber-surgeons, midwives, and bleeders on the one hand, and the educated, theoretical understanding of formally trained doctors on the other.[3]

In 1827 the Crown, aware that Brazil's newly independent status would require an improved infrastructure for education, recommended further reorganization and expansion of the early courses into a school with a curriculum and faculty modeled after the medical schools in Paris and Montpellier.[4] The changes were adopted in 1832 in the midst of the crisis of Pedro I's abdication and the initiation of the liberal federalist experiment during the Regency (1831–40).[5] Initially, therefore, institutions of higher education had a good deal of autonomy in the allocation of their resources, the election of their directors, and the recommendations for changes in the content of the curriculum.[6] However, once the Regency gave way to the increasingly centralized rule of Emperor Pedro II (1840–89), school autonomy was ended. Indeed, the creation of medical education by governmental decree determined that medicine would become a more or less centralized enterprise, depending on the relative power of the royal bureaucracy and the strength of local challenges to that power. On the whole, this control stifled moves for innovation and reform.

Gradually the imperial government came to dominate all aspects of medical school life. An educational reform in 1854—the Bom Retiro law, named after the presiding prime minister—formally ended the autonomy of the medical schools. The stated purpose of the new law was to bring Brazilian medical teaching more into line with the latest developments in the leading medical schools in Europe. Thus it called for greater practical training, for better laboratory and clinical facilities, for maternity centers, for adequate autopsy facilities, and for botanical nurseries to carry out research into Brazilian plants with medical properties, all improvements that were virtually unaddressed for another thirty years.[7] However, the underlying purpose of the law, that is, the attack on the autonomy of institutions of higher learning, was rigorously implemented. As a result, the imperial government controlled the finances of the schools, nominated the directors, and, although professors were selected by competitive examinations, was known to overrule the outcome of a competition and appoint its own candidate.[8] Another source of regulation over the schools was the annual reports dealing with all aspects of the schools' business, which were written by a different professor each year, read to the faculty congregation, and forwarded to the central government. In 1875 the government further tightened its control by deciding that adjuncts were no longer to compete for full chairs but to be appointed by government decree.[9]

Throughout most of the nineteenth century, the medical schools continued to draw on the French example in shaping the curriculum, choosing examination topics for vacant faculty posts, selecting subjects for student dissertations, and deciding what to publish in Brazilian medical journals. Indeed, many Brazilian doctors preferred to publish in France and in French. Ironically, the most original Brazilian medical work in the first half of the nineteenth century came from a French physician, Joseph Sigaud, a resident of Brazil from 1825 to 1856, who wrote an epidemiological work focusing for the first time on illnesses most common in Brazil. His book, *Du climat et des maladies du Bresil; ou statistique medicale de cet empire* (1844), remained the most innovative medical approach in Brazil until the advent of the Tropicalistas in the 1860s.[10]

As the century progressed, the numbers of graduating doctors increased dramatically and advancement in medicine became far more competitive. In the early decades of the new nation's history, the number of physicians graduating per year in Rio de Janeiro and Salvador was sufficiently small so that the doctor/patient ratio was favorable to the physician.[11] Thus Robert Dundas, a British doctor who resided in Salvador from 1819 to 1842, noted that the Brazilian physician "is characterized by a great liberality of feeling; is little disposed to jealousy, and *altogether devoid of professional intrigue*."[12] But this sort of comment contrasted starkly to the common complaint later in the century that some doctors unethically undercut others with discount rates. Moving from graduation into a successful career, a thriving practice, and a prestigious position on the medical faculty always depended on patronage, but as the numbers of graduates grew, competition for patronage was greater and the sought-after posts relatively fewer.[13]

After midcentury, the higher number of doctors graduating from the two medical schools in Brazil not only created competition among the doctors within the two cities but also exacerbated the differences between the two medical communities. Increasingly, the rewards for physicians in Rio de Janeiro were much greater than in Salvador. This was in part because of the much larger European and Europeanized population that demanded the services of Western medicine. The array of medical institutions in Rio was also greater: the medical school had more students and thus there were more professors; a successful medical association formed in 1829, which became the Imperial Academy of Medicine in 1836; and the academy had its own journal, originally titled the *Anais de Medicina do Rio de Janeiro.* But undoubtedly the most important factor for the advancement of the individual physician in Rio de Janeiro, as well as for the status of the medical profession, was that Rio, as the capital of the Empire, was the seat of the court and of royal patronage. Thus, for example, in theory the medical school in Rio de Janeiro lost as much autonomy as the Bahian school under the centralizing tendencies of Dom Pedro II's government. But, in fact, the school in Rio de Janeiro could compensate for this loss of autonomy much more successfully than the Bahian school simply because it had close connections with the high echelons of power. Rio benefited from the emperor's personal interest in medical affairs. Fascinated by the development of nineteenth-century science, Pedro II often attended sessions at the Imperial Academy of Medicine, Rio medical school theses defenses, and graduation services.[14] He was thus personally known to a number of doctors.

The outcome of the Rio medical community's proximity to the seat of power can be clearly seen in the more liberal financing of the Rio de Janeiro school and main medical institutions. It was also evident in the unbalanced dispensation of noble titles for the two medical communities. Of the forty-nine noble titles Pedro I and II granted doctors, only one was given to a Bahian physician.[15] The whole theater of royalty in Rio de Janeiro also gave the capital's medical community a glitter and sophistication that, as the century wore on, contrasted more and more with the provincial, backwater nature of the Bahian one. Whereas early in the century numerous Bahian physicians had managed to become nationally prominent, by midcentury the Bahian medical community played second fiddle to that of the capital.[16] The justification was that Rio de Janeiro attracted more brilliant minds. Ambitious Bahian physicians who could do so moved to the capital to pursue their careers.[17] Those who remained behind began to air their grievances.

It is understandable, therefore, that those who managed to position themselves well in the system had little incentive to rock the boat by fostering change. This may have been especially true at the Bahian medical school, where a medical education was often prized primarily as a means of entering the ranks of power and less as a scientific endeavor. Local grandees, when they could, preferred to send their sons to the law schools of Recife and São Paulo, from which the highest proportion of imperial civil servants was drawn.[18] As the medical historian Cassiano Gomes asserts: "Medicine, at least in Salvador, was the profession of poor people, of the sons of merchants with small amounts of capital, or even the sons of workers, of the petty bourgeoisie; herein lies the great social function of the school."[19] Numerous examples in Salvador bear this out. Antônio Pacífico Pereira and his brother Victorino were of humble Portuguese immigrant stock, as were José Francisco da Silva Lima and Manoel Joaquim Saraiva. Pedro Severiano de Magalhães began his studies at the orphanage school of São Joaquim. All of these men became prominent as doctors, as civil servants, or as politicians.[20]

The Bahian medical school, like the other institutions of higher learning in Brazil, was also a vehicle for the rising social status of the mulatto.[21] The fact that the government provided scholarships for poor students to enter the professions, regardless of color, was one of the underpinnings of the elite's complacent belief that in Brazil, in contrast to the United States, there was no "Negro problem."[22] Brazilians noted with pride, and foreigners recorded in amazement, the many prominent mulatto Brazilian intellectuals and professionals in the Empire. This was true of medical graduates and faculty in Salvador. The professor Lino Coutinho, for example, was of a poor, mulatto background, and Domingos Carlos da Silva, Luis Anselmo de Fonseca, and Raimundo Nina Rodrigues, students and later teachers at the medical school, were mulatto.[23] The values of most young men entering the medical school, therefore, led to the passive acceptance of medical education as a general, philosophical training rather than as a functional and practical profession. As Gilberto Freyre has noted, the value system of culture and knowledge in the Bahian medical school, certainly until the last decade of the Empire, subordinated the "scientific study [of medicine] to the study of classical literature, oratory, rhetoric, elegance, and purity in speaking and writing, to debate over questions more grammatical than physiological, and to dissecting problems closer to the pathology of literary style than human anatomy."[24] It was unlikely, therefore, that the impetus for change would have come from within the Bahian medical establishment.

The Tropicalistas, more than any other group of doctors in nineteenth-century Salvador, first articulated a critique of Brazilian medical teaching and practice. As foreigners, the founding Tropicalistas were excluded from the existing network of patronage so crucial to the advancement of medical careers; none of them, for example, ever taught at the Bahian medical school. The fact that they were on the periphery of imperial power and patronage allowed them more room to develop questioning and sometimes controversial ideas than if they had been in the capital city, close to official medicine, where such an autonomous group would have faced serious obstacles. At the same time, they were aware of the important medical strides being made in Europe and were especially interested in German advances. Clearly, for these men, audacity, daring, and original investigation would pay far greater dividends in possible fame and personal satisfaction than adherence to the local Western tradition of medicine, which, they saw, was failing to move into the new era of scientific medicine. They pushed, therefore, to make full use of the research arsenal of European medicine such as, for example, medical statistics, new clinical methods based on measurement and applied physiology, the application of chemistry in analyzing bodily fluids, an increased understanding of hematology, animal experimentation, and, most important, microscopy, which they pioneered in Salvador and through which they began to question hallowed theories about the etiology of Brazilian ailments.[25] Above all, they insisted on looking at disorders of primary interest to Brazil.

The "scientific" form of medical knowledge that the Tropicalistas proposed was, at first, intrusive and unsettling. Their outspoken belief that it was time for a "shake-up" in local medicine threatened to upset the accommodation of Bahian physicians within the Empire, especially as the Tropicalistas drew on new German ideas of scientific and social medicine that were initially viewed in Rio de Janeiro as rivals to the older French environmental approach to disease.[26] Over time, however, because the Bahian medical establishment did increasingly poorly within the system of royal patronage—a fact it resented more and more bitterly—the Tropicalistas ended up becoming allies in the Bahian doctors' struggle to secure greater munificence from the central government. Between 1866 and 1890, therefore, the medical school in Salvador became transformed, a transformation initiated by the Tropicalistas' criticisms and propelled by the larger social changes unfolding during this crucial period in Brazil's history.

The Founding Tropicalistas

The three most important founding members of the Escola Tropicalista Bahiana were Europeans who made their home in Brazil. Two of them, Otto H. Wucherer and John Ligertwood Paterson, became well known in Salvador rather suddenly as a result of two epidemics that ravaged the city at midcentury: yellow fever (1849) and cholera (1855).[27] Certain events in the two epidemics are worth highlighting for they were important precursors to the formation of the Tropicalista movement and in creating the early perception of the Tropicalistas—in the opinion of some—as disruptive outsiders. Soon after a puzzling epidemic arrived in Salvador, Wucherer and Paterson, the latter the physician to the British community in Salvador, diagnosed the disorder as yellow fever, in opposition to the opinion of most of the members of the medical school and several of those on the Council of Health (Conselho de Salubridade). They stated it was contagious, although the manner of contagion was unknown.[28] The practical implications of this position, which called for quarantines in a port city and the likely disruption of trade, were highly unpopular. So, too, was the assault on the prestige of the Bahian medical elite. The latter retaliated with offensive articles in the local press against the foreign doctors, arguing that the disorder was one of local origin and that the epidemic was neither as contagious nor as frightening as had been made out. "The serious cases that have occurred," they stated, "were caused by the predisposition of patients to the disorder, to the panic that has taken hold of them, and to the use of unreasonable cures."[29] However, as the cases multiplied in an alarming manner, it became clear that the Europeans were correct in their diagnosis and that yellow fever had indeed struck and was spreading in a manner suggesting contagion.

In 1855 the animosity between the foreigners and some of the leading Bahian doctors was reinforced when a similar confrontation developed over the arrival of cholera in the city. When called to minister to the ailing captain of a British frigate, an English doctor, Edward G. Fairbanks, declared the illness was cholera.[30] The provincial governor urgently summoned Wucherer, Paterson, and Fairbanks to discuss the situation. As in 1849, most local doctors and authorities opposed the view that cholera had struck, blaming the epidemic on the sale of rotten codfish and meat.[31] When the Europeans proposed that three special centers be set up to treat cholera patients and limit its spread, officials opposed the notion. Once again there were scathing articles in the press about the foreign doctors, and for a second time, events proved local physicians wrong.

The two incidents damaged the prestige of some of the most preeminent local physicians while enhancing that of the Europeans. The Council of Health, for example, several of whose members had opposed the Europeans, fell into disuse and finally ceased to exist in 1876. After 1851 the main sanitation body was the Board of Public Hygiene (Junta de Hygiene Pública), run almost single-handedly by José Goes Siqueira, who became inspector of hygiene.[32] The foreign doctors gained in prestige among the highest administrative authorities and in later years were asked to serve on a number of health commissions.[33] Their help and courage during the epidemics also earned them praise from wide sectors of the population.[34] There was a good deal of sympathy for Wucherer, for example, who lost his wife in the yellow fever epidemic after he opened an infirmary in his home for poor patients. The two episodes also led to a crisis of confidence in the then prevalent Bahian medical theories that, strongly derivative of outdated French medical ideas, pointed to a vague and fatalistic notion of climatic miasma derived from the combination of poor living conditions and the humid heat of the tropics, rather than a specific source of contagion.[35] Wucherer and Paterson's insistence that yellow fever was contagious suggested that they believed that even if unhygienic conditions and a tropical climate were important factors in the outbreak of disease, these were not the whole explanation. They wanted to be much more specific in pointing out how the peculiarly Brazilian social factors impinged on disease, as well as how the special conditions of a warm climate interacted on a human constitution to produce disease. Thus they provided a new approach to disease etiology in Salvador at a time when traditional explanations were being undermined. It took another decade for the foreigners—and a handful of Bahian physicians who recognized the deficiencies of the state of local medicine—to get together and organize themselves into a group interested in the exploration of new approaches. Undoubtedly the two epidemics and the role of Wucherer and Paterson acted as a catalyst for that effort.

Wucherer, who was born of German parents in Portugal and then moved with them to Brazil when he was eight, became the most renowned of the

Tropicalistas and was the crucial link between advanced European medical ideas and local medical concerns.[36] With his studies of Brazilian snakes and their poisons, his finding of the hookworm in Salvador, and his discovery of the embryonic filaria, Wucherer, more than any other of the Tropicalistas, forged the group's identity, set its program of research, and made it visible in the European press. Wucherer brought to Salvador the newest ideas of laboratory medicine and parasitology—a knowledge he acquired at the University of Tübingen, from which he graduated in 1841—at a time when Germany was beginning to play a leading role in laboratory medicine.[37] He was particularly influenced by the brand of German medicine espoused by Rudolf Virchow, who, even as he moved away from bedside medicine into the laboratory and greater specificity, remained one of Germany's strongest medical advocates of social reform. Indeed, Virchow's axiom, "medicine is a social science," can be seen as central to Wucherer and the Tropicalistas' approach to the profession.[38]

Wucherer's exposure to advanced European medicine increased during his time as a medical assistant at St. Bartholomew's Hospital in London before his return to Brazil in 1843. In 1847 he took up the position of physician to the German community in Salvador.[39] After the epidemics mentioned above, he continued to run his own infirmary, where he tended to all classes. Although he never received an official appointment to the main charity hospital, the Santa Casa de Misericórdia, he worked there closely with a handful of colleagues, particularly Paterson, José Francisco da Silva Lima, and Manoel Maria Pires Caldas. They performed operations and autopsies together and consulted one another on their cases. Wucherer supported the idea of weekly meetings of those physicians in Salvador interested in keeping up-to-date on new developments in medicine, and he was one of the founders of the prestigious *Gazeta Médica da Bahia,* to which he contributed a handful of seminal articles. His best-known work was in the field of parasitology. In 1865 he isolated hookworm parasites for the first time in Brazil; he was the first person ever to isolate the embryonic filaria, the parasite that leads to hematuria and elephantiasis. He was also a pioneer in the study of Brazilian herpetology, with two of his papers on snakes read at the London Proceedings of the Zoological Society in 1861 and 1863.[40]

The approach to medicine that Wucherer brought to Salvador was reinforced by the Scotsman Paterson, who graduated from the University of Aberdeen in 1841. At the time, Scottish medical schools were deeply interested in the idea that it was the government's task to safeguard the health of the public, and that questions related to housing, sanitation, sewerage, the water supply, and the adulteration of food were all within the purview of government. Moreover, they believed that such a government could act practically and legislate wisely only if it considered the advice of the physician.[41] After graduating, Paterson was accepted into the Royal College of Surgeons in London. He went on a medical tour of the best-known hospitals in France, Switzerland, Italy, and Vienna until, encouraged by his older brother, Alexander, who had set up practice earlier in the British community in Salvador, he traveled to Brazil. By then in his early twenties, John Paterson planned to settle in Paraíba do Norte but succeeded unexpectedly to his brother's practice after the latter succumbed to a paralyzing stroke in 1843. Except for a few years from 1869 to 1872, and 1879 to 1881, during which he returned to Britain, Paterson remained in Salvador until his death, at which time his practice had become the largest in Salvador.[42] Like Wucherer, Paterson was dedicated to the treatment of the poor. In a biographical article on Paterson written in 1887, Silva Lima told how, from the beginning of his work in Salvador, Paterson had reached out to more than just the British community. He worked from early sunrise in a small infirmary attached to his house and at the Santa Casa Hospital, serving not only British sailors but needy Bahians, some of whom he never charged for his services. At noon he would start paying sick calls on horseback, often until after nightfall. When the infirmary ran low on the contributions on which it survived, he subsidized it for a time from his own pocket before reluctantly closing it down. Although other foreign doctors also attended Brazilian patients, none had the large numbers of poor patients that Paterson did. Thus, in his adopted town, wrote Silva Lima, he came to be fondly known as *pai do povo* (father of the people).[43]

Paterson was important for Bahian medicine in two ways. First, he marshaled the interests of the early Tropicalistas by proposing that they hold informal meetings in order to exchange ideas, talk about their own cases, and keep abreast of developments in medicine and surgery. The suggestion led in 1866 to fortnightly meetings of about fourteen Bahian doctors and, eventually, to the birth of the Escola Tropicalista. The meetings, at which there were earnest discussions on the work in parasitology of Angelo Dubini, Theodor Bilharz, and Wilhelm Griesinger, among others, emboldened Wucherer to write about his own findings. Here, too, the third member of the initial Tropicalistas, José Francisco da Silva Lima, first raised his interest in beriberi. There were talks about advances in surgery, an area that particularly attracted Paterson. From these interchanges also came the idea of starting a medical journal; the *Gazeta Médica da Bahia* was not the first medical journal founded in Salvador but it became the most successful, privately financed Brazilian medical journal in the nineteenth century.[44]

Second, as a result of his sojourns in Europe, especially in Scotland where he learned about antisepsis, Paterson was instrumental in introducing Lister's method into Bahian medicine. During these visits, sometimes extended due to family reasons, Paterson spent time at the most advanced hospitals in Britain and attended the lectures of some of the most famous physicians of the time. In 1869 he worked with Joseph Lister in Edinburgh. This was a turning point in Paterson's professional life, for he was rapidly won over to Lister's method of antisepsis.[45] In 1871 the Bahian physician Antônio Pacífico Pereira visited Paterson in Edinburgh. Paterson took his friend to have a lesson in antiseptic measures from the master himself. In 1879, once again on leave in Scotland, Paterson received a visit from Antônio's brother, Victorino Pereira. He too was introduced to Lister and made familiar with his antisepsis. Paterson and the two Pereira brothers were sufficiently impressed with what they had learned from Lister to introduce the method into their Bahian medical practice. In subsequent reports on surgery in the *Gazeta Médica da Bahia,* whether by Paterson or his colleagues, the antiseptic preventions taken are usually noted.

The third in the triad of founding members of the Escola Tropicalista, José Francisco da Silva Lima, provided the perseverance and continuity that led to the group's success. Born in Portugal, Silva Lima moved at the age of fourteen with his parents to Salvador, where his father was a merchant and his uncle a pharmacist. He graduated from the medical school in Salvador in 1851. Between 1853 and 1881 he made five trips to Europe in part to advance his medical knowledge.[46] One of the founders and long-time editor of the *Gazeta Médica,* he contributed some two hundred articles to the journal. His range of interests and activities within medicine was enormous. Like Wucherer and Paterson, he was a clinician who made his original contributions to the school from cases in his sizable practice. He was the first Bahian doctor to report on what he considered the beginning of an alarming epidemic of beriberi in the city. He was the first to describe ainhum, a disorder that caused the growth of a tumor on the small toe of a person's foot and that, according to Silva Lima, struck only Africans.[47] He worked closely with Wucherer and others on hookworm, filariasis, and schistosomiasis. But it would be misleading to classify Silva Lima as interested only in what we now term tropical disorders. A scan of his writings in the *Gazeta Médica* reveal him as a doctor concerned with a whole range of clinical problems including heart disorders, diabetes, tumors, stigmata, surgery, hygiene, and legal medicine. He was very interested, too, in the latest developments in gynecology and obstetrics and sought to expand these specialties in Salvador.

Regarding medicine in Salvador, Silva Lima had two objectives. He wanted to professionalize medicine in Salvador, and he wanted to see the Bahian medical community contribute to the patrimony of international medicine and be given its due credit for it. By "professionalize" I refer to Lima's attempts to set boundaries around the medical profession in Salvador, excluding the "irregular" healers and including physicians and pharmacists trained in Western medicine and pharmacopoeia. To do this he worked to forge a spirit of solidarity among physicians, and also between physicians and pharmacists, so that they should agree on ethical standards of practice and behavior. He also endeavored to draw more physicians into medical scientific research. Physicians united in this way, he believed, would be in a stronger position to force the authorities to recognize their importance as experts in the nation's decision-making processes. To this end, Silva Lima was tireless in his efforts. Although he never held a paid official position, he helped create and chaired numerous professional bodies, such as the Doctors' and Pharmacists' Mutual Aid Society (Sociedade Médico-Pharmacêutica de Beneficência Mútua), formed in 1868; the Bahian Medical Society (Sociedade Médica da Bahia), formed in 1888; and the Medical and Surgical Society of Bahia (Sociedade de Medicina e Cirurgia da Bahia), formed in 1894. He pushed for a national medical congress to be held in Salvador (it finally was held there in 1890) and sat on commissions to promote vaccination, to contain yellow fever epidemics, to improve the sanitary conditions of the city and of the port, and to look into the spread of beriberi in the province.[48]

Together, these three men spearheaded changes in Bahian medicine that led to their national and international recognition. Their vision led to the formation of a small research community in Salvador informed by some of the newest European ideas in medicine that provided an important precedent of original research and experimentation in Brazil yet never altogether shed the idea of the importance of environment in understanding disease.

The Making of a School of Tropicalistas

Although existing sources do not give an exact figure for how many men formed the Escola Tropicalista, a rough estimate is possible.[49] In 1887 Silva Lima provided a list with the names of fourteen men whom he recalled started meeting regularly at Paterson's house.[50] The approximate correctness of this figure is confirmed by an examination of the doctors who published regularly in the *Gazeta Médica*, and who were on its editorial board up until the fall of the Empire in 1889. Further data can be gleaned through a careful examination of the Tropicalistas' clinical papers published in the *Gazeta Médica*, which reveal the names of doctors who assisted, observed, and commented on their work as well as the lists of members of the professional associations formed by the Tropicalistas.[51] A prosopographical analysis of all these sources together suggests a "core" group of Tropicalistas that, though never numbering more than about twelve members at any one time, was surrounded by a larger circle of identifiable supporters of about twenty to twenty-five men. Among the Tropicalistas were five foreigners: the three founders I have already mentioned, and two supporters, Dr. Thomas Wright Hall, who worked with the British community, and Dr. Alexander Paterson, John Paterson's nephew.[52] The rest of the Tropicalistas, core or supporters, were Brazilian-born and trained, although a number of them made visits to European centers of medicine after their graduation.[53] Since there was an average of thirty doctors on the faculty of the medical school and possibly as many as eighty-six to one hundred and fifty regular practitioners in the city, the Tropicalistas constituted a sizable minority of the total medical community.[54] Moreover, because they were such an active minority in teaching (albeit extraofficially), in the creation of the city's medical institutions and commissions for the improvement of hygiene, in the main charity hospital, and in the establishment of the only successful medical journal in Salvador, they exercised an influence upon the whole medical community that belied their numbers.

Because in their first decade nearly all the core Tropicalistas operated outside the existing Bahian medical establishment, and rapidly became a forum for its critique, they needed an institutional framework if they were to be a successful, innovating force in Bahian medicine. Of the fourteen men Silva Lima recalled at the early meetings held first in Paterson's house, only two were on the medical school faculty at the time.[55] Over the next two decades the Tropicalistas had considerable success in winning over adherents from the medical school, and many of their earliest supporters moved into teaching posts in the medical school. Thus, by the late 1880s, their teachings had become mainstream. But in the 1860s the two institutions that became pivotal to the success of the group, the Santa Casa de Misericórdia Hospital and the *Gazeta Médica da Bahia,* were outside the medical school.

The Santa Casa de Misericórdia Hospital was a charity hospital administered by nuns that provided many social services under the aegis of the historic "Brotherhood of Our Lady," a part of the Portuguese colonial legacy.[56] The hospital attended to the poor who were reputed to have a "horror of the hospital," so that they sought out its services only when they were already extremely ill.[57] It also attended to sailors, prostitutes, those afflicted by venereal disease, and women with birthing problems. Other charity services provided by the Santa Casa included the provision of burials for the poor, dowries for poor female orphans, a "roda," which was a foundling wheel made from a little revolving door to the side of the main door, or elsewhere, where unwanted babies were left, a retirement house for "wayward" women, and another for orphaned girls. At the time of Emperor Pedro II, the province of Bahia had six charity hospitals run by the Santa Casa.[58] The largest was the Santa Casa de Misericórdia in the city of Salvador, which from 1833 was housed in the old Jesuit quarters in the Terreiro de Jesus next to the medical school. It operated largely with donations and legacies made to the order by wealthy members of the community, and through the years it had amassed considerable wealth. In the course of the century its expenses mounted as a result of a rising population and growing expectations in social services. Moreover, the economic decline of the province that exacted its toll on the generosity of donors and the mismanagement of its finances led to hard times for the order.[59] Already in 1853 João Maurício Wanderley, then president of the province, had pointed to a litany of woes plaguing the Santa Casa hospital, such as overcrowding, filthy conditions, and a deficit. He suggested solving these through the sale of properties and the acquisition of a separate building to house the insane.[60]

By 1868 the Santa Casa hospital seemed to be in better shape. An official noted that, although the overcrowding of the institution was still a serious problem, its finances, under a new stewardship, had improved. In fact, by the 1870s expansion and reforms in the hospital were such that some Bahian doctors hoped the city might finally boast of a "modernized" hospital.[61] The provincial government promised to purchase a place for the insane and repairs were carried out in the hospital.[62] An important aspect of the reforms was the separation of patients with different ailments. Thus a separate infirmary was established for smallpox victims in 1874–75, an insane asylum inaugurated in 1874, and a ward for women in labor set up in 1876.[63] The push to expand was in part a response to the increase in the numbers of patients entering the Santa Casa de Misericórdia Hospital from the 1870s on, an increase related to the growth of the city's population.[64] The modest expansion of the facilities and staff carried out in the previous years, therefore, was barely adequate to cope with the increasing numbers, and demands continued to be made for the building of a new Misericórdia hospital, demands finally heeded in 1886.

The changes to improve the hospital were also the result of pressures from the Tropicalistas, as can be seen from their repeated calls for reforms in their writings in the *Gazeta Médica*.[65] If the statement made in 1876 by the president of the province, Luís Antônio da Silva Nunes, that "in its conditions of cleanliness, health, abundance, and order, [the Santa Casa hospital] can compare to the best [hospitals] of other countries . . ." was an exaggeration, he certainly captured some of the optimism in a decade when the Tropicalistas were shaking up the lethargic medical establishment in Salvador.[66] Not only were they attempting, with some degree of success, to get the Santa Casa hospital, dominated as it was by nonmedical administrators, to be organized according to modern, expert medical criteria, but they were also managing to use the hospital as a platform for their own career advancement. Thus the Santa Casa hospital became a forum for the teaching of the Tropicalistas, a meeting place for competition and camaraderie, and a testing place for new surgical methods and therapies.

The hospital had its own physicians, surgeons, and interns. Appointments to the hospital were prestigious but not lucrative.[67] Eight physicians were appointed to the "medical" and the "surgical" clinics. In 1879 seven of them were Tropicalistas. They were assisted by one paid faculty intern, who had to remain at the hospital all day and deal with emergencies when none of the appointed physicians was present.[68] As well as the regular appointments, there were a number of medical school faculty holding professorships whose teaching included practical instruction in the hospital.[69] There were also other physicians who, although not formally linked to the Santa Casa, were well connected with those who were, and they too attended patients in the charity hospital.[70] This was the case with Wucherer and Paterson. The latter was given an honorary appointment by the sisters of the Santa Casa in 1867 in recognition of his services. Between 1860 and the fall of the Empire, all the core Tropicalistas, and many of their supporters, practiced at the Santa Casa hospital. Some combined appointments at the Santa Casa with teaching at the medical school, as did Antônio José Alves; some worked first at the Santa Casa and only later moved into the medical school, as did José Luís D'Almeida Couto, Victorino Pereira, and Augusto Freire Maia Bittencourt. A number of doctors never taught at the medical school but worked long years at the Santa Casa hospital. In this last group were Silva Lima, Paterson, Wucherer, Joaquim dos Remédios Monteiro, Manoel Maria Pires Caldas, Paulino Pires da Costa Chastinet, and Francisco dos Santos Pereira. Of twenty-five doctors identified as working at the Santa Casa hospital during this period, twenty were core Tropicalistas or their supporters.[71]

If the Santa Casa hospital was a centerpiece in the emergence of the Tropicalistas, this was because it provided a mechanism for centralizing their otherwise isolated inquiries and energies. Here they could experiment with new surgical methods and therapies that they read about in European and North American literature. Not only were they able to pool their experiences with novel methods, but they could do so in a relatively unrestrained manner, which was not possible with their middle- and upper-class patients. This restraint with upper-class patients existed because such patients were cared for in their own homes, a fact that physically dispersed the doctors and gave patients greater control over the conditions of their treatment.[72] Moreover, the Tropicalistas, like all doctors at the time, were dependent on the better-off classes for their livelihoods; thus their practice with them was subject to the market considerations of building up a clientele. This led to a more conservative medical approach that honored the accepted and established methods over the risks of novelty and experimentation. Particularly in a place like Salvador, where patronage played a crucial role in securing civil service, teaching, and hospital appointments, as well as clients, it was unwise to incur the wrath of a powerful family lest the means of a physician's advancement be jeopardized.[73] This explains why a large majority of the cases in which surgery was performed by five core members of the Tropicalistas involved patients from the poorest classes.[74] It also accounts for why the Tropicalistas used innovations in gynecological and obstetrical methods first among the poorest patients.[75] These were patients on whom they could use the full gamut of their technologies, and experiment with new ones they had so far only read about. As the *Gazeta Médica* noted regarding the use of poor patients, "We do not lack hospital patients; but we must use them for teaching. [A polyclinic for the poor] would be the best way to teach, and would also be extremely useful for the poor."[76] A further incentive to treat poor patients at the Santa Casa was that, as Pacífico Pereira noted, private patients did not allow their bodies to be used for autopsies.[77]

But Tropicalista interest in the lower classes as patients went beyond a desire to carry out experimentation unimpeded. It was also a result of still being very much part of a European medical tradition, prevalent in the first half of the nineteenth century and revitalized and—to a point—radicalized by German physicians like Virchow. This tradition, like the French, stressed environmental and populational explanations, arguing that the improvement of people's health and progeny could be achieved through the betterment of social and physical environments. Virchow added the importance of improving the working environment of the laboring classes. Thus when Wucherer's work on parasitology was announced in the *Gazeta Médica*, for example, the journal claimed excitedly that his discovery would surely become a milestone in the improvement of the health of the lower class, particularly that of agricultural workers and slaves.[78] Other disorders that targeted the poor, like tuberculosis and leprosy, were central to the concerns of such Tropicalistas as Wucherer, Pacífico Pereira, and Nina Rodrigues. Beriberi, which Silva Lima discovered in Brazil, hit middle-class sedentary people but was most rife among the least well-off who lived and worked in the poorest of hygienic conditions.[79]

In the operations they performed at the Santa Casa, the Tropicalistas were able to experiment with some of the latest procedures. In 1869, for example, Alexander Paterson, a recent graduate from the University of Edinburgh and licensed to practice in Brazil, performed a successful operation at the Santa Casa for the partial removal of a tumor on the lower jawbone of a black woman. He performed the operation together with his uncle and Pires Caldas, and received Wucherer's help in the postoperative period. The most interesting aspect of the operation was the young Paterson's reference to the application of carbolic acid as antisepsis during the operation to the wound and the needle used for suturing.[80] Although it would be erroneous to conclude from this single event that henceforth the Tropicalistas were diligent in antiseptic precautions, it certainly does demonstrate just how interested they were in the latest European developments and in experimenting with them. The real breakthrough in the use of antiseptics in Salvador was, as mentioned above, John Paterson's association with Lister, which began in 1869. Not only did he facilitate introductions to Lister for several traveling Bahian physicians, but when Paterson returned to his adopted city he began to apply antiseptic methods.[81] Other Tropicalistas followed suit in the 1870s. By the 1880s antisepsis and then asepsis were widely used in Brazil.[82] Other examples of the Tropicalistas' pioneering new techniques include the first Bahian use in 1866 of Richardson's method of anesthesia, a method the three leading Tropicalistas and Pires Caldas used on a patient who had a thumb amputated.[83] Wucherer was also the first doctor in Salvador to use the hypodermic needle in 1867. A year later he used it to inject patients with quinine, apparently thus curing them of malaria.[84]

The Santa Casa de Misericórdia Hospital was not only an arena for medical experimentation but also became the Tropicalistas' forum for disseminating the new approaches to medicine among the young medical students. Even though a number of the core Tropicalistas never taught at the medical school, they taught informally at the Santa Casa hospital, where many of their cases and operations were observed and assisted by interested young students. That the charity hospital became a center for Tropicalista teaching was due in part to the fact that the three Tropicalista leaders were foreigners. After the educational reforms of 1854, foreigners were not allowed to teach at the medical schools, and thus none of the three Tropicalista founders ever held an official teaching position in Salvador.[85] Students were also drawn there because, although all agreed that the practical teaching facilities at the medical schools, especially the poorer Bahian one, were abysmal, the few facilities and reduced equipment at the disposal of faculty professors were poorly used. For example, even though microscopes were available at the medical school, only a handful of professors actually made use of them in their teaching; most professors preferred to deliver their same lectures year after year with no use whatsoever of practical aids.[86] Moreover, when professors did use the hospital as a practical teaching clinic, they usually had their assistants perform the necessary operations, deeming it below their dignity to get physically involved.[87]

The Tropicalistas' practice was in marked contrast to the hands-off approach of the traditional Bahian physician-professor. Despite the fact that conditions in the Santa Casa left much to be desired, the Tropicalistas stretched what few facilities there were. Years later Pacífico Pereira, who was instructed in the use of the microscope by Wucherer himself, recalled the Sundays and holidays he had spent as a student with the initial core Tropicalistas, huddled over one of the autopsy tables at the Santa Casa, or over some operation or clinical case.[88] The Tropicalistas were generous toward such avid young students. For example, they encouraged their assistants to write up some of the interesting cases in which they were involved and these reports were published in the *Gazeta Médica*.[89] Victorino Pereira assisted the elder Tropicalistas in many of their operations as a student, and when he graduated in 1876, rather than going straight into private practice or into teaching, he chose to enrich his medical education by spending time at the charity hospital working alongside the innovators.[90] In the latter part of the 1880s the most ambitious and promising young students and recent graduates, such as Alfredo Tomé de Britto, Braz H. do Amaral, Ezequiel Cândido de Souza Britto, Antônio Pacheco Mendes, Domingos Pedro dos Santos, and Rio de Janeiro graduate Raimundo Nina Rodrigues, all associated with and became strong supporters of the Tropicalistas, either working with them at the Santa Casa hospital, or developing interests inspired by the Tropicalistas.[91]

By the 1880s the original "Tropicalista" topics for research, developed outside the medical establishment, had been taken into the medical school by early Tropicalista supporters who had, by then, become part of the school faculty. Nina Rodrigues, physician and father of Brazilian ethnology, recalled the challenge proffered by the Tropicalistas in the 1860s and 1870s to the medical status quo in Salvador:

> Early last century, medical teaching was started in Salvador. . . . The teaching was detestable. It was a copy of [medical] science made for other races and other climates. . . . One day the remarkable German researcher Wucherer . . . and the British clinician Paterson led a meeting of notable doctors. . . . [T]hey resolved to break their routines and study medicine, not from the European books, but with their own patients. And so was formed the renowned school, guided by Silva Lima, which studied filariasis, schistosomiasis, . . . beriberi and other disorders common to our climate.[92]

In several ways, therefore, the Santa Casa hospital helped focus the incipient research activities of the Tropicalistas and mold the direction of their clinical practice. It provided them with an institutional framework that gave structure to their movement, and a base from which they could experi-

ment and disseminate ideas, and also gain social legitimization even though
many were outsiders to the established network of medical patronage. The
charity hospital was not left unchanged by the Tropicalista movement. It
underwent improvements in its physical structure as well as in its organization. The hospital authorities agreed to divide up patients according to
their disorders, to open a ward for birthing women and another for the
insane, and to promote greater hygiene. Doctors slowly began to use antisepsis and anesthesia in surgery, and introduced surgical innovations that
alleviated some patients.[93]

A second institution crucial to the success of the Tropicalistas was the
Gazeta Médica da Bahia. The journal was founded as a result of the meetings held by the first Tropicalistas at Paterson's house and then at other
physicians' homes. The first issue of the journal, which was published regularly every two weeks, appeared in July 1866. Except for some breaks in 1870
and 1871, and an eighteen-month hiatus between July 1874 and December 1875, both due to financial problems, the journal ran continuously into
the twentieth century and, with a few gaps, right up to 1934. The *Gazeta
Médica* started out and remained throughout the Empire years the journal
of the core Tropicalistas. In its first years the board of editors was made up
of Silva Lima, Pacífico Pereira, Demétrio Ciríaco Tourinho, and Virgílio
Clímaco Damázio. The latter was the director of the journal until 1867
when, on the plea that he was overburdened with work, he resigned in
favor of Pacífico Pereira, who remained in the post throughout the Empire
years.[94] When the journal reopened after its eighteen-month closure from
1874 to 1875, it was run by a board of five editors instead of a single director and, as the journal became more successful, the board increased to
seven and finally to nine editors by the end of the Empire. On the whole
the editors, who were drawn from a total of fifteen men, held their positions for many years.[95] Some key figures, such as Wucherer and Paterson,
never served on the editorial board, but they had been among the initial in-
stigators of the project and were a crucial influence on the journal. Indeed,
Wucherer's articles in the journal became the foundation of its fame abroad
and Paterson was always a faithful contributor who wrote on a wide array
of topics, including the latest surgical procedures.

The *Gazeta Médica* contrasted sharply with virtually all other attempts
to start scientific or literary journals in nineteenth-century Brazil, which
floundered hopelessly.[96] It was financed by private subscriptions and by
commercial advertisements that proprietors of the leading pharmacies in

Salvador and the bookstores carrying medical textbooks and foreign journals placed in its pages.[97] The journal's remarkable success had a great deal
to do with its clearly articulated interests and consistent objectives. The first
issue stated that the journal's aim was

> To join together the most . . . active members of the medical class . . . ; to
> disseminate medical knowledge gained through doctors' observations,
> near or far; to keep abreast of the scientific developments of the most
> advanced countries; to study the questions that are of most interest to
> our country; to ensure the union, dignity, and autonomy of our profes-
> sion. . . . Colleagues, from [Bahia] and other provinces . . . will always
> find these columns open to their work [provided they] are serious [and
> adhere] to the high standards to which the *Gazeta Médica* aspires.[98]

The Tropicalistas, therefore, intended to forge a cadre of informed, united
doctors who might augment the medical profession's legitimacy and authority among Bahian patients. A guiding principle in their medical practice was the focus on disorders relevant to the health of Brazilians. Thus
they looked primarily at the disorders they believed were most common in
warm climates, at disorders to be found as a result of poor living conditions in Brazil, and at disorders that resulted from the existence of African
slavery in Brazil.

The boundaries the Tropicalistas wanted to set around the medical profession in Salvador concerned the construction of a particular kind of physician. They wanted to move away from the medical tradition in Salvador
whereby a medical degree was mainly a cultural acquisition that translated
into social mobility.[99] As Gilberto Freyre says, the Tropicalistas "had the
temerity to intrude on [the] Bahian tradition of cultivating the classical
and liberal arts behind a facade of medical studies." [100] They wanted to
introduce the authority of scientific and positivistic knowledge into Bahian
medicine because they believed that progress in Brazil was intricately linked
to this approach, and they also understood that their own advancement
in the medical field, their chance for recognition at home and abroad, depended on their contributions being presented within the most advanced
scientific medical canon of their day. It was this scientific authority, a "universal" and positive form of knowledge, purged of the discordant elements
of competition, politics, and religion, that the Tropicalistas hoped would
be the cement of the medical class.

The contrast between the traditional Bahian doctor and the modern scientific doctor was vividly portrayed in Silva Lima's own writings. In 1908, as an octogenarian, Silva Lima reminisced about mid–nineteenth century Salvador, and recalled the pompous figure of the grandly dressed and perfumed Bahian physician riding in a slave-borne litter, supervising heavy bleeding treatment to his patients—a treatment the physician himself did not perform, deeming it beneath his dignity.[101] This image was in stark contrast to the one Silva Lima gave of his friend Dr. Paterson, who, somberly dressed, was always to be seen riding his own horse, on his visits from patient to patient, and was closely involved in his patients' treatment.[102] After working long hours, according to Silva Lima, Paterson returned home to study and investigate late into the night using his microscope to help his diagnosis, and medical books on the diseases of warm climates to find clues about the disorders he found locally. The existing portraits of the Tropicalistas show them as serious and sedate Victorian figures, and the story told in their writings is one of highly dedicated doctors who, as clinicians and scientific investigators, were personally involved at all stages of their patients' illnesses, including at their autopsies when the outcome was unfavorable.[103] The image they sought to portray was one of doctors who were interested not in medicine as conducive to conspicuous consumption, classical erudition, and political posts, but in medicine as conducive to scientific excellence.

As part of their attempt to forge a strong medical profession in Salvador, the Tropicalistas advocated an alliance between doctors and pharmacists against irregular healers. In the pages of the *Gazeta Médica* they cajoled Bahian doctors and pharmacists to agree on the ethics and the scientific nature of their work, and to end the flirtations of some doctors and pharmacists with homeopathy.[104] In inviting the pharmacists to join them the Tropicalistas were calling for a cleavage between "serious" pharmacists and those who were not. Underlying the call was the fear that the changing nature of pharmacy, rapidly becoming a much greater source of competition to doctors, would encroach on the physician's territory and lead to the sort of rivalry that would detract from the image of scientific doctors and pharmacists above all polemics. This was because, from the second half of the nineteenth century, drugstores—hitherto very modest stores with a very small range of medications—started to become more commercial as they imported greater quantities of patent medications from Europe promising near miraculous cures, which they boldly advertised in the daily press.[105] In Brazil, as in other places, the apothecary had long played a central role in dispensing health care, but now apothecaries, who also had the authority of a degree in pharmacy from the medical school, threatened to reinvigorate this traditional role by becoming rivals to doctors bent on enlarging the scope of their authority.[106]

The Tropicalistas used the *Gazeta Médica* to counter the threat by proposing that doctors and pharmacists should each accept clearly defined boundaries and ground rules. Doctors should not sell medication, and pharmacists should restrict their task to fulfilling doctors' prescriptions faithfully.[107] In return for an alliance with the doctors, the pharmacists were promised association with the higher-status physicians such as membership in the Doctors' and Pharmacists' Mutual Aid Society (Sociedade de Beneficiencia Mútua) and a platform of support in the *Gazeta Médica* should they need it.[108] In a subtle attack on the influx of European patent medicines, and in keeping with their Brazilianist stance in medicine, the Tropicalistas constantly suggested that research be carried out on Brazil's immensely rich flora. They reminded their readers of the Brazilian origin of various contemporary medications used widely in European medicine such as araroba (ringworm powder), quinine, ipecacuanha (an emetic), and papaya (used for digestive purposes). They paid homage to Brazilians who in centuries past had studied Brazilian plants for their possible therapeutic qualities.[109]

Very important in the attempt to professionalize medicine was the breach the Tropicalistas tried to forge between the layman and the scientist. The Tropicalistas were deeply affronted when doctors reported on their work in the regular press.[110] They were even more offended when doctors aired their "dirty linen" in the laymen's press instead of closing ranks and keeping the disputes of physicians away from public view. This was one of the central issues underlying the lengthy debate in the *Gazeta Médica* over the notorious "Questão Braga" of 1878.[111] The case concerned a Bahian doctor who had reportedly raped his young bride on their wedding night and then declared the wedding annulled on the plea that she had not been a virgin when he married her. Expert medical advice was called in to determine the status of the woman's virginity, a decision central to the legal outcome of the case, but, as the experts could not agree and bitterly attacked each other, the case grew ever more sensational and was avidly reported in the daily press. The Tropicalistas railed against this reporting not only because they believed the aggrieved husband was guilty of personal misconduct and of attempting to twist the objectivity of science for his own personal gain, but, above all, because they held that the public should be screened from such professional disputes.[112]

By proposing to make the ranks of doctors impermeable to other areas of society, the Tropicalistas challenged the heart of the Brazilian medical tradition in which there had always been a close association between the medical, literary, and political worlds. I have already noted how a medical degree was often a means to enter the civil service or politics. Traditionally, physicians made ample use of the press, and often pursued medicine together with a career in journalism.[113] To ask them to avoid the layman's press and to keep to the specialized, medical one represented an important break with precedent. But this was crucial to the Tropicalistas, who wished to see the status of the profession as a whole raised by becoming "scientific," rather than continue to see individual men make use of medicine for their own rise up the social and political hierarchy. A united and highly esteemed profession would be much more successful, in the Tropicalistas' view, in persuading and pressuring the government to allow the profession to take its rightful place within the civil service and the national bureaucracies and have a clear impact on government legislation.

Another aim of the *Gazeta Médica* was to create informed professionals who drew on a common pool of scientific knowledge. To this end the editors reported assiduously on new European and North American therapies and surgical techniques and kept their readers updated about medical publications through articles, book reviews, and notices of books. The journal also included Tropicalista articles on the results of therapies and techniques they learned about in literature and then tried out locally. Thus they engaged in the current medical debates arguing for one medical approach or technique over another.[114] In addition, the journal reproduced seminal writings of the main pioneers in medicine, often with remarkably little time lag. In 1884, for example, it reproduced Pasteur's writings on his in-progress search for the microorganism involved in rabies and his attempt to develop a vaccination against it. Pasteur achieved his remarkable breakthrough only a year later. In 1884 the *Gazeta Médica* ran two long articles on Koch's crucial visit to Egypt and India in 1883 that led to the discovery of the cholera vibrio. The journal also reproduced articles by Virchow, Lister, and Charcot along with local and foreign commentaries on their contributions.[115] Through their journal the Tropicalistas wanted not only to inform local physicians about the developments in the outside world but also to inform the world, outside Salvador, about the innovating trends taking place in that city, trends that, the periodical believed, could lead to Bahian physicians' playing a role on the world medical stage. Just as Bahians had much to learn from Europe, so, they believed, Europeans could learn from Bahians.

Throughout the period the European sources of knowledge the Tropicalistas drew on shifted from primarily French to include German and Austrian. In the early years of the *Gazeta Médica* the editors relied heavily on a Portuguese naval medical publication, *Escholiaste Médico,* as their source of information for international medical news. This journal, founded in 1843, was wholly oriented toward French medicine. After the *Escholiaste Médico* folded in 1870, the editors—no doubt emboldened by their first years of success—looked for information from a broader variety of sources, including Austrian and German medical news.[116] The German-trained Wucherer was always an important link in Salvador to German medicine but other Tropicalistas also looked to Germany and Austria for medical models. Antônio Pacífico and Victorino Pereira, for example, not only became proficient in German, but on their medical tours of Europe in 1872 and 1879–81 respectively, Germany was a crucial stop. Victorino Pereira spent almost two years attending the classes of Virchow and Robert Koch in Germany, and working under the direction of the surgeon Theodor Billroth in Austria. In 1877 Pacífico Pereira also spent time at the polyclinic in Vienna. The Germanophile spirit of the *Gazeta Médica* was evident in the series of articles published from 1881 on medical education in Germany and Austria, as well as the "Variedade" selections in 1885, which were largely from the German medical press.[117] Rudolf Virchow's influence runs through its contents. Wucherer's articles are filled with references to the doctor-scientist and statesman, concerning him as both a scientist and a social reformer.[118] In 1877, after his return from Vienna, Pacífico Pereira wrote a series of seven articles to the current legislators outlining his agenda for the reform of medical teaching. As a centerpiece he demanded the sort of consolidation between university teaching and research achieved by German and Austrian schools. Moreover, a most effective way of improving medical training, Pereira argued, would be to set up a free polyclinic that would benefit the poor and also be a training ground for students, providing them with opportunities to examine and treat patients and perform minor procedures.[119] The idea of the polyclinic, an ambulatory and inpatient clinic, attached to a medical school, was taken from the German teaching model.

The Germanophile tendency, so often noted in terms of the Recife school and Tobias Barreto, and for a later period Rio de Janeiro and São Paulo, has hardly ever been linked to Salvador. This is part of the tendency to identify Salvador with colonial traditions and the monarchy, and to gloss over the attempts of some groups to break the mold. The Germanophile influence of the Tropicalistas was probably able to flourish in Salvador precisely because it was far from the capital, Rio de Janeiro, where the government kept a closer hold over the introduction of new currents of thought that could undermine the Empire.[120]

The counterpart to the creation of a professional medical corps was the creation of the "right" type of patient. Thus in 1882 Victorino Pereira, reporting admiringly on the medical schools he had seen in Austria, wrote in the *Gazeta Médica:*

> In clinical study . . . the patient is a robot [*automata*]; almost devoid of will power, submitting to everything. During the examination, in the presence of the professor or his assistant, he never rebels against anything the students may want to do with him no matter how . . . uncomfortable. Even in the absence of the professor or assistant, it is rare for patients to resist being observed by medical students, as do our patients.[121]

That Bahian patients provided a sharp contrast was a problem that had to be addressed. Not only did patients refuse to allow students to observe them, but patients also challenged the doctor's authority to make decisions concerning their treatment. Thus, for example, of twenty-one cases Pires Caldas related he had attended at the Santa Casa hospital in November 1866, nine refused to submit to the treatment proposed and either left the hospital or forced the doctor to adopt an alternative. In the treatment of women this was particularly common.[122] When doctors were called in to help with labor emergencies or other crises pertaining to women's disorders, they often found that a midwife barred direct access to the patient, or that the patient herself refused to be examined.[123]

Although the doctors did not discuss reasons for the contrast, some suggestions may be made. First, there was no tradition in consulting doctors throughout the colonial period and much of the nineteenth century, when the numbers of doctors were so paltry. Second, partly as a result of this dearth, there was a well-entrenched tradition of consulting folk healers who drew on European, African, and Indian traditions. One foreign observer

noted in 1883, "there is perhaps no part of the world in which a larger proportion of irregular practitioners are found than in Brazil and, even in cities
where civilization is most advanced, the quack is fostered and supported
by the credulity of . . . the population."[124] Even when a trained doctor was
called in, patients often consulted several doctors so they could get an array
of opinions.[125] One of the fundamental aims of the *Gazeta Médica,* therefore, was to allow physicians to construct a scientific medical authority that
could be used to undermine the control that laypeople still exercised over
illness and its treatment.[126]

As well as helping to disseminate Western medicine in Brazil, the Tropicalistas set out to claim that there was something medically distinct about
practicing medicine in the tropics. The Tropicalistas wanted to set their
own agenda of priorities in medicine, which they held was different from
the European because of the climate and other social factors peculiar to
Brazil. As an 1872 editorial in the *Gazeta Médica* put it, "We always pre-
fer to [report] on our own investigations rather than to transcribe articles
on foreign medicine because our main objective is to clarify and develop
the study of Brazilian medicine."[127] The Tropicalistas, therefore, primarily
investigated and described locally occurring disorders. Between 1866 and
1899 the *Gazeta Médica* published more than three hundred articles discussing local Bahian, or other northern Brazilian, clinical cases. They asked
questions that became central to tropical medicine by the turn of the century. Was there a geography of disease with specific illnesses confined to
tropical regions? Did heat and moisture favor the multiplication of harmful microorganisms thus making a tropical climate per se have a deleterious
influence on human beings, regardless of whether a person lived within
a milieu of good sanitation and followed a sound diet and a regimen of
healthy exercise? Did tropical climate affect various races differently? Was
acclimatization possible for whites? Could Brazilians be healthy? The complex relationship between the Tropicalistas' desire to provide a Brazilian
option to European stereotypes about disease in the tropics while remaining within the framework of European scientific authority is the subject of
later chapters. What I want the stress here is the degree to which this call to
Brazilianize medicine was also a call both to reinvigorate local Bahian medicine and, subtly, to critique the longtime hegemony that Rio de Janeiro
had held over medicine in Brazil. By calling for contributions to their journal from the four corners of the Empire, the Tropicalistas presented the
Gazeta Médica as the alternative medical journal in Brazil, especially for

northerners, who would find the *Gazeta* more accommodating than the high-handedness of the *Anais Brasilienses de Medicina*.[128]

The Politics of the Tropicalistas

The founding Tropicalistas held that in an ideal world, active political participation as a result of personal ambition and the exercise of the medical profession and research were incompatible. For example, of his friend and colleague Almeida Couto, who was president of São Paulo and later of Salvador, Silva Lima observed:

> His activity, . . . is divided into teaching at the medical school, [working] at the hospital, his large private practice, and politics. He is irresistibly . . . drawn to the latter . . . which leads to the question, . . . whether politics and medicine exercised together are incompatible: . . . There is no doubt whatsoever that this [man's] great activity would be more fecund if it concentrated on only one of those realms.[129]

Silva Lima had a similar lament about his son-in-law, Victorino Pereira, who entered politics and paid for it by sacrificing his early great promise as a physician and researcher.[130] The demand to refrain from politics went very much against traditional expectations of physicians. As one French observer put it, "It's rare for Brazilian doctors to dedicate themselves to only medical practice or science; they engage actively in politics."[131]

Despite such reservations, the Tropicalistas can best be understood as a politically engaged group. Indeed, as well as a medical journal, the *Gazeta Médica* must be read as an inherently political journal. Although they disapproved of using a medical career to attain individual political advancement (a number of them did just that), the Tropicalistas were articulate spokesmen of a new and expanded role for doctors within any nation that would embrace progress. In other words, the Tropicalista pursuit of the creation of an excellent physician was related to furthering the power of the profession, not that of individual doctors. In contrast, therefore, to the traditional Brazilian doctor who "wheeled and dealed" in the business of patronage and connections for personal advancement, these "new" men believed that a doctor's entry into politics should be the result of his excellence as a doctor-scientist and that the object of entry into politics should be related to the simple yet radical idea that the solutions to illness in Brazil were as much political as medical. What then were their politics?

The Tropicalista journal became a platform for demanding change and, ultimately, an important local participant in the political struggles in the final decades of the Empire. Their arguments resonated with those of other new groups emerging in the final decades of the Empire among urbanizing and modernizing sectors of Brazil, groups made up of immigrants, merchants, bureaucrats, professionals, and army men. It would be a gross oversimplification to say that these groups were always in opposition to the emperor and in agreement with each other, but, ultimately, in the face of a changing economy and the grave crises over slavery and church-state relations, they began to view imperial centralization as the key obstacle to Brazilian progress.[132] Tropicalista demands for change focused both on health and medicine, and, eventually, on broader political changes.

On one hand, the Tropicalistas viewed doctors as agents of improvement who had a duty to influence public legislation to impose health. As they put it in the *Gazeta Médica,* "In these pages we have censured the lack of scientific criteria with which key issues of hygiene and medical teaching are resolved, and we have lamented that the prime minister does not have, as in Prussia and Austria and other countries, a special body made up of experts to deal with such vital matters."[133] Thus they began to raise issues that would not be fully addressed until after the turn of the century when national and local authorities finally moved beyond the concern of the health of ports and port-cities to spread the net of public health to encompass all classes and populations, urban and rural. As early as 1868, for example, the *Gazeta Médica* stated that the main significance of Wucherer's breakthrough in hookworm disorder was that it would lead to the improvement of the health of slaves and agricultural workers, indicating their belief that this was a neglected group that should be made the concern of the modern doctor and state.[134] They also suggested ways of improving the delivery of health, asking, for example, that health measures taken for ships and the port of Bahia be coordinated with those for the city at large, that the city's sanitation be improved, that more efficient institutions be set up to regulate health on an ongoing basis instead of a reactive one—all demands for an enlarged medical purview that threatened to dilute the power of local strongmen.[135]

On the other hand, by the 1880s Tropicalista demands for health measures began to broaden into overtly political areas. Swept up in the turmoil of the final imperial years that saw the demise of slavery in 1888 and of the monarchy in 1889, the Tropicalistas came to believe that a principal obstacle to their vision of advanced medicine was the increasingly centralized power of the monarchy, the high-handedness of its decrees, the favoritism, the unfair distribution of resources among regions, and the continuation of slavery. Indeed, by the 1880s it was clear to some young Tropicalistas like Victorino Pereira and Braz do Amaral that the struggle for scientific medicine was indistinct from the struggle against a controlling and encroaching monarch.[136] They argued that the Tropicalista movement was an attempt to bring progress to a backward nation by introducing scientific knowledge and practices, in much the same way that the projects for political reform and the abolition of slavery in Brazil were attempts to purge the country of its backward and colonial institutions. Ultimately, the force of the political events of the 1880s pulled many of these men into political action and some of the leading Tropicalistas neglected their research rather than resist the call to politics.

Of nineteen Bahian doctors who sat in the Provincial Assembly over the nineteenth century, five were core Tropicalistas who were also editors of the *Gazeta Médica,* and another three were Tropicalista supporters.[137] The core Tropicalista Almeida Couto and supporter Sodré Pereira were also presidents of the provinces of São Paulo, Salvador, and Sergipe.[138] On a national level, there were seventeen Bahian doctors who served in the Chamber of Deputies over the course of the century. Of these, one was a core Tropicalista, Almeida Couto, and two were supporters, Goes Siqueira and Sodré Pereira.[139] With the exception of Goes all were either members of the Republican party or proabolition liberals. Almeida Couto was an abolitionist and active in the Liberal Party for many years; Victorino Pereira was one of the leaders of the Liberal Party in Salvador and a fervent abolitionist; Virgílio Clímaco Damázio was the founder and leader of the Republican Party in Salvador; Luís Álvares dos Santos was a liberal and an abolitionist; Jerônymo Sodré Pereira, a liberal and an abolitionist.[140]

Even when the records do not positively identify the Tropicalistas with the Liberal or Republican Parties, the positions taken by the *Gazeta Médica* show clearly that the journal sided with the forces of reform and innovation. Not only did the Tropicalistas criticize the medical establishment from early on, but in the final decade of the Empire, when they realized that few of their enlarged professional demands would be met under the current political structure, they took increasingly combative positions against the imperial government. From the mid-1880s on, the *Gazeta Médica* became vigorous in its criticism of the government over such issues as its ineffective attempts at educational reform and its favoritism toward the medical establishment linked to the court. Two factors allowed the journal to become bolder in its criticism of what it saw as unfair governmental practices working to the detriment of the Bahian medical community. One was the successful reception of the *Gazeta Médica* in the European medical press, which gave it prestige at home; the other was that the *Gazeta* had built up a more secure local following, thus ensuring its financial survival.

Within Salvador, therefore, the *Gazeta Médica* came to wield considerable influence in local politics. Articles constantly derided local and central government, pressured for the reform of schools so that the caliber of the incoming medical students could be improved, and argued for the reform of medical teaching, especially practical teaching. Moreover, they favored provincial autonomy in these matters. By taking on the imperial government, the *Gazeta Médica* was taking a stand in the regional rivalry between the medical establishment surrounding the court and the Bahian one. As the *Gazeta* became more and more successful, it became a significant ally in this rivalry; it won over Bahian physicians who, once annoyed by the critical outsiders, now had to admit to the political value of the group and their journal. By allowing the *Gazeta Médica* to become a platform for criticism that could be used by the Bahian medical school in its struggle for greater autonomy against imperial encroachment, the Tropicalistas gained increasing influence within the Bahian medical establishment.

Even in Rio de Janeiro the Tropicalistas' influence can be seen in the attempts made there to revitalize medicine: the aims of the most innovating physicians who formed the Rio de Janeiro Medical Society (Sociedade Médica do Rio de Janeiro) in 1876 and the Medical and Surgical Society of Rio de Janeiro (Sociedade de Medicina e Cirurgia do Rio de Janeiro) in 1886 resonated with those of the Tropicalistas. For example, the Bahians applauded the idea of producing a bibliography of Brazilian medical contributions and the decision to hold an annual medical congress.[141] Carlos Costa, founding member of the 1876 society, had the installments of his bibliography published to much praise in the *Gazeta Médica,* and in 1888, when the First Brazilian Medical Congress was held in Rio, the journal published the papers presented and lobbied to get the congress to meet in Salvador. In the 1880s new medical journals in the capital city challenged the *Anais Brasilienses de Medicina*'s virtual monopoly of medical publishing. The opening editorials of journals like *União Médica* (1881), *Brasil Médico* (1887), *Progresso Médico* (1887), *Revista Brasileira de Medicina* (1888), and

the Rio de Janeiro student-run *Revista Médica do Rio de Janeiro* (1873) repeated the Tropicalistas' long-held objectives of focusing on original investigations related to the disorders of tropical climates, disorders that, "like
the immense riches of our country," were almost unknown. The new journals published work on ainhum, beriberi, filariasis, hookworm, and other
parasitological investigations; they noted the importance of carrying out
research on Brazilian flora and of shrugging off European tutelage. The
União Médica explicitly named the *Gazeta Médica* as its model, noting that
it aspired "to play a similar role as the *Gazeta Médica da Bahia*, . . . a journal that has raised the most interesting aspects of tropical disorders, that
has announced the most important discoveries made among us, and that
has helped to elevate the name of Brazilian [doctors] in countries scientifically far in advance of ours."[142] Júlio de Moura (a parasitologist and one of
the earliest of the Tropicalista supporters in Rio de Janeiro), Silva Araújo
(a core Tropicalista who moved to the capital city), and Pedro S. de Magalhães (a younger-generation Tropicalista supporter who also moved to Rio
de Janeiro) are found in all the new medical ventures of Rio de Janeiro.
Júlio de Moura and Silva Araújo were editors of the *União Médica;* Moura
also edited the *Revista Médica do Rio de Janeiro* and *Brasil Médico;* Magalhães was an editor of the *Revista Brasileira de Medicina* and at the forefront
of parasitological investigation through the turn of the century. The work
of Nina Rodrigues, Pacífico Pereira, and others was published in the new
Rio journals. Of course, the changing medical discourse in Rio de Janeiro
cannot be attributed simply to the Tropicalista influence; there were other
significant sources of change, local and foreign. But as the earliest group to
develop a new medical discourse in Brazil that later became "typical," the
Tropicalistas were a model to emulate, and their members in Rio de Janeiro
had the energy and influence to successfully disseminate Tropicalista approaches.

By 1889 the Tropicalistas were happy to report in an editorial on some
of the changes medical practice in Salvador was undergoing. A large new
training hospital was being planned according to the most updated ideas on
hospital building (ideas filtered into Salvador largely through the Tropicalistas). Medical teaching had undergone a profound reform with a reorga-
nized school curriculum and the building of laboratories for teaching. New
disorders and medical topics, several of which had been first introduced
by the Tropicalistas themselves, were being studied. The *Gazeta*'s editor
proudly noted of the journal,

This issue marks the twenty-first year of the *Gazeta Médica*. Such a long existence is almost unique in the annals of the Brazilian medical press. . . . In its early years the journal was kept going by erudite professionals . . . , hardworking and enthusiastic for progress. . . . And today there is no lack of support [for the journal].[143]

A few years later another editorial was even more forthright in enumerating the group's achievements, among which were

original investigations on tropical medicine that received national and international recognition and contributed to the resolution of important etiological questions; . . . efforts to improve public health; improvements in medical teaching; the publication of the most interesting national and international works on pathology, hygiene, and therapeutics, and the defense of . . . our professional interests.[144]

It was clear to the Tropicalistas that many of the changes in local medicine were the result of their own political perseverance and the platform of their medical journal.

Conclusion

In considering the emergence of the Tropicalistas several factors should be noted. First, there was little hope for foreigners outside the network of patronage in Salvador to satisfy their personal ambitions as doctors within communities of foreign traders and entrepreneurs. Moreover, they had trained as doctors in Europe at a time when medicine had emerged out of the eighteenth-century morass of grand theories and abstract systems and turned to clinical observation and detailed autopsies.[145] The 1840s through the 1860s was a particularly fruitful period in the development of Western medicine, a period often eclipsed by the later triumph of the germ theory. But for those alive then, these earlier decades must have been pathbreaking in many ways. The Tropicalistas were very self-conscious of themselves as an innovating group and they positioned themselves squarely within the new medicine. As they noted about the medicine they espoused, "clinical and therapeutic observation, microscopic investigations, chemical analyses, and animal experimentation are the bases of today's medicine. [Abstract medical theories] may be ingenuous, but they only satisfy dreamers. We will not follow that path."[146]

Second, the movement's initial enthusiastic reception by some Bahian physicians and students was reinforced in the 1870s when the development of bacteriology opened up a new era in the prevention and treatment of illness. The new germ theory of disease, with its stress on the laboratory method of research, combined with older notions of hygiene and sanitation, began to make real gains in the fight against such longtime scourges as cholera, smallpox, rabies, and tuberculosis. What could have been a brief burst of innovation in Salvador, in fact, became a sustained movement as it was reinforced by the trends of innovation, discovery, and success from abroad. The Tropicalistas drew supporters from among both established physicians attracted to the idea of original research and ambitious young doctors and students lured by the Tropicalistas' fruitful investigations and eager embrace of the newest developments, such as the use of microscopic examinations in clinical medicine.

Finally, the Tropicalistas' success cannot simply be explained by the fact that they were a handful of ambitious and resourceful foreigners with leadership qualities, or that European medical science was making pathbreaking strides in the nineteenth century. All of these factors were crucial, but they were not enough to explain the rise of the Tropicalistas as the most successful research-oriented doctors in nineteenth-century Brazil. In the course of the century there had been other notable foreign doctors working in Brazil and many Brazilian doctors eager for more scientific approaches to medicine.[147] What differed now was that the criticism of the status quo in the medical establishment initiated by the Tropicalistas, the striving for innovation, the doctrines of "progress" and "science" all dovetailed with a broader social and political agenda for change that, from the 1870s on, was slowly being defined within pockets of discontent all over the Empire.

CHAPTER TWO

The Politics of Disease

A central theme that has preoccupied historians of nineteenth-century medicine has been how practicing physicians dealt with the barrage of new knowledge accumulating as a result of positivistic approaches to illness, and the deployment of far better technical methods to view pathology than had ever been available. Not only was there a good deal more information to digest in many areas of medicine, but the increasing understanding called into question old paradigms of disease, most particularly the humoral theory that, under one guise or another, had been dominant for more than two millennia in Western medicine. However, even as a more specific understanding of the causes and processes of disease unfolded, undermining the humoral edifice, it failed to provide much in the way of answers to help the physician involved in the practical, daily task of trying to cure an individual of his ailment. What was a physician to do regarding the practical delivery of medicine once the protean and infinitely flexible humoral theory of disease was called into question by "scientific" results emerging from laboratory investigations, which, for a considerable time, offered nothing in the way of therapeutic solutions?[1]

The rise of greater specificity in the understanding of pathology also made the therapeutic search narrower as doctor-scientists cast about for a series of magic bullets, discarding the broad, community-oriented directives that looked to such remedies as the removal of miasma, and changes in lifestyle to cure and prevent sickness. Sometimes the new demarcations blurred, for a doctor-scientist might push ahead with his discoveries in the laboratory but continue in his practice to invoke old causes and call on old therapies that were familiar and reassuring to his paying patient.[2] The changes in medical knowledge upset in other ways. Those who were influential and authoritative in the old knowledge were no longer so in the new. Established boundaries were questioned, new demarcations formed, often acrimoniously. The many varied responses to these dilemmas for the nineteenth-century doctor have proven grist for the historian's mill. They were dilemmas that the Tropicalistas also faced.

In Brazil the Tropicalistas were among the pioneers of the new form of knowledge that by the turn of the century had transformed medical thinking, making way for institutions that supported biomedical sciences, such as the Oswaldo Cruz Institute and Butantã.[3] Confronting a medicine steeped in early-nineteenth-century French traditions, the Tropicalistas discovered new disorders and asked new questions about medical practice, threatening to displace powerful physicians whose authority rested on the old.[4] Eschewing both the rigidity of outdated medical practice and an unthinking imitation of European medicine, they advocated the use of the new scientific medicine to study questions of specific interest to Brazil. Theirs was an innovative position that pitted them against established authorities and led to controversies both among physicians in Salvador and between the medical communities in Bahia and Rio de Janeiro. Ultimately, the Tropicalistas were a significant influence on Brazilian medicine in several ways, most importantly because they were the first group of nineteenth-century doctors in Brazil who dared challenge the way medical authority was constructed. Leading Rio doctors could not ignore the challenge the Tropicalistas proffered, especially once the latter became linked to an international network of geographically scattered doctor-scientists interested in similar themes. Moreover, the Tropicalistas gained acceptance because their search to produce a medical science relevant to the special circumstances of Brazil, and especially the country's northern regions, was very much in line with a rising Brazilian nationalism that stressed regionalism over imperial centralism, and looked for a national identity that would move Brazil away from a deferential imitation of Europe.

What made the Tropicalistas even more palatable was the way they juggled concepts from a dying era in European medicine with those of a nascent one. The Tropicalistas are best understood as a transitional generation. Thus, even as they pioneered parasitology and led the shift in Brazil toward greater etiological specificity, they held on to environmentalist explanations of disease and remained believers in the melioration of humanity through environmental reform. That is, the thrust of their medical theory was toward greater specificity, and thus they accompanied the general direction of Western medicine from mid–nineteenth century on, but they never altogether shed a view of disease as inextricably interwoven with broader social conditions. This blending is common to most shifts in medical paradigms, especially given the problem of the time lag between discovery and therapeutic solutions. However, the Tropicalistas' reluctance to let go altogether of an older environmentalism was because the theory—with its practical advocacy of a strict adherence to programs for sanitation and hygiene—provided them with an easy way to argue in favor of the possibility of progress in Brazil. As such, the Tropicalistas' voice must be added to those other contemporary voices who refused to altogether accept European ideas about degeneration in the tropics.[5]

Beriberi: Constructing a New Disorder in Brazil

One of the key disorders that came to define the Tropicalistas was beriberi. In 1866 José Francisco da Silva Lima warned of an epidemic outbreak in the city of Bahia in an article published in the *Gazeta Médica da Bahia*.[6] Between 1863 and 1866 Silva Lima attended thirty-two patients who presented such similar symptoms of weakness, numbness in the extremities, edema, degeneration of muscular tissue, and paralysis related to a dysfunction of the nervous center that he strongly suspected he was dealing with a specific disorder. As he made inquiries among his colleagues, he found that they too had recently treated such cases. His close friend and colleague Dr. Paterson directed Silva Lima to a reference in Dr. Copland's *Medical Dictionary* that described a disorder known in India as *barbiers* or *beriberi*. To Silva Lima, the description sounded remarkably like what he had been treating. In his subsequent reading, Silva Lima became convinced he was dealing with beriberi, a conclusion further validated for him in his correspondence with the French naval physician and beriberi expert A. Le Roy de Méricourt.[7] As a result of Silva Lima's "discovery" of beriberi in Bahia, an editorial in the *Gazeta Médica* in November 1866 warned other doctors of the danger of this new illness reaching epidemic proportions in the state of Bahia.[8]

Declaring an epidemic was always problematic because various groups could be harmed by the announcement. Commercial interests feared for their businesses, poor sectors of the society feared the state's increased search and quarantine powers, and the authorities had to consider the problems of panic and social disorder that such a declaration might lead to among the general population.[9] From the physicians' point of view, however, the declaration of an epidemic could have some favorable consequences. The label "epidemic" was a way of acknowledging the importance and seriousness of a disease. In such a case, a government might be forced to call on the expertise of physicians not only to treat patients but to formulate preventive and emergency policies. The Tropicalistas, whose first leaders had gained fame and influence in the two great Bahian epidemics of yellow fever (1849) and cholera (1855), well knew that an epidemic could give them the sort of clout they never commanded during the routine treatment of endemic ailments. It is likely, therefore, that underlying Silva Lima's use of the term "epidemic" was the desire to make a strong statement about the importance of focusing on this ailment in Brazil. But in doing so he must have been aware that he was going outside the accepted channels for such a declaration.

It is instructive to look at Silva Lima's attempt to decipher the problem of the etiology of beriberi in order to gain a sense of his place regarding contemporary ideas of epidemic disease in the tropics both within and outside of Brazil. He held the disorder to be a blood intoxication caused by miasma in the tropics. Miasma, a common theme in Western medicine, believed to emanate from filth, stagnant water, churned-up soil, and rotting vegetation, was held to be particularly lethal when found in the tropics.[10] It seemed clear to Silva Lima that the blood intoxication he believed led to beriberi was caused by some agent that relied for its existence on the climatic conditions of the tropics. But he was aware that the concept of tropical miasma was so general as to be almost irrelevant in the explanation of disease etiology:

> The great kingdom of tropical disorders to the north and south of the equator contains a large number of disorders peculiar to these regions. . . . Unfortunately, . . . we know only that climatic conditions favor this or that tropical disorder, without knowing the actual cause of the disorders. . . . So long as science does not disclose those mysteries . . . let us be content with investigating what are the most favorable conditions [of the disorders].[11]

As a pragmatic physician working in the tropics, Silva Lima wanted to go beyond the blanket term of "tropical miasma" to search for causes. Working within long-established European etiological traditions of topography and climate, he attempted to tease out which might be the most dangerous topographical and climatic conjunctures for those predisposed toward the disorder. There was little novelty in the conclusions he reached. For example, he considered sudden climatic changes to be an important contributing factor. Even more dangerous were long periods of heat combined with humidity and unhygienic conditions. An individual's constitution weakened as a result of former illness, or a life of vice and debauchery, increased the chances of contracting the disorder, as did pregnancy in the case of women. Silva Lima believed that hygienic conditions were vital. He was not wholly satisfied with these explanations, however, and for the next two decades he continued to mull over the possible causes of beriberi. Attuned to the debates of his time, he was willing to consider the possibility of a narrower and more specific cause. He was intrigued by the diet-deficiency theory proposed in connection with the Dutch East Indies and the Japanese navy, but he was unable to reconcile this theory with the fact that people with apparently good diets were known to have succumbed to the disease.[12] In the end he continued to adhere to the broader miasmatic/environmentalist explanations, professing that "for the moment most of the evidence supports the miasmatic theory."[13]

For a well-informed doctor like Silva Lima it was difficult to shift from a multicausal theory of disease (in which predisposition, diet, and habits combined with miasmatic factors and climate to lead to illness) to a bacteriological theory or a diet-deficiency theory (in which a single cause was responsible for a specific disease). There were too many questions left unanswered, particularly concerning why some persons became ill while others, in similar conditions, did not.[14] But beyond the general difficulty many nineteenth-century physicians had in making this theoretical shift was the particular situation of the Tropicalistas, who were uncomfortable about giving up environmentalist ideas because they provided a confident and activist view of man's ability to manipulate the milieu. By preserving the complex interplay between health, morality, environment, and (soft) heredity, the Tropicalistas were able to continue to believe that if people's free will (often exercised in error and ignorance) had brought them to illness, then free will (exercised according to the "scientific" prescriptions of physicians) could reverse or prevent illness. Retaining a broad conception of etiology also enabled a doctor like Silva Lima to have a more forceful political impact in his demand for social reform than if he adopted a monocausal theory of disease. That is, the polluted conditions that produced miasma pointed clearly to the need for social reforms, reforms that updated doctors, like the Tropicalistas, were most qualified to pilot.

Silva Lima's writings on beriberi show him to be a doctor well within the European medical tradition. But he also represented a spirit of reform in Brazilian medicine. He was willing to challenge European doctors by questioning accepted geographical frontiers for a disorder such as beriberi, long held not to be found in Brazil.[15] He stressed the importance of Brazilian doctors using their practice as the prime source for the discovery of illnesses of warm climates, and although he accepted that a tropical climate was the fundamental context for beriberi outbreaks, he wanted to investigate exactly how a tropical climate was relevant to the disorder. His position was not unlike those European sanitarians who were aware that although filth was the context of many diseases, it did not adequately explain those diseases.

The declaration of a beriberi epidemic in the pages of the *Gazeta Médica* drew fire from health authorities, in particular José Goes Siqueira, a physician who dominated public health in Bahia from the 1840s until his death, and who not only disputed the declaration of an epidemic but also argued that there was no such disorder as beriberi.[16] Indeed, the clash between Silva Lima and Goes Siqueira can be seen as a dispute over how medical authority was to be constituted. Son of an ennobled father, the Marquês de Araújo Goes, and a graduate in 1835 of the medical school in Bahia, Goes Siqueira became the most powerful sanitary officer in Salvador, heading the Board of Public Hygiene, which was created in 1851 to oversee the health and hygiene of the port-city. Inspired by nineteenth-century French and English sanitarians, and with only a skeleton staff, he worked indefatigably toward better sanitation in Salvador.[17] He inspected the quality of food sold to the public; advocated the removal of the slaughterhouses away from the center of the city; and pushed for the cleaning up of the streets, for drainage systems to be installed, for an official body to be set up to compile medical statistics, and for physicians to have more than merely advisory roles in the government. He continuously criticized the municipal government for its slovenly performance in sanitation and in 1871 vehemently denounced the provincial governor, Araújo Freitas Henriques, for the latter's refusal to acknowledge an outbreak of yellow fever in the city and take the necessary precautions against its spread.[18] Goes Siqueira was also a member of the Council of Health, a council of venerable physicians who had opposed the "foreigners'" diagnoses in the yellow fever and cholera epidemics. In 1854 he joined the Bahian medical school as professor of the newly created chair in general pathology and the imperial government named him the director of the Council for Public Education (Conselho Superior de Instrução Pública) in the province of Bahia. He headed the lepers' Hospital dos Lázaros in Salvador, had a large and successful private practice, and wrote numerous articles for medical journals, medical treatises, and his own memoirs.[19] He managed to combine all this activity with a political career first as a deputy to the Provincial Assembly and, from 1848 to 1856, as Bahian representative in the National Assembly. In 1855 the central government awarded his services with the title of Official e Commendador da Imperial Ordem da Rosa and the Ordem do Christo.

Why Goes Siqueira opposed Silva Lima over the question of a beriberi epidemic in Bahia offers a brief glimpse into how the Tropicalistas threatened the existing means of distributing power and influence in Bahian society. As I have noted, Goes Siqueira was actively involved in the attempt to expand the realm of professional medicine within his society. In this respect he was like the Tropicalistas, and his strong advocacy of hygiene and sanitation impressed the latter.[20] He himself was sufficiently interested in new trends in medicine to attend the early meetings of physicians at Dr. Paterson's house and to contribute to the first issues of the *Gazeta Médica*. However, whereas the Tropicalistas represented a transition between the French medical environmentalist tradition and the Pasteurian age, and mixed their French influences with large doses of German ones, Goes Siqueira remained firmly planted within the older French tradition, a tradition intertwined with the most prestigious sectors of Brazilian medicine, to which Goes belonged. When he took up new ideas, he borrowed from France, not Germany. Thus, for example, he became increasingly interested in French ideas on the treatment of the insane and pushed for setting up a special institution for the insane in Salvador.[21] The Tropicalistas, even while they promoted hygienism and policies of sanitation, moved toward the German variant best exemplified by Virchow, who, even though he continued to be interested in the environment and saw disease as a social phenomenon, also sought to understand and describe its processes through the investigation of the cell and an understanding of physiology and physiopathology, activities that drew him into the laboratory.[22] But even more important than these ideological differences regarding European influences was the fact that while Goes represented the establishment in Bahian medicine, the Tropicalistas were outsiders. It was the authority of his position that Goes defended when he attacked the Tropicalistas.

In January 1867 Goes Siqueira included in his annual health report to the provincial governor a long section that scathingly rebutted allegations of a beriberi epidemic.[23] Intimating that the epidemic was a fiction of the medical press, he proceeded to question both the use of the term "epidemic" and the veracity of the existence of beriberi as a specific disorder. Epidemics, he wrote, involved large numbers of sick, which was not the case in this instance, since the mortality rates for the province had remained stable. Using various descriptions of beriberi given by physicians in different countries, he showed there was little agreement among them on the symptoms of the disease. A central symptom, the disorder of the nervous system, was not peculiar to the so-called beriberi disorder. "In order to explain the frequency and gravity of the disorders of the nervous center, . . . it is not necessary to resort to beriberi," Goes Siqueira affirmed, "when all around us we have a complexity of causes which act [to produce] multiple pathological states."[24] Quoting approvingly from the French doctor and positivist Émile Littré, he argued that specific disorders characterized different epochs.[25] The present epoch was particularly prone to disorders of the nervous centers, found mostly among those professions wholly concerned with amassing money. The desire for enrichment together with excessive pleasure-seeking made for the high incidence of nervous disorders.

> In a period when desires are exorbitant, when the imagination is exalted by man's great feats, when change is constant, when illusions are rapidly destroyed, when family life is weakened, this period cannot but lead to the . . . deterioration of the nervous centers.[26]

According to Goes Siqueira, it would be better for Bahian physicians to turn their attention to these sorts of disorders rather than waste their time on a highly questionable sickness like beriberi.

The debate between the public health administrator and the Tropicalistas revealed several fundamental differences. Goes Siqueira showed in his arguments how strongly entrenched he was within the French tradition of medicine and culture. He was very much part of an older generation of Brazilian physicians who believed that in order to bring progress to Brazil, it was necessary to replicate European institutions in the new nation. Consciously or not, Goes Siqueira was also importing French anxieties grounded in urbanization, early industrialization, and rapid change that lay at the root of the French passage quoted above. While the city of Salvador certainly underwent urbanization in the nineteenth century, its population almost doubling from 45,600 people in 1805 to 81,544 in 1850 and then rising to 144,959 in 1900, this growth was due not to industrialization but to an influx of immigration from the surrounding countryside, as well as natural increase. To some extent, the city was therefore spared the most acute miseries of the back streets of London and Paris in the nineteenth century.[27] The Tropicalistas, with their emphasis on Brazilian themes, were far less interested in the anxieties imported from Europe than in the disorders occurring locally as a result of *local* social and climatic conditions. Thus while Goes Siqueira found evidence in Brazil of how similar (upper-class) Brazilians were to Europeans, the Tropicalistas preferred to show that Brazilians were "like" Europeans by providing evidence of original scientific discovery. Goes Siqueira rejected the existence of beriberi in Brazil and asked doctors to focus on the "nervous" disorders of the epoch; Silva Lima ignored this call and encouraged doctors to look at disorders occurring within their clinical practice that were more directly relevant to Brazil.

The debate over whether an epidemic existed or not also revealed the stresses between a well-appointed civil servant guarding his position and the challenge of a group of doctors who spoke with no authority other than that of "science." What Goes Siqueira particularly resented was that the Tropicalistas, through the platform of their journal, had taken it upon themselves to be the judges of the state of health in the city and province, thus challenging Goes Siqueira's own official authority.[28] Having made his disagreement public, Goes Siqueira never again published an article in the *Gazeta Médica* nor, in his subsequent health reports, did he ever make reference to beriberi again. In 1873, when he was appointed by the president of the Province of Bahia, Antônio Cándido da Cruz Machado, to serve on a commission to look into beriberi, he asked to be excused from serving on it.[29]

Upon Goes Siqueira's death in 1874, one of the first actions of his successor, Luís Álvares dos Santos, one-time editor of the *Gazeta Médica* and a close associate of the Tropicalistas, was to declare beriberi epidemic in the state of Bahia. From then on, in official circles, beriberi received as much attention as yellow fever, cholera, or smallpox, and a special hospital was opened in 1874 for beriberi victims on the island of Itaparica. In 1879 the imperial minister, Barão Homem de Melo, set up commissions to inspect incoming ships with suspected cases of beriberi and to gather information on the disease by sending out questionnaires to physicians in the afflicted provinces.[30] From the 1870s the interest in beriberi also grew in the Bahian medical school, where an increasing number of doctors and students came to accept the Tropicalistas' argument that beriberi was a crucial illness to study in Brazil and chose to write their dissertations on it.[31] Some professors, like Januário de Faria, soon to become head of the medical school, moved from a position of early skepticism (which Faria confessed he had endeavored to pass on to his students) to the conviction that Silva Lima was correct.[32] Thus, even though the initial reaction of the Bahian medical establishment to Silva Lima's discovery of beriberi and his warning of it reaching epidemic proportions had been negative, after Goes Siqueira's death, Silva Lima successfully placed beriberi on the noso-logical map of northern Brazil and received official support for preventive measures against the disorder. The reason for this is linked to the recognition the Tropicalistas began to receive for their work internationally, which boosted their prestige in Brazil.

It was Silva Lima's younger colleague Antônio Pacífico Pereira, another key figure among the Tropicalistas, who took up the challenge of further unraveling the puzzle of beriberi. In the end, however, he too fell back on environmentalist explanations. Indeed, the Tropicalistas' juggling of concepts from a waning paradigm in European medicine with those of a nascent one, and their tendency to straddle the older miasmatic/environ-mentalist approach with the newer parasitical/bacteriological one, is par-ticularly well illustrated in the work of Pacífico Pereira. In 1879–80 Pacífico Pereira carried out original research into beriberi, focusing on the patho-logical anatomy of the disorder and the hematological alterations in the blood of beriberi patients in particluar.[33] He performed autopsies on more than sixty beriberi victims and made detailed examinations of their diseased tissues, blood, and urine. The report on the work that Pacífico Pereira pub-lished in the *Gazeta Médica* shows how influenced he was by the model of German biomedicine that began emerging from the 1840s on. In the study, Pacífico Pereira, operating with the new concepts of histology devel-oped by Virchow and others, shifted from a reliance on naked-eye autopsies to microscopical anatomical examinations, asked questions regarding the pathological alterations of the cells and blood in beriberi, and, using the results of German experimentation with animals on body temperature and respiration, posed questions about how those results could be adapted to understand the influence of warm climate on beriberi.[34] From his reading on beriberi, his clinical observations, and his autopsies, Pereira arrived at the conclusion that the cause of beriberi was "anoxemia," or a lack of oxygen in the blood.[35] What then caused anoxemia? The common denominator Pacífico Pereira found in all his reading and his own clinical experience was tropical climate: "It seems irrefutable that . . . beriberi is a disorder of the tropical zone, and especially of hot and damp areas."[36]

Like Silva Lima, however, Pacífico Pereira sought to probe exactly how the damp and heat affected a person. For an answer he turned to the work of the German hygienist Max von Pettenkofer and his student Carl von Voit.[37] According to their studies, in a cold climate, more activity producing heat was required to keep the body's temperature even and this activity was intricately linked to the oxygenation of the body and the expelling of carbon dioxide ("carbonic acid"), and, thus, to the regeneration of the body's tissues. In a hot climate, where less activity was required, the processes of oxygenation were also reduced. The worst problem arose in a hot climate with excessive humidity in which, according to Pereira, the body was the least able to expel carbonic acid, severely inhibiting the whole process of oxygenation. An extreme form of this condition caused anoxemia, which, he believed, gradually led to beriberi.[38]

Had Pacífico Pereira left it at that, his theory on the etiology of beriberi would have been profoundly damning to the possibility of a healthy population in Brazil and to the relevance of a doctor's role in the tropics. However, he also held that beriberi could be exacerbated or ameliorated according to "many causes combined, external and internal, inherent to the [place of residence] of the individual, to climate, to habits, to [types of] profession, age, etc."[39] Sedentary professions in which a person was forced to spend long hours immobile in humid conditions, the lack of an adequate diet, the lack of exercise, living in a house or city with a dangerous topographical exposure to damp air or in the proximity of toxic soil—all of these environmental conditions predisposed an individual to the disease. Above all, Pacífico Pereira blamed crowded, damp places with a lack of ventilation such as, he contended, were found on Brazilian ships, in prisons, in seminaries, and in the merchants' offices of the Lower City. As he put it, "the crowding of individuals in hot places, especially when they are damp and poorly ventilated, is a predisposing cause of major importance."[40] Indeed, the question of ventilation became a key theme pursued by Pereira in many of his writings. In this way, he always retained the ability to argue that there were certain practical measures on which a doctor could advise in order to ensure adequate oxygenation in the tropics. Even as he courted the newest physiological theories and applied them to Brazil, Pereira did not abandon the malleability of the environmentalist paradigm of disease.

Influenced by the pathbreaking discoveries then being made in Western medicine, Periera was also interested in exploring the possible bacteriological cause of beriberi. In his investigation of the pathological anatomy of beriberi, he reported that he had found a particular microorganism in the blood of almost all the beriberi patients he had examined.[41] Despite this finding, Pereira resisted concluding that the microorganisms were the cause of the disease. The microorganisms, he explained, also existed in the blood of patients suffering from other disorders. Moreover, although he was able to cultivate them according to Pasteur's methods, he had not been able to generate the disease in laboratory animals. Pereira's caution in this area of his research can be attributed to the simple fact that as a good scientist he recognized that he had not proven the bacterial cause of beriberi. Nevertheless, his caution cannot simply be ascribed to his excellence as a scientist. It was also a measure of how far he was wedded to older medical theory.[42]

Even though Pereira himself never pursued further research along the lines of bacteriology, he proposed a way in which both the microorganism and environmentalist factors might be harmonized in the etiology of beriberi. He hypothesized that the process of anoxemia—for him the main cause of beriberi—created the conditions in the blood of the victim for microorganisms to carry out their harmful effects.[43] In other words, by proposing that a microorganism was able to become pathological only in combination with a certain environment, and by giving primary etiological weight to that environment, Pacífico Pereira sought a balance between two approaches to disease etiology.[44] He encouraged his younger colleague Antônio Pacheco Mendes to continue the bacteriological investigation along these lines.[45] Pereira himself felt far more comfortable with the older theories of environment, and the transformative powers of hygiene and sanitation on a malleable population—theories that had pushed him to become an active and visible member of the Bahia community. In this case, Pereira was on the cusp of a conceptual shift in medicine from a generalized notion of disease dependent upon many ambiguous variables to a search for specific causes and treatments in each particular disease.[46] Pacífico Pereira's fundamental concern was to show that sanitary changes and progressive social policies could address the problems of achieving a healthy population in a tropical milieu. He had spent many years translating this concern into practice, and although we know that bacteriology ultimately did much to remove the stigma of "tropicality" from Brazil, Pacífico Pereira continued to perform the task of removing that stigma primarily as a sanitarian.

As a result of the work of doctors like Silva Lima and Pacífico Pereira, within Brazil Salvador became known as the place where the study of beriberi was started and, throughout the imperial years, as the center for information on the disorder.[47] When doctors from other areas of the country, including Rio de Janeiro, began to study the disease, they always turned to the Bahian writings as the main point of reference. The Tropicalistas occasionally griped that they were ignored by the court physicians, but, in truth, they jealously guarded their expertise on beriberi, one of a handful of disorders that became crucial to their identity and international recognition. Just how vigilant the Tropicalistas were of any encroachment upon their expertise from physicians in Rio de Janeiro can be seen in a biting exchange between João Baptista Lacerda and Pacífico Pereira in 1883–84.

In 1880 Lacerda, a restless young physician who had graduated from the Rio medical school in 1870, was appointed as researcher and subdirector to the physiological laboratory of the recently reinvigorated National Museum in Rio de Janeiro.[48] He was interested in promoting Brazilian medicine and carried out research on the possible therapeutic uses of curare and several types of snake poison. He was especially interested in the search for germs and carried out investigations on the bacillus of yellow fever and of beriberi.[49] In 1883 Lacerda examined the passengers of the frigate *Nitheroy* reported to be suffering from beriberi. He obtained blood samples from six patients in order to test them for microorganisms and to grow cultures from the ones he found. In August of that year he published his conclusions in the *União Médica* and asserted: "[We] do not want to be over hasty in our conclusions. . . . However, all the facts lead us to believe that [the cause of beriberi] is not humidity, or diet, or any other of the banal factors so often invoked. . . . The cause appears to be a foreign entity, a microorganism."[50] Even before the publication of his findings in the medical press, he allowed the main daily newspaper in Rio de Janeiro to report his "discovery." The paper claimed emphatically that a microorganism "is the true and only cause of this disorder," hailing Lacerda's findings as an important contribution to science.[51]

The response from Bahia was prompt. In the October issue of the *Gazeta Médica* Pacífico Pereira reprimanded Lacerda for breaching medical etiquette by publicizing his "discovery" in the popular press before the matter had been conclusively settled by physicians.[52] Caustically, Pereira noted, "We will not review the scientific quality of the diligent Dr. Lacerda's work from a single news item . . . , but we cannot allow certain statements to go unchallenged, not because of the desire to assert our rightful priority to [this discovery], for we do not attach much importance to such things, but in order to set the facts straight."[53] Then, indicating that he himself had found such a microorganism, Pacífico Pereira questioned the originality of Lacerda's investigations as well as the inferences he made from his data. Not only did Pacífico Pereira question some of Lacerda's methods in isolating the microbe, and the small number of blood samples involved (six as opposed to the one hundred Pacífico Pereira had by then examined), but above all he was not persuaded that the microbes, if they were connected to beriberi, were not the result, rather than the cause, of the disease. He himself still felt that tropical climate was crucial, and that the role of microbes had to be more thoroughly investigated.[54]

Lacerda responded by depicting Pacífico Pereira as overly concerned with being acknowledged as the "first" in this medical area in Brazil and as being technically incompetent in laboratory methods. "Refusing or forgetting to review the paper [I sent him of my work], Dr. Pacífico preferred to publish a long article in which . . . he tries to prove that there is nothing in my work on the parasitological nature of beriberi that has not already been discovered in Bahia."[55] Denying the charges, Pereira countered with Lacerda's sloppy scientific methods and deplored the haste with which he had jumped to conclusions in marked contrast to Pasteur's extreme caution.[56] He concluded, "The inconsistent proofs offered by Dr. Lacerda lead us to be dubious about [his work on beriberi]. We hope he will continue his investigation and when his evidence is clear, we promise . . . to receive his work enthusiastically."[57]

The exchange represented more than a clash between two individual physician-scientists drawing different conclusions from their data. On one level, it can be viewed as a clash between two physicians who, in an age of rapidly changing medical paradigms, chose to prioritize different systems of thought. As indicated above, Pacífico Pereira hesitated to fully embrace the new bacteriology. Lacerda, in contrast, was very much one of those scientists who, fascinated by the recent bacteriological breakthroughs and willing to believe that nearly all disease was caused by bacteria, was happy to be drawn into the isolation of the laboratory where the most significant discoveries were being made.[58] Thus, with hardly more than a handful of cases in his study, he made bold inferences. Pereira, whose laboratory work was balanced with clinical practice, was more cautious, more aware of the confusing nature of beriberi and less ready to believe he had found its cause. Also at stake for the ambitious Lacerda were his career prospects in a country where few opportunities for research and scientific posts created many rivalries.[59] His aggressiveness in attempting to "discover" the cause of a disease common in Brazil and rampant in other tropical areas would have paid handsome dividends at home and rewarded him with fame abroad.

On another level, the interchange between Lacerda and Pacífico Pereira, which came at a time of heightening tension between the Bahian medical school and the imperial government, was about intensifying regional rivalry. By the 1880s the *Gazeta Médica* had begun to champion the cause of the local medical school and to criticize the government's apparent favoritism toward the Rio de Janeiro medical school, as well as its patronage of research institutions like the National Museum, where Lacerda worked, which were nonexistent in Salvador. After years of struggle by the Tropicalistas to have their contributions to science recognized and their efforts supported financially, to see an apparently well-provided-for newcomer like Lacerda try to usurp the Tropicalista "patrimony" of beriberi must have been a bitter pill to swallow. This was particularly so when Lacerda came from Rio de Janeiro, where, according to the Tropicalistas, the medical establishment had never volunteered much enthusiasm for their work. In 1890 Raimundo Nina Rodrigues confirmed that there had been a "great schism" among Brazilian doctors on the question on beriberi. The schism, he said, was between the doctors of the north who had long concentrated on the study of beriberi, and had placed many forms of paralysis under its umbrella, and the doctors of the south who tended to be skeptical about the disease. Nina Rodrigues was referring to the different medical theories of two communities of doctors. However, the physicians of Bahia and Rio de Janeiro differed not merely because they had varying interpretations of the content of "scientific" facts. The competing interpretations of two updated physicians who embraced the new medicine were dependent on regional differences and professional rivalries, both of which came most clearly into play in the case of Wucherer's discovery of the hookworm in Brazil.[60]

From Tropical Anemia and Tropical Hematuria to Parasites

On December 13, 1865, Dr. Otto Wucherer received an urgent call to go to the monastery of São Bento to attend to Delfino, a very sick slave from a sugar plantation in Santo Amaro. Wucherer described the man:

> The patient was of the dark race, thirty years old, married, average height with a well-built and strong body. The skin was pale, but there was no notable emaciation; the face was swollen, mostly in the eyelids, and there was edema in the hands and feet. The skin was dry, and the body temperature was low, especially in the extremities. The patient was lying down, and his features expressed great anxiety since his respiration was exceedingly difficult, particularly when he made any movement.[61]

Wucherer learned the patient had had seizures, that he did not drink alcoholic beverages, and that he had a habit of eating mud. He diagnosed the patient as suffering from an extreme case of what Brazilian doctors then called *hypoemia tropical, opilação,* or *cansaço,* but he was unable to help him, and the man died that night. The next day Wucherer insisted on performing an autopsy, which revealed numerous worms in the victim's small intestine. Wucherer identified them as *Ancylostoma duodenale.*

By mid-1866 Wucherer had performed another six autopsies, all of which revealed large clusters of the parasite. The *Gazeta Médica* hailed the finding excitedly, calling it an important breakthrough. It stated that Wucherer had demonstrated that slaves and agricultural workers, the main victims of the disorder, suffered from anemia due to loss of blood because of the action of the parasites, a fact that completely changed the understanding of the pathology of the disorder.[62] As Wucherer noted, climate, poor diet, alcoholic beverages, and unhygienic conditions could not account for the disorder as satisfactorily as the presence of the parasites, which, he speculated, were carried in water. What had to be established were the conditions in which the parasite thrived, how these were related to climate, and how the worm was transmitted. These were all questions that Wucherer and his colleagues subsequently investigated.[63] For example, using the experiments of the German parasitologist Leuckhart as his model, Wucherer tried to reproduce hookworm disorder in dogs. He learned that the *Ancylostoma* grew well in damp earth and although he was able to find the parasite in a dog's stomach after it had ingested the infected soil, he could not discover how the parasite might be conveyed into the stomach of a human host.

Significantly, Wucherer did not discard factors such as poor diet and lack of hygiene, holding that they weakened the body and so predisposed it to illness.[64]

The disorder Wucherer encountered has been identified as hookworm disease and it was another of the disorders that became central to the identity and research agenda of the Tropicalistas.[65] Like beriberi, the case of hookworm illustrates the pull in opposite directions of the Tropicalistas as they contributed to the new parasitological theories of disease but continued to find the environmental paradigm a powerful tool with which to confront health in the tropics, and to frame demands for improved social conditions. It also depicts regional and professional rivalries within Brazil as new knowledge upset old power brokers.

As early as 1838 Angelo Dubini in Milan found the hookworm, *Ancylostoma*, but it was not until 1853 that Theodor Bilharz and Wilhelm Griesinger, using Egyptian data, pointed to causal links between the worm and Egyptian chlorosis. European doctors did not pick up this insight for a long time because they were not particularly interested in the findings. European doctors began to seriously focus on hookworm disease only in 1880 as a result of the building of the St. Gotthard tunnel between the Italian and Swiss Alps, when scores of workers succumbed to an unknown chlorosis.[66] Despite the lack of interest in mainstream European medicine, a number of European colonial physicians were always interested in the disorder, as were Wucherer and his colleagues, and they recognized it as a major health hazard in the regions where they worked. This group of widely dispersed doctors corresponded with each other, exchanged specimens, and generally kept alive investigations into the hookworm disorder for many years. By the time the mysterious chlorosis that hit the St. Gotthard tunnel workers had been diagnosed as hookworm disease, a bank of information on hookworm-related disorders had been accumulated, an important part contributed by the Brazilians.

While advancing the shift over to a theory of medical specificity, Wucherer was reluctant to relinquish the environmental; in the writings and research of his disciple, Manoel Victorino Pereira, we see a blatantly eclectic bundling of disease etiologies in order to satisfy his own political agenda for social reform. Of all the Tropicalistas, Victorino Pereira was the most politically engaged and the most active campaigner against slavery, an institution he despised as a measure of Brazil's backwardness.[67] In reviewing Wucherer's work on hypoemia tropical, Victorino Pereira extolled the former's contribution of highlighting the parasitical nature of the disorder.[68] But he did not shed older notions of its etiology. He wrote that environmental factors determined the reproduction of the worm in the host and a particular individual's becoming that host. After blaming environmental factors for the presence of the worm, if not for the cause of the illness, Victorino Pereira moved on to a scathing attack on the institution of slavery. Enumerating the abysmal social conditions likely to promote the spread of the worm, he noted:

> Africans are undoubtedly the main victims of the disorder. It is not that the disorder is peculiar to their race but [that they fall victims] because of their servile condition. . . . The best preventative measure that I know of . . . is to return to those miserable captives the liberty they were robbed of, and to hand over to the robust arms of free labor the prodigious fertility of our lands [*matas*], and the incalculable wealth of our mines. . . . "Hypoemia" is a disease of the poor, of the slaves, of the wretched.[69]

Victorino Pereira illustrates well the Tropicalistas' attempt to retain environmental factors as molding influences on people's health. Certain environments or bad institutions operating within the tropics, tolerated by a lax and ignorant government, were conducive to the sickliness of the population. This approach placed the Tropicalistas squarely within the abolitionist camp on the question of slavery.[70] To the abolitionists' argument that slavery was a sign of backwardness and an obstacle to higher progress, the Tropicalistas added that slavery was an obstacle to the advance of civilization, for slavery provided a milieu in which all the dangers of tropical climate, and thus unhealthiness, were exacerbated.

The Tropicalistas were by no means the only physicians in Brazil who took this critical line on slavery and the government that endorsed it. What was new about the Tropicalistas was that, together with an older approach to disease and medicine, they juggled with a new and "scientific" model that was shifting the focus of their scrutiny from the environment to individual and specific disorders. The new aspect of their work made them internationally known and, in turn, gave them a more forceful identity as a medical movement to be taken seriously back home. But in their critique of domestic problems the Tropicalistas remained close to social medicine, viewing disease and social conditions as inextricably interwoven and calling on the government to be more active in the removal of tropical miasmatic condi-

tions, such as slavery. In the writings of the Tropicalistas, therefore, was a
constant tension between the doctors as part of an older tradition of medicine focusing on populations and conditions and the doctors as participants
in the ongoing shift toward specificity focusing on specific exotic entities
producing specific disorders in the individual.[71]

That Wucherer's work on hookworm signaled a marked departure from
traditional Brazilian medicine can be seen in the degree of controversy his
work generated in the capital city. The debate pitted those who argued with
Wucherer that the helminths he had found in the gut of victims of cansaço
were the cause of the disorder against those who argued that the worms
were another symptom of the ailment. The debate was not only about a specific medical etiology but about larger social and political questions emerging to the fore in the second half of nineteenth-century Brazil, in particular,
questions about who was to determine (medical) truth in a changing nation
and what the nature of medicine was to be. Would medicine in the tropics
remain largely Western and, as such, continue to replicate European medicine and institutions as closely as possible? Or would it primarily address
issues of Brazilian concern and, as such, use European methods, theories,
and techniques to promote original research? Could medical knowledge be
harnessed to make "civilization" and progress possible in the tropics?

Wucherer's main opponent was José Martins de Cruz Jobim, court physician and the leading expert on hookworm at the time. Jobim's expertise
on the disorder rested on his description in an 1835 paper on the most prevalent ailments among the poor in Rio de Janeiro.[72] In the paper, he had
singled out the disorder as one of the most serious because of the large
numbers of people it affected. Jobim had provided highly detailed and remarkably accurate descriptions of the disorder, its evolution, and its pathological anatomy, noting the victim's altered skin color, extreme lethargy,
and, often, an uncontrollable desire to eat soil.[73] Internally, he stated, the
disorder caused an obstruction or blockage to digestion and a "marked
alteration of the blood, which, in turn, dammed all the organs."[74] Jobim
renamed the disorder *hypoemia intertropical* (anemia caused by the airs of
the tropics that "altered" the blood) because he believed it was caused by
the unhealthy airs of the tropics.[75] Although climate was seen as a principal cause, Jobim, following the French sanitarian school, considered local
meteorological conditions and topography as important secondary circumstances determining the onslaught and course of the disorder—as were the
hygienic negligence of the poor, their habit of sleeping out in the damp

night air, and deficient diet, including the abuse of alcoholic beverages.[76] Jobim's presentation made him the acknowledged expert on the disorder in Brazil and in Europe. His description entered European annals in *Schmidt's Jahrbücher* and August Hirsch's early edition of the *Handbook of Geographical and Historical Pathology*.[77] In Brazil and elsewhere, Jobim's explanation of the disorder stood as definitive until Wucherer shifted the emphasis from the unhealthy airs of the Brazilian climate to parasites and social conditions.

When this happened, the medical establishment in Rio was clearly affronted. Soon after Wucherer's discovery was published in the *Gazeta Médica,* Dr. Torres Homem, a colleague of Jobim's, a baron, and one of the preeminent physicians in Rio de Janeiro, presented a report on Wucherer's work at the Imperial Academy of Medicine in Rio de Janeiro. An animated debate led by Jobim followed, after which the academy put Wucherer's parasitological theory to the vote, a vote that went against Wucherer. The worms, the academy decided, were the result rather than the cause of the disorder. At most, it was willing to grant that the worms might present a hindrance to a patient's full recovery.[78] Scathingly, Wucherer retorted that scientific issues could not be settled by being put to the vote.[79] As a result of the academy's decision, most members of the medical community in Rio shunned Wucherer's discovery, and Jobim's etiological explanation continued to hold sway among doctors in Brazil. In 1882 Dr. Júlio Rodrigues de Moura, ever the loyal spokesman for the Tropicalistas in Rio de Janeiro, noted that it was unfortunate that almost the entire faculty at the Rio de Janeiro medical school still rejected Wucherer's findings and clung anachronistically to Cruz Jobim's theories.[80] As late as 1883 Torres Homem continued to give lectures to his students arguing that the worms were the result rather than the cause of the disorder.[81] For Brazilians the controversy ended only after the St. Gotthard phase in the history of hookworm, which clearly established the parasitological cause of the disorder.

What were some of the underlying issues in the controversy between Jobim and Wucherer? First, it was about a prestigious court physician being challenged by an unknown provincial and immigrant doctor on how medical authority was to be constituted. Part of an older generation of physicians who had trained abroad, Cruz Jobim graduated in medicine in Paris in 1828 at a time when that city was on the cutting edge of medical advance. After spending almost a decade in Paris, he returned to Brazil and went on to have a very successful career, fostered in no small part by his closeness to the royal family. As well as physician to the rich and powerful, he

POLITICS OF DISEASE 69

was a clinician at Rio de Janeiro's main charity hospital, the Santa Casa de Misericórdia, a teacher, a sanitarian, a senator, and one of the five founding members of the Society of Medicine in 1829, which seven years later became the officially supported Imperial Academy of Medicine. Jobim was made the society's president and in 1842 he became director of the Rio de Janeiro medical school, a post he retained for thirty years. The only reason that Wucherer's discovery came to the attention of the Rio physicians was because he had published it in the journal he had helped found; otherwise, this unknown doctor would have had no forum. Wucherer, therefore, did more than upset a well-known doctor from Rio. He was challenging the hierarchical way medical authority was constructed in Brazil.

Second, the confrontation between Cruz Jobim and Wucherer was between an older theory of disease and a newly evolving one, between old methods of clinical observation and new technical ones. Jobim's point of reference was grounded, as I have noted, in French medicine of the 1820s. Even though much had changed by the 1860s, Jobim remained very much planted in the past. He seems not to have been familiar with the new techniques in medical investigation. For example, he never referred to the need of observing the disputed parasites under microscope; he does not seem to have carried out any experiments with animals the way Wucherer and the other Tropicalistas did; he did not publish much. Moreover, although he was clearly influenced by the French hygiene movement and its belief in the relationship between disease, poverty, and a lack of sanitation, he never criticized the Brazilian authorities. Indeed, he was a prominent member of the authorities. As such, he tended to blame the poor rather than the government for the lack of sanitary conditions, and tropical miasmas rather than specific entities.

Wucherer, in contrast, returned to Brazil filled with the latest concerns and interests of the new medicine to which he had been exposed in Germany, armed with his microscope, determined to employ the newest European techniques in clinical practice, and also interested in research with little immediate application to medicine, as can be seen in his studies in herpetology and parasitology. He believed in the importance of communicating his findings in writing so that his work could reach a broad specialized audience and was a regular contributor to European, mainly German, journals.[82] Wucherer's factual and narrowly descriptive language contrasted with Jobim's rambling tones. Moreover, Wucherer's interest in and familiarity with Darwinism placed him not only outside the mainstream of Bra-

zilian doctors in the 1860s, but in complete opposition to the medical establishment in Brazil, which staunchly resisted the entry of Darwin's ideas.[83]

The shift in medical ideas also meant the two physicians were linked to
different networks of European doctors. Wucherer recognized the hookworm because he was familiar with the work and interests of men like
Wilhelm Griesinger, Rudolf Virchow, Rudolph Leuckhart, Theodor Bilharz, T. Spencer Cobbold, and Le Roy de Méricourt, among others.[84]
Indeed, it can be argued that the Tropicalistas were part of an informal
network of geographically isolated doctor-scientists, working in warm climates, often focusing on parasites, who corresponded with each other,
exchanged specimens, kept informed of one another's work through the
medical journals, and who also, as one historian has suggested, met up
occasionally on their trips to European capitals and were able to com-
municate because of their lack of specialization.[85] Wucherer, for example,
quickly understood the significance of his discovery because he knew that
the relationship between tropical anemia and the *Ancylostoma* had first been
posited by Griesinger in 1854.[86] Indeed, the importance of Wucherer's contribution regarding the hookworm was that he was able to make the connection between all the different sightings of helminths and the profusion
and confusion of names that had been appearing in the medical literature
for years, and to realize that they probably all referred to the same phenomenon. Wucherer, in fact, suggested that Jobim's description, reproduced in Hirsch's popular book on the geography of disorders, had retarded a full understanding of the importance of Griesinger's findings.

One of the most salient differences between an earlier generation of
Brazilian doctors, such as Cruz Jobim, and a later generation of doctors,
such as the Tropicalistas, was that the former preferred to replicate European medicine and institutions as closely as possible as a sign of Brazil's
advancement, whereas the latter preferred to use European methods and
theories to promote original research. Thus, whereas Jobim's gaze was primarily European, importing wholesale a growing European fatalism about
tropical climate—a fatalism that stemmed from European fears and experiences—the Tropicalistas asked that medicine address Brazilian problems
and fears. This novel approach can be seen in the articles they chose to reproduce in their journal. They were far more interested in the findings of
a then relatively unknown Patrick Manson or Joseph Bancroft than in the
leading exponents of European medicine. They found the former, working
in warm climates, more relevant to their own situation. Thus, even while

the Europeans' temperate medicine continued to be crucially important, the Tropicalistas chose to privilege some aspects of European medicine over others, according to what they deemed most relevant to the requirements of their country. Like Europeans, this generation believed in science, but they looked to science produced in the tropics, about the tropics, to help them confront what they saw as the distinctive problems of health and civilization in a torrid zone.

In their search for relevant medical models and approaches, Wucherer and the Tropicalistas looked beyond the French, turning toward those emerging out of German medicine, and used German ideas and innovations together with the French in an eclectic manner, but often highlighting the German. This was not simply a case of the competition between French and German medicine being played out on the European periphery. Rather, the extolling of German medicine over French responded to a Brazilian issue. That is, in order to gain visibility and effect the changes they deemed necessary for Brazilian medicine, the Tropicalistas used German scientific medicine to displace an older, French tradition within Brazil, a tradition in medical knowledge on which the medical establishment, led by the Rio elite, had built its power and authority. And they did this in the 1860s, some two decades before various "Germanisms" became fashionable among Brazilian doctors.

Finally, the differences between Jobim and Wucherer were also indicative of who was to be "blamed" for poor sanitary conditions. When Jobim addressed social environmental causes, he tended to lay the blame on the poor.[87] He saw the poor as part of the urban or rural landscape; at least in Brazil, he noted complacently, they were better off than in Europe, where they were subject to periodic famine. Wucherer and the Tropicalistas, in contrast, made pointed and biting criticisms of the government as they pointed to the deterioration of living conditions for the poor. Indeed, Wucherer moved toward a concept of the poor as socially constructed, and saw diseases like hookworm disorder as social in nature. That is, overarching his investigations into hookworm disease was an understanding that the disorder was related to a disgraceful poverty that government and elites tolerated. For example, where Jobim blamed diet, Wucherer analyzed why the poor ate badly in Salvador. He noted that the diet of the poor had deteriorated because of the rapidly rising cost of living, so that the poor were reduced to eating bad meat sold at markets that the authorities failed to inspect adequately. He noted, "in Brazil there is not a true proletariat class . . . but there is a great deal of poverty that [in the last twenty years] has increased. . . . Today people work harder but live worse."[88]

Thus, on one level, the confrontation between Jobim and Wucherer can be understood as a statement from a provincial group, on the periphery of medical power, that was demanding its "place in the sun" and a say in shaping the contours of Brazilian medicine. On another level, the controversy was symbolic of a clash between a younger generation of medical men who, although they believed Brazil had many problems of race and place, also believed science offered solutions, and an older generation who believed that Brazilian problems were irreversible. For Jobim, who as a member of a small elite was probably content with the state of his world, the prevalence of "unhealthy air" meant that little could be done about the poor, who, like the airs, were naturally "dirty" and diseased. For Wucherer and his colleagues, men impatient to see a new era of progress, reform was key and they demanded changes based on new scientific understanding.

In the early 1860s Griesinger asked Wucherer to contribute to his work in Egypt on schistosomiasis by looking for the eggs of the schistosome parasite (*Bilharzia*) in the bloody urine (hematuria) of patients in Brazil. For the next two years, Wucherer tried unsuccessfully to find them in the urine of hematuric patients. On August 4, 1866, however, he examined the urine of one of Silva Lima's patients and found "threadlike worms that were very thin at one end and blunt at the other."[89] Despite consulting lists of known parasites, Wucherer could not identify the parasite. Today we know it as *Wucheria bancrofti,* the cause of filariasis.[90]

Wucherer was slow to appropriate his findings and to spell out their full implications. He was cautious in attributing to the worms the role of causative agent of any particular disorder and he never discussed the possible relationship between filaria and elephantiasis. "It seems rash," he stated, "to hazard conjectures on the occurrence of these worms in cases of hematuria and on their etiologic significance; therefore, I will refrain from doing so until I have made new investigations."[91] He asked questions about whether the threadworm was a cause or effect of hemochylous urine and, if a cause, what other symptoms were linked to the parasite, what other fluids in the body contained the parasite, how its life cycle was structured, and how it was transmitted. Wucherer and other Tropicalistas proceeded to investigate all these questions.[92] Finally, two years later, encouraged by the recently formed group of Tropicalistas, who not only discussed his work but also urged him to write about it, Wucherer published his findings in the

Gazeta Médica da Bahia and initiated a whole cycle of investigations into the filaria.[93]

Once the news of Wucherer's discovery reached the European medical press, the Brazilians were seemingly left behind. In 1868 Le Roy de Méricourt, a personal friend of Wucherer's, quoted from his colleague's writings, and two years later the French journal *Archives de Médecine Naval* published Wucherer's findings.[94] In 1876 the same journal gave a summary and commentary on subsequent Tropicalista work on the filaria and by 1883 one French journal was referring to the Bahian doctors as the Bahian school of parasitology.[95] In England, T. Spencer Cobbold, the leading British parasitologist, informed the Linnean Society in London on March 7, 1878, and a branch of the British Medical Association in May 1872 of the discovery, and in Germany it was communicated in the medical journal *Deutsches Archiv für Klinische Medicin.*[96]

Although the French first reported the findings in Europe, the British rapidly moved to the forefront of the investigation into the human parasite.[97] As early as 1868 an Englishman working in India, Dr. Timothy Lewis, had duplicated Wucherer's findings, and presented proof of the link between elephantiasis and hemochyluria by locating the parasite in the urine and lymph of the victims of elephantiasis. In 1872 Lewis made a further breakthrough in the investigations on the filaria by finding the embryonic worms in the blood of persons suffering from chyluria, diarrhea, and elephantiasis.[98] In 1876 Dr. Bancroft, in Australia, found the adult filaria and suggested an independent vector might be involved in the transmission of the filaria and that the vector could be the mosquito.[99] Between 1875 and 1876 Dr. Patrick Manson, a British colonial physician based in China, was home on leave in England, where he learned about the developments concerning the filaria.[100] Armed with this information, Dr. Manson, the father of tropical medicine, returned to China and in 1878 confirmed Bancroft's hypothesis about transmission. Manson's work led to the idea of a vector or intermediate host in the transmission of disease, a cornerstone of modern tropical medicine.[101]

How did the Tropicalistas react to the British achievements? Far from seeing themselves as passive recipients of the advances of European doctors, the Tropicalistas portrayed themselves as very much a part of an international network of doctors working on the disorders of the tropics.[102] They replicated and confirmed the British findings, working to verify the identity of various microorganisms by exchanging specimens with European scientists and publishing comparative illustrations of helminths from Brazil and other parts of the world.[103] They discussed hypotheses on the parasite's life cycle and modes of transmission, helped trace the related disorders, and experimented with therapy.

Thus, for example, Victorino Pereira, Júlio de Moura, Felício dos Santos, and Silva Araújo replicated Bancroft's work in Australia by finding the adult filaria in Brazil in 1877; Silva Araújo also advanced knowledge about the filaria by locating the parasite in the scrotal tumor of an elephantiasis patient where it had not been seen before.[104] Silva Lima sought unsuccessfully to confirm Manson's finding regarding the presence of the filaria in a mosquito's stomach, a finding that Silva Araújo replicated in 1878.[105] Silva Araújo also confirmed the suspicion that filaria could lead to a variety of disorders by finding filarias in a single patient who suffered from chyluria, scrotal elephantiasis, craw-craw, and erysipelas. He reported that electrotherapy was a particularly effective cure.[106] In 1886 Pedro S. de Magalhães found two adult specimens of the filaria in the heart of a patient. He searched for the filaria in water as a possible mode of transmission.[107] He and Paterson engaged in a debate in the *Gazeta Médica* over whether Lewis had correctly described the life cycle of the embryonic filaria.[108] In 1878 Paterson and Thomas Hall—the latter, like Paterson, a British doctor resident in Bahia and very much a part of the Tropicalistas—tried to determine how much of Salvador's population was infected with the parasite by testing some three hundred of their patients over a two-month period. They reported that more than 8 percent of their patients were infected and that when one broke this down by race, blacks and mulattoes had a higher incidence of infection than whites.[109]

Every advance made by Brazilians or by doctors abroad was reported in the *Gazeta Médica da Bahia*. The journal told a story about the Tropicalistas in which they emerged as an intricate part of an international cadre of doctors at the forefront of the investigation into a newly discovered parasite. That this was not an altogether false presentation can be seen in an article by Bancroft, summarized in the *Lancet* in 1885, regarding the case of a patient with scleroderma in whose blood Bancroft had found the filaria. In the article he not only called on his British colleagues Manson and Lewis to carry out "further inquiries into the nature of this complaint," but he also singled out for help "the practitioners of Brazil."[110]

The *Gazeta Médica* portrayed each new filaria-related discovery as embedded in the broader context of the Brazilian contribution with reference to the starting point, Wucherer. As Júlio de Moura noted, "Manson, Bancroft, Lewis, and our [Brazilian] pathologists are simply the tillers of the great tree that our dead colleague [Wucherer] managed to grow."[111] Although the journal reprinted all the important writings on the subject from around the world, its focus remained fixed. An 1880 editorial reminded its readers that "in the [Gazeta Médica] are found all the conquests won [over filariasis] through the diligence of many observers in many countries, and not a few [of these conquests] have been due to the work of our own countrymen."[112] Moreover, the editors avidly picked up on European references to the Brazilian contributions. They reacted very quickly to threats to ignore Brazilian participation. In 1876, for example, Silva Lima annotated an article by the French naval doctor J. Crevaux on filariasis that he believed was an important contribution to understanding the ailment. Silva Lima asked the author to correct his facts about its discovery, however, giving priority to Wucherer rather than to Lewis.

The discovery of the filarias in urine is generally attributed to Dr. Lewis. As he has already justly received great honor for having discovered the filarias in blood, and the lymph of elephantoid tumors, it will not hurt him to acknowledge the priority of Wucherer's discovery of the filaria in hemachylous urine, and [to recognize] that it was our humble journal [the Gazeta Médica da Bahia] that announced the important discovery.[113]

Silva Lima also complained that Cobbold did not give Wucherer his rightful due. In July 1877 Cobbold informed the Lancet about a communication he had received from Dr. Bancroft in Australia, describing the latter's discovery of the adult filaria and enclosing specimens for Cobbold's inspection; but in his discussion on what was known about the helminth, Cobbold failed to mention Wucherer. When Silva Lima read the report in the Lancet, he wrote in an incensed tone about the omission.[114] Wucherer, he stated, had been the first to reveal and fully describe the worms, and although others had since made important advances, it was grossly unfair that the efforts of "one of the most dedicated and patient contributors of science in Brazil" were being ignored.[115]

Silva Lima's article, reproduced in the Archives de Médecine Navale, came to the attention of Cobbold and in a subsequent meeting at the London Society of Pathology, Dr. Cobbold made amends, establishing Wucherer as the discoverer of the filaria.[116] In his 1879 book on parasites, Cobbold went further and not only described Wucherer's work but also wrote about the work of other doctors in Brazil, such as Silva Araújo, John Paterson, Júlio R. de Moura, Felício dos Santos, and Pedro S. de Magalhães, among others.[117]

Cobbold's recognition of the Brazilian contribution, however, was the exception. On the whole, the British did not consider the Brazilian doctors' work to be of any great import.[118] Even when Brazilian findings were clearly part of the whole body of filariasis research, the British medical press tended to report, appropriate, and then ignore the source of the information while keeping a complete record of British contributions.[119] Thus the detailed accounts of Patrick Manson's work on filariasis written by his son-in-law, Philip H. Manson-Bahr, include no mention of Wucherer's work; they credit Timothy Lewis with the early discoveries.[120] Manson's colleague and rival Ronald Ross, who wrote his own recollections of Manson's work, mentioned Wucherer but noted that he had never read Wucherer's writings.[121] The British were far less concerned about the origins of the discovery, perhaps because they were rapidly moving on to new ones; perhaps, too, they did not believe that Brazilians could make good medical researchers. The Brazilians, in contrast, accentuated their role because they had so much at stake, both for the successful development of a distinct medicine and for European recognition of their efforts.

What was the significance for the Tropicalistas of the portrayal of themselves as a part of the community of doctors actively involved in framing the idea of tropical disease and medicine? The Tropicalistas' recognition by European physicians of the stature of Spencer Cobbold and Le Roy Méricourt, and by medical journals as prestigious as the *Lancet*, the *Journal of the Quekett Microscopical Club*, and the *Archiv feur Pathologische Anatomie und Physiologie und fuer Klinische Medizin* (always referred to by the shortened name, *Virchow's Archiv*), was no small coup. It was one way of moving from obscurity to influence in Brazil, forcing the medical community in Rio de Janeiro to open at least some doors to their colleagues from the provincial medical community. Thus, from the mid-1870s on, several of the Tropicalistas were made correspondent members of the prestigious Imperial Academy of Medicine.[122] Two Tropicalistas who moved to Rio de Janeiro continued to research and publish in accordance with the Tropicalista agenda.[123] They became prominent figures in the capital city, founding the *União Médica,* modeled on the *Gazeta Médica* and emphasizing original work. The latter journal was an inspiration for other journals, like *Brasil Médico* and *Progresso Médico,* which acknowledged the Bahian journal and also exchanged articles with the *Gazeta Médica.* In so doing they assaulted the dominance of the academy's official journal, the *Anais Brasilienses de Medicina;* as the *Gazeta Médica* noted somewhat bitterly in 1887, "We don't know if the court doctors know yet of the existence of the *Gazeta Médica* even though we are in our eighteenth year of publication."[124] Thus by the 1880s the Tropicalistas' work was being discussed in journals in the capital city, their research agenda taken up by the main research laboratory, the National Museum, and papers on "their" topics given at the first two medical congresses ever held in Brazil.[125] The third medical congress was held in Salvador as a result of hard lobbying by the Tropicalistas Pacífico Pereira, Nina Rodrigues, and Silva Lima, and the latter was the key speaker at the conference.

But the significance of international acclaim for the Tropicalistas went further. First, unraveling of diseases like filariasis, hookworm, and beriberi, among others, was clear evidence that the ubiquitous menace of the torrid zone was something that could be rationally understood, deciphered, described, and combated. Even if the high numbers of persons suffering from filariasis was sobering, ultimately, the doctors viewed the discovery of the parasite in their midst with profound optimism. The Tropicalistas' experiments on their patients with electrotherapy and high dosages of purgatives, their experimental use of Brazilian pharmacopoeia like gameleira, their energetic demands that the government intervene to improve public health, their analyses of the sources of water the population consumed, were as much attempts to resist the idea of the menacing tropics as to cure a disease.

Second, the story of the Brazilian role in the unraveling of tropical disorders was also a way of demonstrating that good science was possible in the tropics. This, in turn, was another way of resisting the stereotype of Latin American doctors as passive recipients of European knowledge. Silva Lima, for example, presented Wucherer as an initiator and an active agent in pursuit of knowledge: "Wucherer's investigations shaped the course of further studies of this curious disorder. . . . He showed us the way and he must be followed with perseverance so that the mysteries of [filariasis] may be unraveled."[126] The Tropicalistas wanted to portray themselves as being on the cutting edge of a new kind of medicine focusing on the tropics, and as key actors in the process of reconceptualizing Brazil as a newly civilized and advanced nation, a nation able to socialize its people into civilization, in part by the intervention of its doctors.

Conclusion

The decade after the Tropicalistas coalesced as a group saw some of the most significant developments in the history of medicine. As the germ theory of disease emerged out of the doldrums in which it had lain for much of the century, "scientific" doctors slowly began to understand the relation between filth and disease. They also came to recognize the importance of biomedical research and of new techniques such as the ophthalmoscope, larynoscope, and especially microscopy to reveal processes hitherto concealed. Some physicians working in the tropics and inspired by the advances turned, with new lenses, both cultural and technical, to the special problems of tropical disease. Rejecting the notion of tropical heat and moisture as the direct causes of illness in the tropics, and therefore of tropical disorders being beyond the help of medicine, they looked for specific causative agents and found parasitology to be a particularly fruitful line of inquiry.

In Salvador a group of physicians intellectually stimulated by developments in Western medicine found little space within the Bahian medical establishment to accommodate their interests. The leaders of the group, who were foreigners and thus outsiders to the establishment, had little to lose and much to gain by taking risks to advance their careers, establishing their fame abroad, and securing greater influence locally. It was still possible, in an age when the ambition of a single entrepreneur could redraw the map of the British Empire, or when the serendipity of a lone scientist could discover the relation between fermentation and bacteria, for isolated doctors, working with their microscopes in homemade laboratories, to seek a breakthrough, and fame, in medicine. As one historian has noted, it was a period when "the biomedical sciences constituted a common or unspecialized scientific culture. It was easy to move from one subject to another, with considerable academic and geographical mobility. The whole approach was what we would now call interdisciplinary."[127]

From the late 1870s, however, biomedical advances proceeded so fast and spectacularly that increasingly the roles of clinician and researcher were less likely to be found in the same person. Research now began to require far more than enthusiasm on the part of individual doctor-scientists. These were the decades when there was a split between amateurs and professionals as a result of the growth of specialization and the development of a stringent code of professional techniques and standards. A few European centers, such as the well-financed Pasteur Institute of Paris (1889) and others in Germany, became trendsetters in the science of bacteriology, which emerged at the forefront of the medical breakthroughs, molding a whole generation of medical scientists, enabling them to compare the results of their research and to become part of a web of select doctor-scientists initiated into the culture of bacteriological knowledge.[128] Now the development of parasitology and bacteriology in the laboratory, and later the "alliance between field-work and laboratory," required funding, most coming from governments.[129] In Brazil, this change was formally recognized in 1900, when the government for the first time turned health into a national question and agreed to set up a tropical medicine research institute, later known as the Oswaldo Cruz Institute. By the time of this heightened concern for "national efficiency," many of the Tropicalistas had died, others were old men, and although they had attracted younger doctors into their ranks, the Tropicalistas, working from home laboratories and amid informal groups, had never trained up a cadre of disciples single-mindedly pursing a research agenda. However, they played an important role in opening a path for the new paradigm in medicine that took hold in Brazil.

In the early decades after they set out on their journey of medical discovery, the Tropicalistas discerned new disorders in Brazil, they posited new etiologies for old ones, they challenged Brazilian canon regarding local disorders, a canon closely derivative of the French, they looked to the newest German sources of medicine as models questioning the long hold of French medicine over Brazilian, and they investigated the ways in which the latest discoveries in histology and physiology were relevant to the tropics. They chose to highlight parasitology as particularly relevant to their warm milieu and they yoked their evolving ideas and discoveries to an older, meliorist, environmentalist approach to disease that was always forward-looking—an attitude derived from their profound faith in science and progress. As a result of the Tropicalistas' work, the lead in Brazilian medical innovation and discovery came, for a few crucial decades in the nineteenth

century, not from Rio but from Bahia. As a result, the Tropicalistas became embroiled in controversies essentially about the primacy of place and
hierarchy in the construction of medical knowledge in Brazil.

For all their novelty, the Tropicalistas retained aspects of environmentalism. This eclecticism was deliberate. On the one hand, it enabled them to
keep up with the forefront of European developments; on the other hand,
it allowed them to retain a malleable conception of human beings molded
by their environment, a crucial underpinning to their faith in the possibility
of progress through general sanitation and the creation of a civilized nation
in Brazil, and crucial to their belief in the relevance of the role of the doctor
in a nation with a tropical climate. It was also a conception central to the
Tropicalistas' strategies of resistance in the face of the negative portrayal of
the problems of "tropicality" as defined by European and North American
science.

CHAPTER THREE

Race, Climate, and Medicine:
Framing Tropical Disorders

In September 1888 the First Brazilian Medical Congress was held in Rio de Janeiro. Júlio de Moura, the lead speaker at the congress and an early Tropicalista supporter, recalled how he had first raised the idea of such a congress in the pages of the *Gazeta Médica* as early as 1868.[1] At the time, he said, the apathy and indifference of the medical community in Brazil meant that doctors had ignored his call. The fact that such a conference was now being held, stated Moura, was a sign that Brazilian medicine was finally emerging from the inertia and torpor that had long been its hallmarks.[2] For this reason, Moura held, there was much room for satisfaction. However, a great deal still remained to be done. In particular, doctors in Brazil had to ask themselves, "What do we want? What are our ideas? . . . What [future] directions do we envisage?"[3] In answer to his own questions, Moura posited:

> What preoccupies us now is . . . tropical pathology [*pathologia intertropical*]. . . . There is no other area of medicine in which we can so readily . . . establish . . . the value of [Brazilian] research. . . . The French have already instituted the study of exotic disorders . . . to improve the health of their naval personnel. Such an initiative should have started in our country. . . . How greatly would the reputation of Brazilian medical professors grow . . . if they clarified what is most doubtful about the disorders of the tropics and established the basis for a . . . course in [tropical pathology].[4]

Moura called for the creation of a chair specializing in tropical medicine in Brazilian medical schools and outlined how he thought Brazilians could most effectively carve out a special niche for themselves in the annals of international medicine. This idea had always been the backbone of Tropicalista medical thinking, and it was no wonder that they reprinted the full text of Moura's speech in their journal.[5] Clearly, the Tropicalistas were proud that their journal had been publicly praised at the most important medical gathering that had ever taken place in Brazil, but even more, they sympathized with the direction that Moura sought to give the conference. Indeed, with their emphasis on the importance of studying disorders relevant to Brazil, the Tropicalistas were the most important precursors of tropical medicine in Brazil.

However, the issue of institutionalizing tropical medicine in Brazil was by no means as clear-cut as Moura would have it. The Tropicalistas themselves constantly came up against the question of what exactly the new approach to medicine in Brazil should be. Should tropical pathology be concerned with such orders as ancylostomiasis, filariasis, malaria, beriberi—in other words, those disorders that appeared to be largely exclusive to hot and humid climates? Or were all the disorders of Brazil to be considered tropical in the sense of being universal but subject to peculiar exacerbating factors in the tropics? If one defined tropical medicine in the first sense, then a case could be made for a separate chair in tropical pathology; if in the second sense, then there was little room for a separate chair specializing in tropical disorders.[6]

Indeed, questions about what defined a tropical disorder, and whether there could be such a thing as tropical medicine, run through the writings of the Tropicalistas just as they do through those of many physician-scientists who, over the last century, attempted to define the ever elusive and changing field of tropical medicine.[7] One historian who recently proposed some answers noted that embedded within the idea of tropical medicine are competing strands of conceptual thinking "jostling with each other for priority amid a good deal of confusion."[8] When, for example, did malaria—a recurring onslaught for centuries in Europe—become defined as a tropical disorder? Is tropical medicine to be defined as dealing primarily with parasitology, or the geography of disease, or tropical hygiene, or poverty and malnutrition? If tropical medicine is unique among medical specialties because it is defined "by the part of the world where the illness was acquired," does hookworm cease to be tropical when it is acquired building a tunnel in Switzerland rather than in the hot Brazilian *sertão?*[9] Michael

Worboys has examined how the European idea of diseases in the tropics—with its concern for naval medicine, and the health of Europeans living in hot climates—evolved, by the turn of the century, largely through the parasitological work of such British Empire doctors as Patrick Manson, into a new specialty of tropical medicine with a focus on "vector borne parasitic infections."[10] Today, the definition of tropical medicine has moved so far beyond the study of parasitic infections—ironically returning, to some extent, to the broader vision of nineteenth-century doctors like the Tropicalistas—that some have advocated discarding the term "tropical medicine," replacing it instead with "medicine in the tropics" in order to emphasize that these are diseases to do with communal poverty and socioeconomic underdevelopment.[11]

Tropicalista tentativeness, and even contradiction, about the idea of tropical medicine and the distinctiveness of tropical disorders places them within a long line of people who have tried to mark out the boundaries of this sphere of medicine. The history of the rise of tropical medicine has usually been studied from a European point of view.[12] In particular, historians have focused on European imperial expansion, with its need to deploy more troops and administrators in the colonies, as the underpinning of the rise of tropical medicine. Once the breakthroughs in bacteriology explained more fully the processes of contagion and the causes of epidemics, then, it is argued, Europeans were able to understand tropical disorders and develop tropical medicine. The problem with this approach is that it ignores earlier, nonformally institutionalized interest in tropical medicine that came from physicians living and working in the new nations in the tropics, such as Brazil. The modern idea that led to the rise of tropical medicine as a specialty—namely, that nothing inherent to tropical climate or peoples inevitably caused disease and moral and physical degeneracy—was already present in the work of many of these doctors. From this perspective, the rise of tropical medicine, and the groups with vested interests in such an enterprise, becomes an even more complex and ambiguous process than European historians have portrayed it. For British, French, and Portuguese imperialists, for example, the rise of tropical medicine may have signaled the chance to perform the tasks of domination more efficiently. For physicians in Brazil, like the Tropicalistas, the elucidation, differentiation, and demystification of "tropical" disorders were a means of fending off the mounting pressure of European literature on degeneration that relegated

Brazil and the Brazilians to backwardness. The rise of tropical medicine in Brazil, therefore, must be viewed as a response to a specifically Brazilian set of problems concerning fears of cultural, racial, and biological inferiority.

The Tropicalistas not only attempted to develop an understanding of the disorders they dealt with daily, but also sought to construct a theoretical framework about the relationship between disease and the tropics. In so doing, they were frequently contradictory, lurching back and forth from the notion that there was no disease peculiar to the tropics, to the idea that the tropics, if not a ubiquitous incubator of mysterious disorders, certainly was a formidable ally of pathological agency. Overall, they tended toward the idea that most disorders were universal but that the heat and humidity of the tropics exacerbated disorders in such a way as to make them distinctive.[13] Exactly how the tropical heat and humidity affected disease and decay was what they intended to elucidate. Central, always, to this puzzle was the link between social conditions and disease. Thus, if they did not disagree with Europeans about the dangers of "tropicality," they rejected the irreversible nature of decay in the tropics. The Tropicalistas, therefore, initiated a conceptual medical shift in Brazil away from the fatalistic view that the tropics and degeneration were inevitably intertwined over to the assertive view that, through medical and social engineering, Brazil could participate in the march toward civilization.[14]

The Idea of Tropical Disorders

The idea of the tropics as deleterious, in particular to Europeans, had developed in the European mind over the centuries. Early European appraisal had seen the tropics a place of such abundance that it augured a new era in the relationship between humans and nature. In his study of British colonial Africa, Philip Curtin has shown how this shift toward a dread of the tropics was based on the real and very high mortality rate in the region exacted of Europeans, who lacked the immunity native peoples acquired, mainly in childhood.[15] That the immunity was not understood added fuel to the notion that some races were naturally suited to the tropics while others, particularly Europeans, had best keep away. If Europeans were forced to spend time in the tropics, they should function only in managerial positions and take frequent breaks in temperate climates.[16]

James Goodyear has charted a similar shift in opinion in Portugal regarding its colonial empire. In their writings, early Jesuit missionaries and doctors saw Brazil as a place of great salubrity.[17] By the eighteenth century, this favorable view had changed to a very negative conception of the "torrid zone." Donald Cooper places the shift as late as the 1849 yellow fever epidemic, which took more than seven thousand lives in Salvador and Rio de Janeiro and was followed in 1855–56 by an even deadlier cholera epidemic.[18] Whatever the timing of the shift, European doctors began to argue that Europeans could not expect to maintain their health in a hot country like Brazil. The change in attitude meant that Europeans who went to Brazil feared for their health, which prevented large numbers of Europeans from emigrating to that country, selecting instead the more temperate climates of North America and Argentina. A second consequence of the change of attitude toward Brazil's climate was that European doctors tended to believe that whites "degenerated," morally and physically, in the Brazilian climate. Blacks, as natives of the tropics, were considered degenerate; the problem for Europeans was whether they would degenerate too.[19]

By mid–nineteenth century, the concept of the tropics had become an integral part of a North American and European debate on biological degeneracy. Some of the leading figures in the debate, such as the naturalist Louis Agassiz and the writer and diplomat Arthur de Gobineau, had visited Brazil and their ideas were well known to Brazilian physicians.[20] The debate dealt with whether different physical racial characteristics were correlated to distinctive intellectual qualities, whether certain climates were more conducive to social progress than others, and whether the crossbreeding of different races led inevitably to degeneration. The backdrop to this debate was the belief in a hierarchy of racial types in which some races, hailing from tropical climates, were posited as being more degenerate than others.[21]

In its original monogenetic version, drawn from the Scriptures, scientists assumed that all races belonged to the same species, but that environmental factors had created a degeneration away from a primordial form to the racial varieties of the world. The softer forms of the monogenetic version allowed a blurring of the different racial ranks because of the belief in the "infinite adaptability of man."[22] At the very moment that slavery in the New World was giving way under economic change and moral pressure, however, European and U.S. racial theory was crystallizing into a "science" with ever more negative consequences for non-Europeans and the denizens of tropical climates.[23]

By midcentury a new group, the polygenists, had abandoned the Scriptures, and reformulated the older theory, arguing that different races were more like different species.[24] Not all polygenists went to the extreme of applying this distinction to blacks and whites, but they argued that variations between races had grown so numerous that, for all intents and purposes, they could be treated as separate. The polygenists provided "evidence" for the biological and fixed differences among the various human species, including testimony from U.S. doctors who, ignorant of the processes of immunity in such illnesses as malaria and yellow fever, believed that blacks had to be medically treated differently from whites because of their physical and anatomical variations.[25] The polygenist school argued that races fared best when they retained their purity and proper topological places; it retained intact the monogenetic scheme of the hierarchy of races, which placed whites at the pinnacle and blacks at the bottom. Racial science became now a "science of boundaries between groups and the degenerations that threatened when those boundaries were transgressed."[26]

By the second half of the nineteenth century the label "tropical disorders" had evolved from a more or less neutral and descriptive category of ailments to an idea fraught with complexity—imbued not only with Europeans' fears and prejudices about their often lethal experience in hot climates, but also with an attempted justification of their long history of enslavement of the peoples from tropical regions.[27] The idea of tropical disease now contained two very fatalistic connotations: it was the inevitable outcome of the combination in the tropics of "airs, waters, and places" that produced a pathological miasma and, at the same time, it was the inevitable disease of the natives, which explained their supposed inferiority. According to this rationale, if African slaves were sick and lethargic, it was because they came from a weak race and a debilitating climate, rather than because of the institution of slavery.[28] But even if Africans were known to resist certain tropical disorders better than Europeans, this merely confirmed Europeans' intellectual superiority, because the energy Africans needed to adapt to the rigors of the tropics made them intellectually less vigorous.[29] The idea of tropical disorders, therefore, contained both climatological and racial variables that left very little hope for progress for the natives of tropical countries. Brazil, for example, presented a

> painful contrast between the grandeur of the external world and the littleness of the internal. . . . And the mind, cowered by this unequal struggle, has not only been unable to advance, but without foreign aid it would undoubtedly have receded. For even at present, with all the im-

provements constantly introduced from Europe, there are no signs of real progress.[30]

Gobineau, who as French minister resided in Brazil from 1869 to 1870, held Brazilians to be a "population totally mulatto, vitiated in its blood and spirit, and fearfully ugly." They were "neither hardworking, active, nor fertile." Rather than blame climate, Gobineau held that there was a genetic "degeneracy."[31]

The implications of such theories for Brazil, with its tropical climate and one of the highest rates of miscegenation in the Americas, were devastating. Of all the countries in the Americas, Brazil most fully relied on African slavery. Since the sixteenth century Brazil had imported Africans, supplied from the Congo-Angolan coast, to work as slaves, and slavery continued to be the centerpiece of Brazilian society for much of the nineteenth century. African slaves in Brazil were the "warp and woof of the economy. . . . The institution of slavery patterned the entire social-economic-political fabric of the nation."[32] Even after the slave trade ended in 1850, the demand for slaves remained high. Although Brazil's first national census in 1872 registered a drop in total slave population of about 500,000 slaves from midcentury, there was still a sizable population of 1.2 million economically active slaves in Brazil out of a total population of 10 million.[33] More than 800,000 slaves were employed in agriculture on coffee, sugar, cocoa, and cotton plantations. The remainder were urban slaves and day laborers allied to plantation work. In the urban areas they worked as domestic servants, textile laborers, masons, porters, street vendors, skilled and unskilled artisans, stevedores, barbers, undertakers. The remarkable boom in coffee production in the Rio de Janeiro–São Paulo regions in the nineteenth century was sustained by slave labor supplied in part by an internal slave traffic from the declining Northeast and from slaves from the urban areas; by 1872 more than half the slaves in Brazil were located in the three main coffee-producing provinces.[34]

Despite the continuing economic importance of slavery, from the 1870s on there were concerted voices in Brazil raised against the institution. In fact there had long been criticism of slavery by some members of the elite. The most prominent among the early critics had been José Bonifacio, the first statesman of the newly independent Brazil who in 1825 had proposed its complete abolition.[35] But after 1870 there were more than isolated voices raised in protest: the Brazilian intelligentsia had by and large come to accept the definition of those European "high priests" of progress who, almost unanimously, saw the institution as a sign of backwardness, and an obstacle to future, superior development.[36] It became clear then that change and social improvement would require the introduction of a "scientific spirit," of an efficient educational system, of criteria of merit and achievement over patronage, of the values of work and thrift associated with a "capitalistic ethos" rather than those of leisure and ostentation associated with aristocratic societies.[37] As long as the United States remained a slave nation, Brazilians could always point to the possibility of slavery *and* progress. By 1865 this was no longer possible and Brazilians found themselves uncomfortably isolated in the hemisphere, with only Cuba for company. International condemnation was loud and Victorino Pereira was by no means the only young medical graduate who returned home burning with shame from his medical tour of Europe in 1879–81, vowing to work for the abolition of slavery, the institution that had caused him so much opprobrium on his travels.[38]

The unsettling feeling that slavery was a measure of Brazil's backwardness was reinforced by the country's disgracefully poor performance in the war against Paraguay (1865–70), won only after the intervention of Argentina and Uruguay on Brazil's side. The inquest on Brazil's participation in the war was carried out amid the inflow of positivist and Spencerian ideas of superior and inferior stages of society and of the survival of the fittest groups.[39] The positivists gained strong support among the younger army officers critical of the emperor's conduct of the war, a criticism that easily moved into a more general critique of the whole system of values associated with the Luso-Brazilian past and a desire to see them replaced with modern patterns of thought as well as modern technology and institutions, such as those in the advanced European countries and the United States.[40] Though few who professed support for the ideas of positivism actually joined the Positivist Church founded in Rio de Janeiro in 1875, many did come to view monarchy and slavery as obstacles to Brazil's progress. Doctors, like many other members of the intelligentsia, condemned the institution of slavery.[41] In Bahia, some of the Tropicalistas, like Victorino Pereira and Jerônymo Sodré Pereira, were among slavery's most outspoken critics. Not only did the Tropicalistas condemn the institution morally, but they viewed it as the cause of the most common disorders from which slaves suffered. Wucherer and Victorino Pereira blamed the unhygienic conditions associated with slavery for the spread of the hookworm among slaves. Wucherer also blamed the heavy death toll that the 1855 cholera epidemic in Bahia had exacted among slaves on the abysmal conditions of slavery, and Silva Lima wondered if the enforced barefootedness of slaves could be one of the causes for the prevalence of ainhum among Africans in Brazil.[42] It was amid this politically critical milieu that fueled republican sentiment, liberal criticism, and a hitherto stalled abolition campaign that the entire political spectrum in Brazil shifted to the left of what it had been in the calm of the decade after midcentury, and that debates on the "social question," by no means new, became ever more compelling.[43]

Such debates were formulated in terms of how to ensure an efficient and orderly free-market labor force as the country moved toward the end of slavery: would men and women trained for generations into a slave mentality work without coercion, and would poor, subsistence agricultural workers, far from the forces of civilization, provide the free labor that Brazil required in order to fulfill her promises of wealth and greatness? Antônio Cândido da Cruz Machado, president of the Province of Bahia in 1873, advocated colonization, by which he meant not only the immigration of Europeans to Brazil (a desirable option but not a realistic one in economically declining Bahia) but also using all individuals, whether Brazilian or not, who wanted to work in agriculture, "teaching them how they can reap benefits for themselves and for the nation."[44] Some commentators implicated race as the cause for the backwardness of the Brazilian laborer, but others looked instead for causes in ignorance and isolation from cities, the source of civilization. As the president of the Bahian Imperial Institute for Agriculture, Barão de Sergimirim, noted in 1871 when discussing the lack of productivity among Bahian agricultural workers, "[the situation of labor] is grave. . . . The problem is the [lack of] education, the misconceptions passed on through generations, the reluctance to change, the isolation from civilized centers."[45]

As early as 1859, the inspector of public hygiene, Dr. Goes Siqueira, analyzed the problem from a hygienist's point of view:

It is certain that good hygienic measures, regularly applied, have a two-fold effect on the population; that is, the stronger a people, the more hardworking they become and the less time they spend indulging in vice. . . . Health not only contributes to the happiness of the individual but it is one of the sources of general wealth. . . . How can we hope for a bright and satisfying future if we do not prepare for a true moral and material progress?[46]

For Goes Siqueira, as for the Tropicalistas, laying the basis for a robust population and for material progress was central to the task of the physician.

In Brazil the various answers given to the question of the place of the free black and mulatto in society always involved some degree of social integration for blacks according to the conditions established by the dominant white society. Such responses differed from those given to the same question in the American South. This was because the processes of manumission had evolved in opposite directions in the two societies.[47] Whereas in North America, from the early–eighteenth century on, whites had greatly restricted the possibility of manumission, making the few black freedmen into pariahs with no place within the social and economic order, in Brazil manumission became an accepted process and freedmen and women had a legitimate, albeit precarious, place within the society.[48] Moreover, the free colored population in Brazil grew so fast that by the 1872 census there were 4.2 million free coloreds out of a total population of 10 million.[49] Even though racial prejudice was widespread in Brazil, it was also true that the free colored population performed an important economic role in the society. Thus, although the free coloreds operated, for the most part, at the lower end of the society and were the most impoverished sector with the highest rates of mortality and the most disease, they were traditionally allowed some social mobility. For example, in the nineteenth century many of the most prominent artists, musicians, writers, and artisans were black or mulatto, as were many professionals, such as doctors or engineers.[50] This was an aspect of Brazilian reality that never failed to amaze travelers from Europe or North America. As Count Alexis de Saint Priest, the French minister to Brazil, noted in 1834:

> When I came here I thought I would find that mulattoes formed a class apart, rejected by whites and dominating blacks. . . . [In reality they] are mixed, interfused with all [groups]; they are to be found among slaves, among the vilest of employments, but also among the high society, and in the senate.[51]

This was also an aspect of Brazilian society some of the elite in the Empire were rather proud of, believing that on the racial question they had a more enlightened approach than North Americans.[52]

The other salient factor in Brazilian race relations, and one that contrasted with North America, was the greater tolerance of miscegenation.[53]

It has been calculated that 75 percent of the colored freedman population in five provinces in nineteenth-century Brazil was made up by mulattoes whereas only 20 percent of slaves were mulattoes. In 1872 mulattoes made up 78 percent of colored freedmen in Brazil.[54] Most mulattoes, therefore, were free. There is a long debate in Brazilian literature as to why Brazil freed more slaves and was more accepting of miscegenation than most other slave societies.[55] The high incidences of racial mixing and manumission, compared to the North American context, gave rise to a particularly Brazilian solution to the "black problem." This was the idea of "whitening" (*branqueamento*), which fit quite comfortably with the prevalent populational and Lamarckian approach to medicine that argued that the improvement of people's health and progeny could be achieved through the betterment of the social and physical environments in which populations lived.[56]

Whitening was a means whereby mulattoes could advance up the hierarchy of racial order, sometimes even enter the upper levels of society, provided they acquired the education and "civilized" manners that white upper-class Brazilians deemed appropriate for their cultural assimilation. Whitening was also a biological form of social mobility for the children of mulattoes who entered into marriages or unions with partners lighter than themselves. Both these forms of whitening were widely used in Brazilian society. The theory of whitening was based on the idea that in the Brazilian context, the notion of "foreclosing" a multiracial society—actively pursued in North America—was unrealistic.[57] It also assumed that whites, through miscegenation, would swamp out blacks, leading to their eventual elimination from the Brazilian "race." This idea became especially important after the 1871 passage of the Law of the Free Womb, which, by declaring free all children born to slaves, virtually doomed slavery and encouraged the Brazilian elite to turn to increased European immigration as a solution to the labor problem. In the fast-growing coffee regions of the south, European immigration was far more feasible than in Bahia and the Northeast, which could not compete with the booming conditions of the south.[58] The tendency would be toward whitening because it was believed that since blacks were more degenerate, and thus physically weakened and socially disorganized, they would easily be overwhelmed by whites. Moreover, it was held that black and colored women preferred lighter colored men. Whitening, therefore, retained the belief in white superiority but provided hope that social engineering could change and mold "inferior" black characteristics to be more like those of the "superior" whites. Two key tenets of North

American and European racial science were conveniently dropped: that racial hybridization must mean degeneration and regression, and that racial differences were only biologically determined and not malleable to social conditioning.[59]

The Brazilian belief in the malleable nature of human beings was the crucial underpinning to the process of whitening, and it gave Brazilian doctors an important role to play in the forging of an improved race. As one medical student put it:

> Among all races, even those reduced by climate and passions to the most abject of conditions, men are capable of receiving an education which improves them and which, when applied to a whole nation, enables [the nation] to receive in the first, or at least the second, generation the traditions, laws, institutions, arts, sciences, in a word, all the general progress the civilized nations possess.[60]

If in Europe sanitation held out hope against the unwieldy problems exacerbated by rapid industrialization, urbanization, and defeat in war, in Brazil hygienic, sanitary, and moral living provided an answer to those who held that the racial and climatological conditions of Brazil must lead to increasing decay.[61]

Nowhere in Brazil were the debates of racial science more pernicious than in Bahia. Not only was Salvador a largely black city, but because it attracted far less European immigration than Rio de Janeiro, much of its middle and upper social ranks were filled by mulattoes.[62] This was notably true for mulatto doctors, who were an accepted feature of Bahian society. Given the present status of research on doctors in Bahia, it is impossible to determine the number of black doctors in the city. However, the impressionistic evidence of nineteenth-century travelers and the few cases with definite information about the racial and class background of physicians indicates that mulatto doctors were an accepted feature of Bahian society.[63] Moreover, if we recall that in the Empire years university education played a role in facilitating limited social and racial mobility, then it is understandable that the Bahian school of medicine, the kernel of culture in the city, was central to Bahian mechanisms of racial and social mobility.[64] Not only was Bahian imperial society in the second half of the nineteenth century a society subject to pressures from below by mulattoes and sons of immigrants seeking to open up for themselves better places in the society, but it was also a society changing from a city dominated by rural plantation owners to a city dominated by professionals and merchants at home with the urbanized culture of nineteenth-century Europe.[65] Thus, while on one hand the institutions of higher education were central for upward social and racial mobility, on the other they were crucial in effecting a horizontal shift of focus in nineteenth-century Brazil from rural to urban, from patriarchal to modern, urbanized social relations.[66] Thus the sons and grandsons of the authoritarian patriarch and (now declining) plantation owner became the doctors and professionals of a changing Brazilian social order. In Freyre's vivid image, the umbrella replaced the sword. Thus at Bahia's school of medicine one would expect to see the descendants of some of the great old families, alongside mulattoes, illegitimate sons, white or mulatto, and the sons of immigrant merchants, mainly Portuguese.[67]

From what we know of the social composition of the graduates of the medical school in Bahia, all these social and racial groups were present. In 1848, for example, Tiburtino Moreira Prates noted in his medical school dissertation:

> there are more than a hundred students in the medical school of this city [and] half of them are indisputably mulattoes; of the others, we know that many are quadroons who have "passed"; of others, we are ignorant of their ancestry; those who are unquestionably of the Caucasian race do not number more than twenty.[68]

Lino Coutinho, one of the earliest prominent physicians, teachers, and politicians in Bahia before midcentury was a mulatto of humble origins. So were the liberal physician and faculty professor Luís Anselmo de Fonseca, the archconservative and pro-slavery physician Counselor Domingos Carlos da Silva, and the physician-anthropologist Raimundo Nina Rodrigues.[69] These men worked and taught alongside physicians from such noble families as Malaquias and Luís Alvares dos Santos, Antônio José Pereira Silva Araújo, and Jerônymo Sodré Pereira, descendant of two prominent families in Bahia and also a grandson of Lino Coutinho.[70] The sons of Portuguese immigrants who came to Brazil to work as traders or skilled artisans were also well represented in the School's ranks. Manoel Joaquim Saraiva, Pacífico Pereira, and Victorino Pereira were all from such immigrant stock, the two latter becoming prominent figures within the school.[71] Yet another success story was that of Pedro Severiano de Magalhães, who came from a humble orphan background and rose to achieve some of the highest medical accolades in the land.[72] It is probable that the racial and social heterogeneity of the medical community in Bahia was a direct reflection of the complex transitions and adjustments that Bahian society was undergoing.

This is the context in which the medical community in Brazil, and especially in Bahia, received European racial science. Racial science was digested here very differently from the way it was in Europe or the United States. If the medical community did not reject outright European imputations, it is possible to see, at least in the Tropicalistas' practice and theory, the use of subtle categories of resistance to unwelcome assessments about Brazil and the Brazilians. These processes of resistance were varied.

Rejecting Tropical Determinism

The theoretical underpinning of Tropicalista medical thinking—like that of doctors elsewhere—was the malleability of human beings. This conception of human nature provided the Tropicalistas with a "flexible, etiological model" that emphasized physicians' need to direct their patients to retain, or regain, their health.[73] The physician, for example, could recognize his patients' particular inherited predispositions and steer them in a safe direction by counseling them to avoid those environments (such as low-lying damp places, unventilated rooms, sudden climatic changes) and behaviors (inadequate diet, stress, overindulgence in sexual relations) most likely to lead to sickness.

In applying this conception to their endeavor of resisting the forecasts of doom for Brazil, the Tropicalistas clearly ascribed to the beliefs of the Lamarckian tradition, particularly to the nineteenth-century version of neo-Lamarckianism (although they never self-consciously referred to themselves as Lamarckians). Neo-Lamarckianism emphasized the importance of adaptation to environmental factors such as diet, sanitation, and climate. It was held that the adaptive or "acquired" characteristics that resulted were then passed on in the procreation of a new individual.[74] As Silva Lima elaborated in 1890,

> *Natura non facit saltum,* says the great naturalist, and the saying is true too for other processes . . . [such as] the achievement of the intellectual, moral, and social perfection of a people and its institutions. . . . [However,] evolution in relation to intellectual culture, . . . [and] to scientific advances can be accelerated by human effort, and that effort, if persistent

and well directed, can often achieve [a jump in the process that] might otherwise have taken centuries.[75]

Neo-Lamarckianism, of course, could be used to fit the more pessimistic, moralist thinking of those who felt helpless in the face of the growing army of wretched poor that seemed to be an inevitable part of industrialization in Europe. European observers often viewed the tropics in a similarly fatalistic manner.[76] It was also possible, however, to appropriate neo-Lamarckianism for more optimistic ends; it allowed room for human intervention to manipulate the environment and thereby to improve human beings. This idea of the malleability of human beings, of "soft" hereditarianism, was particularly effective in Brazil, where hope existed that through the correct scientific, medical manipulation of the social environment, a "civilized" people could emerge. Júlio de Moura put the idea best when he noted, in an article on tuberculosis,

> The Brazilian family . . . suffers from an organic weakness accrued through successive generations. . . . Without going into a long discussion on acclimatization of Europeans in hot climates and . . . the advantages and disadvantages of . . . the cross between the invading races and the aboriginal, we must admit that the original trunk from which we descend . . . [has lost] physical and moral vigor. It is quite possible that any Darwinist would find in us sadly visible symptoms of a hybrid race that cannot progress.[77]

However, Moura continued hopefully,

> These innate physical tendencies can be modified. . . . They are elements of decadence that have no other origin than the most basic negligence and ignorance of . . . the science of hygiene.[78]

The Tropicalistas resisted the detrimental labels imposed by climate and race by leaning toward the idea that most disorders were universal, but that the tropical heat and humidity exacerbated maladies in such a way as to make them distinctive.[79] Exactly how heat and humidity affected disease and decay was what they intended to elucidate. In examining their writings on these themes, a useful starting point is the work of Pacífico Pereira, who straddled the old and new in medical concepts, partly to retain an optimistic approach to civilization in the tropics.

A recurring theme in Pacífico Pereira's writings was the oxygenation of people's blood in the tropics.[80] I have already mentioned how he believed that anoxemia could lead to such tropical ailments as beriberi, that it underlay most such ailments by acting as a principal "predisposing cause," and that it was the key to explaining tropical decay. He worried that Brazilian physicians did not give this factor the importance it deserved.[81] Pereira agreed with the German physician and hygienist Max von Pettenkofer that Europeans degenerated in the tropics because in a hot and humid climate the body never wholly threw off poisons to accomplish a thorough regeneration of the tissues.[82] As Pereira noted, "In the climatic conditions in which we live, the influence and effects of vitiated air are much more . . . serious and long-lasting than in temperate climates."[83]

Pereira, however, conveniently ignored the fatalism inherent in Pettenkofer's thinking. Instead, he expressed increasing concern about the practical steps to be taken to neutralize the dangers of poor oxygenation in the tropics. In an influential article on the importance of hygiene within Brazilian schools, he presented these concerns in terms of proper ventilation and exercise, noting how children were forced to sit for long hours in crowded, hot, badly ventilated classrooms, their bodies unable to carry out the oxygenation needed for sturdy development.

> In a modern society . . . education not only addresses the cultural, intellectual, and moral [development] of a child, but it must also address his physical development. . . . Physical education is the great, urgent, and vital question of this country, where the race slowly languishes [as a result of] the climatic conditions, and the level of organic activity gradually atrophies with each passing generation.[84]

Even more forcefully he reiterated,

> Physiology clearly shows us that *air and exercise are even more necessary to physical development in a tropical climate* because it is an incontestable truth that the organism lacks an abundant provision of oxygen for respiration and nutrition.[85]

Pereira then turned to the practical considerations to combat the drawbacks of what he called a debilitating climate and a decadent race, making recommendations for the spatial layout of schools and the reduction of passive learning to ensure that correct oxygenation took place. Thus, despite his flirtation with ideas damning to Brazil, Pacífico Pereira contradicted those ideas by never abandoning his faith in the possibility of manipulating the tropical environment to ensure progress in his homeland. It is significant that the other Tropicalistas accepted many of the European ideas about the tropics, in similar fashion, but if they believed in degeneration, they emphasized regeneration.

In 1888 the second-generation Tropicalista Braz do Amaral took up the theme that correct oxygenation would produce a better caliber of Brazilian. He argued that gymnastics were crucial to the development of people's energies in the tropics and should be made an obligatory part of the school curriculum: "Upon this question depends the beauty of the race, the vigor of the worker, the productivity of the intellectual, the energy of the soldier, the development of industry, the advance of science, and the prosperity of our nation."[86]

Wucherer's writings on tuberculosis also indicate the Tropicalistas' endeavor to move out of accepted beliefs of certain illnesses belonging only to temperate climates and others to tropical climates. According to Wucherer, tuberculosis was erroneously held to be distinctive to temperate climates and extremely rare in the tropics. Not only was tuberculosis common in Brazil, but judging from what few records existed since the eighteenth century, it was a disease very much on the rise. As supporting evidence, Wucherer gave his own personal experience and the statistics kept by the Santa Casa hospitals in Rio de Janeiro and Bahia, which, he was quick to point out, provided only the numbers of those who checked in to the charity hospitals and thus were far below the real incidence of tuberculosis.[87] Why, asked Wucherer, was there this rise in the disorder in nineteenth-century Brazil? He considered the hypothesis, held by some doctors, that tuberculosis could be traced to a single specific agent, independent of the organism, as, for example, smallpox could be. But he was not persuaded; so far there was little evidence for this point of view. It seemed more likely to Wucherer that tuberculosis was an illness that could be contrasted to smallpox, for it was multicausal; many factors had to be considered when studying this disease.

Wucherer did not believe, as did some doctors, that European immigration had contributed to an increase in tuberculosis in Brazil. What he thought was crucial to its increase were the changes in people's life conditions, particularly in the previous three or four decades. One of these changes was the rise in the numbers of persons living crowded together in urban areas, a factor that had acted as a spur to the contagious disorder of tuberculosis; another was a result of Brazilians' falling standards of living. Although wages had gone up, Wucherer wrote, the cost of basic necessities had increased even more. As an example, he indicated that the price of fresh meat had risen by 100 percent over the previous twelve years.[88] At the same time there was a higher consumption of alcoholic beverages among all classes. Moreover, Wucherer stated, as a result of the 1855 cholera epidemic there had been a big drop in the number of slaves; thus many families who before the epidemic had lived off the labor power of their slaves had since fallen into dire poverty.[89] Poverty, undernutrition, and unhygienic conditions, therefore, were crucial, according to Wucherer, in accounting for the rise of tuberculosis, particularly among the poorer classes. The message underlying Wucherer's discussion on tuberculosis in Bahia was that disorders were more universal than some climatologists believed. Moreover, even when some disorders were more prevalent in hot climates than others, a tropical etiology per se explained nothing. For European doctors, the label "tropical" tended to be self-explanatory and therefore dismissive; for Wucherer, it represented a critical starting point, the framework within which he investigated an ailment, and within which he wanted to make his contribution to medicine. Paramount in Wucherer's equation were the social conditions in which people lived. In conditions of social misery the incidence of illness would be high; for Wucherer, as for the German doctor-scientists who influenced his thinking, disease—even tropical disease—always had social agency.

As much as they rejected climatological determinism, the Tropicalistas rejected racial determinism; but they addressed the European stereotypes of inferiority associated with race less openly than they did those of climate. It is possible, nevertheless, to get an indication of their thinking on this issue by looking at the writings from their medical practice. These show that the Tropicalistas refused to pick up the polygenist gauntlet of "different species." Disease in the tropics, in their conception, had a good deal to do with poverty, undernutrition, lack of sanitation, and the conditions of slavery—in other words, with poor social conditions that led to disease in similar ways as in the more temperate climates of Europe. Thus, in their clinical work, the Tropicalistas several times raised the question of the relation between race and a particular illness, but they never pursued this line of inquiry, or they deflected it to the social conditions of Africans and Creoles.[90]

Wucherer and his disciples associated hookworm with Africans and Creoles, for example, but argued that unhygienic social conditions enabled the
hookworm to thrive, and that those conditions, rather than race, were ultimately responsible for the disorder.[91] Silva Lima initially viewed the enforced barefootedness of slaves as an important factor in ainhum but then
he observed that *libertos* (freed slaves), who almost always wore shoes, also
suffered from the disorder. Even though he found the problem only among
Africans, he never argued that it was racially inherited. Instead, he professed to be mystified by the disorder.[92]

Another disorder Brazilian doctors thought struck blacks more than
whites was tetanus. But here again the doctors refused to be satisfied with
a purely racial etiology. R. da Cunha reported, for example, the case of a
tetanus patient who died of the disorder, noting that the victim was black,
which "predisposed" him to the disorder. But da Cunha added that the
victim was male, that he had a strong constitution, and that the city had
recently suffered a cold spell, all equally important variables.[93]

Similar reasoning can be seen in a review Wucherer published in 1867
of the work of the German physician and medical geographer Carl F. Heusinger on geophagy.[94] Heusinger argued that geophagy occurred in all climates and that it was found in European countries as well as tropical ones;
he also asserted that Africans had a greater predisposition toward it. Although not wholly rejecting the first part of the hypothesis, Wucherer
found Heusinger's evidence unreliable and therefore remained skeptical of
his claims.[95] But Wucherer roundly rejected the second part of Heusinger's
hypothesis—that Africans had a greater predisposition to geophagy—arguing that the author had by no means proved his case. Only if all other
factors, including living conditions, remained constant could racial predisposition be accepted as a definite cause.[96]

In the debate over whether the "pure-blooded Negro" was immune to
yellow fever, an immunity some observers believed was lost when "hybridization" occurred, Wucherer sided with the skeptics. He noted that yellow
fever occurred less and in a milder form among Africans but he believed
the difference was related to immunity conferred through acclimatization,
not race.[97]

Wucherer's position was typical of the Tropicalistas' work. Indeed, they
never used medical facts to advocate a separate medicine to deal with the
"peculiarities" of blacks as doctors did in the antebellum South and the
West Indies.[98] In Brazil, the racial and climatological explanations of "de-

generation" were not the rivals that Philip Curtin has suggested they were in the West Indian context, where European doctors rejected the idea that tropical climate caused whites to degenerate, arguing that the natives of tropical regions were backward because of their race and not because of climate.[99] The blurring of racial lines through miscegenation and black social mobility, albeit limited, meant that whites could not comfortably dismiss notions of backwardness based on climate and instead blame racial categories. For this reason, the Tropicalistas' writings are largely silent on the racial question. But they clearly would have agreed with Anselmo de Fonseca, who stated in 1887 that it was an error to seek the origins of Brazilian social, economic, and political evils in the "physiology of the Brazilian race" when the "lessons of history" showed that "people whom we today admire, when they were in a more primitive stage, were even less advanced socially than we are at present."[100]

The Tropicalistas' silence is best interpreted as an ambivalence. Like many in the Brazilian upper class, they accepted the assumption of racial science that the white race was superior to all others, but they refused to accept the rigidity that was becoming one of its more prominent features.[101] As members of the Brazilian intelligentsia, moreover, the Bahian physicians were part of the tradition that, in contrast to the United States, had "assimilated the savage races instead of trying to destroy them, thus preparing us to resist the devastating invasion of race prejudice."[102] Practically speaking, they worked alongside numerous mulattoes like Fonseca, so that the reiteration of the inevitable inferiority and sterility of racially mixed people must have rung false.[103]

It is tempting to speculate that the Tropicalistas clung to a nineteenth-century Brazilian etiquette regarding race. Emília Viotti da Costa has described this etiquette brilliantly.[104] At its center was silence, made possible by the particular Brazilian social construction of race, in which biological, social, and cultural perceptions were so entangled that an individual's phenotype ceased to be the salient characteristic. In other words, it was possible for a person of African descent who had achieved the culture and social distinction of an upper-class white to "pass" as white.[105] Such a framework would help explain why although the Tropicalistas accepted European thinking about a hierarchy of races, they also adhered to older notions of fluidity and the belief that it was possible for "inferior" races to better themselves and move up the hierarchy. As Braz do Amaral stated in 1886,

Man improves himself by improving the milieu in which he lives, . . .
by perfecting the conditions of his intimate life, . . . purifying his blood,
by being provided with good schools, hygienic offices, by reducing the
numbers of work hours . . . , by giving children good mothers, by eating
good food. . . . All of this is within the range of the doctor's [work].[106]

Another Bahian doctor argued even more optimistically,

The racial mixture [in Brazil] will not be an obstacle to progress but
will lead to a definite national type with the resistance needed to dominate the tropics. . . . Our civilization will certainly differ from that of the
European because it will have evolved in a different environment but by
no means will it be inferior.[107]

By the 1880s and 1890s, as the waning of the Empire and the rise of the
Republic made questions of national identity more urgent, Brazil also received a barrage of new currents of thought. Many Brazilians were moving
away from the confident belief in the power of scientists like the Tropicalistas to manipulate the environment and improve the caliber of citizens toward a much greater pessimism about biological determinism.[108]
One such thinker who emerged from the Escola Tropicalista Bahiana and
moved into a close embrace of the new European ideas was Raimundo
Nina Rodrigues.

Beyond the Tropicalistas: The Response of Raimundo Nina Rodrigues

As a young physician in Bahia, Raimundo Nina Rodrigues was much taken
with the Tropicalista approach to medicine in Bahia, seeing an alternative
to what he viewed as the "sterile and banal medicine, of doubtful scientific value, coming from the Bahian medical school."[109] Eventually, however, Nina Rodrigues, most likely a mulatto, began to transcend Tropicalista thinking on the question of whether susceptibility to disease was
racially determined. Not only was racial inheritance a key variable in the
predisposition to certain disorders, he came to believe, but Africans and
racially mixed peoples were also more predisposed to criminality, had inferior powers of reasoning, and should not, therefore, be allowed to become full citizens of the nation.[110]

Nina Rodrigues was born in a rural region of Maranhão and, like many
Brazilians, was steeped in the culture of his family's slaves from an early

age. He grew up on the family estate, associating with the children of sixty slaves, learning to read with a slave woman known as Madrinha Mulata, listening to the stories about the *quilombo* of Pau-da-Estopa (a runaway slave community) and the lepers of Anajatuba.[111] He started his medical training in Bahia but in 1884 he transferred to Rio de Janeiro and graduated there in 1887, returning to his native province to practice medicine. In 1889 he returned to Salvador, where he practiced, taught at the medical school, and carried out the bulk of the anthropological work for which he later became famous.

Already known in Bahian medical circles, and highly praised by Silva Lima for his work on leprosy in Maranhão, which the *Gazeta Médica* published in 1887, Nina Rodrigues soon became active among Tropicalista circles. He worked alongside Tropicalistas at the Santa Casa de Misericórdia Hospital; he joined the fledgling Bahian Medical Society (Sociedade Médica da Bahia), founded by Silva Lima and Victorino Pereira in 1888; and, together with two other Tropicalistas, he organized the Third Brazilian Medical Congress, hosted in Bahia in 1890.[112] Beginning in 1888, he published copiously in the *Gazeta Médica* on subjects within the Tropicalista agenda, such as beriberi, leprosy, the demand for statistical information on those ailments that most afflicted Brazilians, and the need to reform the Bahian health system. By the 1890s Nina Rodrigues had become one of the principal contributors to the journal, and from 1890 to 1893 he became its editor-in-chief.

Links of marriage and friendship sealed his professional association with the Tropicalistas. He married the daughter of José Lima D'Almeida Couto, one of the *Gazeta Médica*'s chief editors. His brother-in-law, Alfredo Tomé de Britto, was a younger Tropicalista. He became close friends with Virgílio Clímaco Damazio, another *Gazeta Médica* editor and a medical school professor, to whose chair Nina Rodrigues succeeded in 1891.

Because he is best known for his later pioneering work in Afro-Brazilian ethnology and Brazilian legal medicine, Nina Rodrigues's early writings have been largely ignored.[113] Yet it is these writings, emerging from his clinical practice, that reveal Nina Rodrigues's early preoccupation with the question of race, a preoccupation that would lead him more and more toward the determinism of nineteenth-century anthropology and racial science. In 1903 Nina Rodrigues recalled how the Tropicalistas in Bahia had provided a challenge to the Bahian medical school's sterile regurgitation of medical science "made for other races and for other countries."[114] He was undoubtedly drawn to the Tropicalista fold because he identified with their emphasis on the importance of original research in medicine. In fundamental ways, however, he transcended the Tropicalistas' belief in the malleability of human nature through social environmentalism. Very early on he began to ask questions about the relationship between race and pathology, a relationship the Tropicalistas had not left unpondered, but which they had always referred back to social factors.

Nina Rodrigues's early explorations in this direction can best be illustrated by two early articles published in the *Gazeta Médica da Bahia*.[115] The articles dealt with a study of leprosy in Maranhão, where he had worked with two physicians collecting data. Leprosy was one of the disorders that became a focus of concern in the years preceding the fall of the Empire. It had acquired international visibility since the Norwegian researcher Gerhard H. A. Hansen had isolated the leprosy bacillus in 1873, even though his findings were disputed for a long time.[116] The disease was endemic in Brazil, particularly to certain geographical pockets in the north.[117]

In his first article, Nina Rodrigues argued that his clinical findings pointed to the importance of contagion in the disorder, although he said he had no positive knowledge about the "infectious agent" or the mode of transmission.[118] Given the uncertainty of the precise cause of the disease, he argued that it was important to consider the factors in predisposition, among which were the familiar atmospheric ones—climate, humidity, sanitary conditions, and diet. Nina Rodrigues, however, went a step further than the Tropicalistas and mentioned the additional factor of racial susceptibility. Drawing eclectically on Darwin's theory of natural selection and Lombroso's concept of atavism, he asserted that susceptibility to leprosy was inherited:

> According to scientific principles of natural selection, the fact that leprosy is caught by some individuals and not other members of the same family in exactly the same conditions, . . . [leads] us to believe that many times these individuals descend from a single genealogical branch which was, at some time, attacked by leprosy. [I]mmunity depends on the laws of alternating inheritance, or atavic inheritance.[119]

Nina Rodrigues, therefore, greatly weakened human agency as a factor in controlling of the disease. Although he still considered hygienic living important, he became far more interested in exploring the ramifications of inherited predisposition. Subsequently, he focused his attention increas-

ingly on this deterministic strand. From the inheritance of the predisposition to leprosy in certain families, Nina Rodrigues moved to the predisposition of certain races. He insisted that racial pathology should be central
to Brazilian medical investigations. Using a polygenist argument, he held
that different human species, constituted by physical and chemical variations and molded by different lifestyles, must offer diverging predispositions to the same illness.[120] The problem to be investigated, therefore, was
the influence of race upon pathology.[121] He lamented the fact that very
little work had been done in this direction in Brazil, and that what had been
done offered no clear statement of what races and race crossings were involved.[122] Devising such a statement, however, was no easy task, for it was
extremely difficult to determine what racial parts went into the formation
of people of mixed racial heritage, such as mulattoes. Nevertheless, said
Nina Rodrigues, it was not impossible. He provided a methodology for
trying to disaggregate the term *mestiço* (by which he meant racially mixed
people in general). Only with such a clarification would it be possible to
elucidate how disorders were racially determined.

Another problem linked to racial hybridization and disease was the apparent contradiction that while indigenous Brazilians were immune to leprosy (as he wrongly believed), those with mixed blood were highly predisposed to it.[123] In the end, Nina Rodrigues was unable to come up with
any meaningful relationship between race and predisposition to becoming
a victim of leprosy. Thus, he concluded that with the exception of Brazilian
Indians (whom he did not number among his cases), all the races living in
Brazil were liable to contract leprosy.[124]

In spite of this conclusion, the question of the relation of race and illness continued to intrigue Nina Rodrigues, and in a second article published in 1890, he entered the realm of racial anthropology, attempting to
break down the racial "types" to be found among Brazilian mestiços.[125] The
search for pure African types among Brazilian mulattoes set the boundaries
for much of Nina Rodrigues's later work. Drawing on the then current
paradigms in European and North American racial science and anthropology, he argued that the inferiority of the African had been scientifically established. In the debate over whether hybridization invigorated the
race or led to further degeneration, Nina Rodrigues sided with the latter
camp.[126] He had already, he thought, added further proof to this view by
noting, in the case of leprosy, that Indians of mixed racial character lost the
immunity of their "pure" ancestors.

By the 1890s, when he moved into the area of legal medicine, Nina Rodrigues's ideas on the "inferior races" had been reinforced so that, in the case of crime and the law, he came to argue that "inferior peoples" should be granted "attenuated" responsibility. Those of mixed races would be ranked according to a hierarchy of greater and lesser degeneration and granted civic responsibility accordingly.[127] Moreover, he warned, it would be a mistake to confuse the cultural value of a race with the laudable qualities of individuals from that race: "If we know black or colored men worthy of our esteem and respect, this does not negate the truth that until now blacks have been unable to build civilized nations."[128]

Some people, Nina Rodrigues continued, believed that the black race would tend to disappear through weakness, sickness, and infertility.[129] But this belief, he stated, "is a manifest error. . . . Racial crossing does no more than retard the elimination of white blood." In no way would racial crossing lead to the disappearance of the black race in Brazil. Thus viewing the question of race mixture and the strong African presence in Brazil through the prism of European theories, Nina Rodrigues was unabashedly pessimistic about the future of Brazil. Civilization in the tropics would, at best, be second rate.

During the following decade, Nina Rodrigues continued to catalog the precise regional and ethnic origins of the colored population in Bahia in Brazil. He differentiated linguistic groups, investigated the African religious cults, collected African artwork—all of which earned him unpopularity among a group of professors at the medical school and the nickname *negreiro* (slaver).[130] Indeed, at the height of his seminal ethnographic work, Nina Rodrigues was bitterly opposed by the medical school. The biggest clash between the school and Nina Rodrigues was in 1897, when the Congregation of the Medical School voted to reject his "Memória histórica," an annual report usually accepted as a matter of course.

Not only did Nina Rodrigues challenge the existing standard of teaching, but his research into race threatened the faculty's attempts to play down African influences in Brazilian culture and highlight European ones.[131] It was well known, for example, that Nina Rodrigues attended such African rituals as *candomblés* as part of his research on Africans.[132] Whether Nina Rodrigues was the only member of the intelligentsia to do so is unknown, but certainly, he did not bother to hide the fact that he thought knowledge about such practices was an important aspect of scientifically understanding Brazil and its people.[133] Indeed, he held that the study of

Africans and African influence in Brazil should be central to the study of medicine and law. Thus he focused on a reality which the Bahian intelligentsia preferred to ignore.

In contrast to Nina Rodrigues, the Tropicalistas kept silent on the question of race and in this they were closer to the traditional Bahian physician. The difference between them may be explained by a shifting over from the imperial racial system that allowed a few mulattoes entry into the ranks of the elite, to a society with a dichotomous racial classification, which, as George Reid Andrews and others have cogently argued, made "passing" from black to white increasingly difficult. The irony is that the position seemingly more accommodating to race—that of the Tropicalistas—was as heavily imbued with ideas of white superiority and black inferiority as Nina Rodrigues's. The Tropicalistas' silence was a way of legitimating the status quo and the manner of dealing with racial difference. While Nina Rodrigues's position would seem more damaging to Brazilians, later historians, seeking to dignify the African contribution to Brazilian culture, were indebted to him for salvaging so much of Brazil's African past, even though they rejected his ideas on the hierarchical ranking of races. Nina Rodrigues's fascination with things African in Brazil, in the long run, laid the foundations for a whole new way of evaluating the African contribution to the formation of the Brazilian nation.[134]

Conclusion

In this chapter I have shown that in Brazil there was a nascent "tropical medicine" several decades before the specialty became institutionalized in Europe at the turn of the century.[135] My interpretation of tropical medicine in Brazil from the 1860s sheds new light both on the history of the rise of tropical medicine and on the transference of scientific ideas and the creation of medical knowledge in Brazil.

Most of the research on this topic has concerned Africa, India, and other parts of the European colonial empire. Indeed, the terms "tropical medicine" and "colonial medicine' are sometimes used interchangeably because it is assumed that tropical medicine was developed almost exclusively by Europeans—joined later by North Americans—due to the demands of empire, which quickened just as the germ theory gained acceptance and provided one of the most successful paradigms for understanding tropical disorders. Early tropical medicine in Brazil, however, developed for different reasons. In Brazil, the tropical medicine of the Tropicalistas was not about more efficient colonial domination, but about softening the harshness of European and North American assessments about the tropics and tropical peoples. If, as in Britain, the "study of tropical diseases [could be seen as] a means of promoting imperial policy," in Brazil the pursuit of tropical medicine was primarily a nationalistic venture to redefine Brazil's place in the world.[136]

So what was the Tropicalistas' view of tropical pathology? As I have argued in the previous chapter, even when the Tropicalistas were well aware of the germ theory of disease, published articles and commentaries on it in the *Gazeta Médica* and had contributed to the related theory of parasitological disease, they remained reluctant to shed the miasmatic theory of infection. But the Tropicalistas were not passive and isolated; they did not hold outdated notions of disease through a lack of information about science in the metropolitan centers and a lack of interchange with other tropical experts. On the contrary, they were well informed, up-to-date, and well connected, and their contributions were seen as valuable enough to be reproduced in European journals and important European texts such as T. Spencer Cobbold's *Parasites* and Hirsch's *Handbook*. Why then did they not abandon the miasmatic theory of disease as soon as they became aware of the role of parasites and bacteria in tropical disorders?

The answer is to be found in the fact that the miasmatic theory of infection, so compatible with the physicians' neo-Lamarckianism and its focus on environment and manipulation, was useful in combating the most fatalistic aspects of the idea of tropical disease. The Tropicalistas' whole practice pointed to their belief that there was no such thing as a *tropical* miasma; rather, there were certain miasmatic sources, linked to the unhealthiness of refuse, of dug-up soil, of stagnant water, of unsanitary housing and street conditions, of the conditions of slavery, that led to disease in the same way all of these conditions did in the more temperate climates of Europe. Thus, just as European physicians pushed to improve these conditions, so physicians in the tropics should do the same. It was, of course, true that for the Tropicalistas a hot and damp climate could provide extra dangerous conditions for the formation and harmful effects of miasma. This was not a reason for fatalism, however, but rather for further vigilance and investigation on the part of the doctors. The environmental concept of miasma, like neo-Lamarckian adaptiveness, provided an ideology to actively manipulate the milieu toward the making of an improved people. The Tropicalistas' framing of tropical disorders, therefore, eschewed the determinism associated with climate and race, and allowed them to retain agency, flexibility, and optimism in Brazil.

However, by the 1880s and 1890s a younger generation of Brazilian medical scientists, ready to break with the more flexible Tropicalistas, began to use medical "facts" to underpin theories about the desirability of excluding certain racial groups from full citizenship, an exclusionary approach that became possible in the face of the new European immigration into Brazil. A good example of this sort of thinking is seen in the writings of Nina Rodrigues. Ultimately, however, Nina Rodrigues's pessimism proved the exception, and the more malleable neo-Lamarckian approach of the Tropicalistas remained a central strand in Brazilian thinking that continued to exhibit novel and inventive ways of adapting European racial science so that it could provide an auspicious outlook to the Brazilian situation. Particularly interesting in this respect was the evolutionary thinking of Dr. Theodoro Sampaio, official orator of the Bahian Geographic and Historical Institute (Instituto Geográfico e Histórico da Bahia) in 1913, who held that human evolution was far from finished and that the mixture of races in Brazil would provide for a new race, specially adapted to the tropics, which would produce civilization in the tropics for the first time.[137]

Finally, it should be noted that the way the Tropicalistas have been defined historically is also, ironically, an illustration of the extent to which science in "peripheral" countries becomes defined by the interests of the leading countries. An important reason for the Tropicalistas' success in the European journals was the rising interest in colonial (tropical) medicine. European editors of medical journals had a highly selective view of the value of Brazilian medicine. When the Brazilians dealt with "tropical" disorders, the Europeans reported on them; they seemed less interested in other aspects of their work. A number of the Tropicalistas, for example, prided themselves on their work as surgeons, and they were avid supporters of the introduction of gynecology and obstetrics in Bahia. They wrote many articles on their experiences in these areas of medical practice, but their writings on such topics were completely ignored by the European press. Rather, they became known as experts in tropical medicine, that is, as experts on certain disorders peculiar to the tropics, a resource for a new European need. Eventually, the broader nature of their work was eclipsed in favor of their contributions to the new tropical specialty so that they were labeled, posthumously, as the school of tropical medicine.

CHAPTER FOUR

Physicians and Women in Bahia

A part of European condemnation of the tropics as unfit was the idea that the tropics were unsuitable for European breeding. Indeed, it was generally believed that European women became infertile in the tropics and that when they did have babies, infant mortality was notoriously high.[1] This was another notion that the Tropicalistas strove to thwart by entering the field of women's disorders, long the preserve of midwives and other healers. They collected, recorded, and published their cases, and experimented with the new operations and treatments they read about in European and North American literature, becoming active participants in the creation of knowledge regarding women's disorders, and attempting to redefine childbearing as a medical event. At the same time, as I noted earlier, the Tropicalistas were very much a part of a horizontal shift in Brazil in which the culture of old colonial hierarchies gave way to a more modern, urban-centered, "bourgeois" culture. This shift involved new ideas about women's position in society, about their ideal roles, and about how they should participate in the production of good citizens—all part of the effort to modernize Brazilian society and take control away from older sources of power such as the patriarchal planter family. At a time when the contours of the medical profession were still fluid, the Tropicalistas pushed to enter the area of women's health because they believed that women's primordial roles—procreation and motherhood—were at the center of any endeavor to build a healthy nation, and that the medical profession had the scientific authority to define that endeavor.[2]

The Tropicalistas were not the first Bahian doctors interested in incorporating women patients within the network of medicine. Even before the formation of the group, Bahian doctors wrote many dissertations on women's disorders and continued to do so throughout the Empire years. The Tropicalistas, however, transcended the wholly imitative, moralistic genre of the older medical tradition in Bahia with their factual, positivistic language, which apparently eschewed moral judgments; their pioneering techniques in surgery and labor; their attempts to overcome the traditional ethics of separate gender spheres; and their tentative support of female physicians. Indeed, the Tropicalistas portrayed themselves as the most rational and advanced alternative that women had in Bahia, and contrasted their practice with the ignorance of the midwife.

Nevertheless, the Tropicalistas were not altogether successful in bringing women under their direction. Traditional mores concerning the separation of gender—which men like the Tropicalistas to some degree bought into—proved too strong, and childbearing continued to be viewed as a natural process. Moreover, in Bahia the idea of a lower-class woman, often Afro-Brazilian, in charge of women's health was deeply entrenched and proved difficult to uproot.[3] Thus although the Tropicalistas did much to advance scientific medicine for women in Salvador, they were less successful ideologically—that is, in persuading women to replace their untrained midwives (symbols of backwardness for the Tropicalistas) with the scientifically trained male doctors (symbols of modernity).

Medicine, Boundaries, and Women

The era of the Second Empire (1840–89) marks the transition from colonial to modern Brazil. As capital, immigrants, science, and technology were introduced from Europe, the dominance of the old colonial aristocracy declined and the texture of Brazilian society, particularly urban, became more varied, complex, and "Europeanized." A part of the process of change was the re-creation of ideal gender boundaries through an examination of gender relations and the role of women in the family. Physicians began turning to the study of women's disorders, advising them on some of the most intimate aspects of their lives and counterpoising traditional Catholic views on the education of women. This was not so much because they were interested in the emancipation of women, but because they believed in the advantages to society of well-educated wives and mothers.[4] From the 1850s on, more and more graduating doctors in Bahia chose to write their theses on women's disorders, concentrating on those associated with pregnancy and childbirth. The theses dealt with puerperal fever, chlorosis during pregnancy, syphilis and pregnancy, cesarean sections, techniques to use when dealing with birthing problems, the advantages of bleeding during pregnancy, the use of abortion when the mother's life was endangered, hygiene during pregnancy, and other topics, such as celibacy and infanticide.[5] The majority of the dissertations used European, especially French, medical dissertations as models, citing European cases and European authorities and, although they tell us little about how women actually behaved in Bahia, they do tell us a good deal about the normative standards and stereotypes of an ideal woman and family perpetrated by an influential group of men.[6]

In the dissertations, the physicians held that women were at the mercy of their reproductive cycle.[7] The key female organ was the uterus with its "mysterious secret of procreation."[8] Women who failed to fulfill this natural and sacred mission of reproduction, through choice (such as nuns), the personal misfortune of not finding a husband, or the inability to bear children, were held to be unhealthy and have shorter life spans than wives and mothers. "Many people erroneously consider pregnancy . . . as adverse to the health of women," wrote Frederico Augusto da Silva Lisboa in 1870, "but are not [sexual] abstinence, . . . certain occult acts . . . leading to the weakness of the virgin [and] . . . chastity considerably more harmful?"[9] Indeed, argued Silva Lisboa, young women needed the legitimate sexual relations that marriage offered more urgently than men. Men could turn to the "arms of love" more freely than women, so unmarried women in fact suffered more from unsatisfied sexual desire than men.[10] If a woman's sexual desire was continuously unrelieved, she could be overcome by a "uterine furor" and "in these sad circumstances . . . she forgets all social ethics and attempts to assuage the frenzy of her passion by all means no matter how indecent."[11] Even worse was the case of the nun, a fanatic, disdainful of the dictates of nature, who withdrew into the sterility of a convent, living sourly and egotistically, with a high probability that she would eventually succumb to nervous palpitations, hysterical hypochondria, and even nyphomaniacal furor.[12]

In complete contrast was the woman who as both wife and mother, surrounded by children and loving husband, dispensed gentle warmth and affection. This woman, when she married, entered with her husband into a "partnership and community of interests, as well as an intimate agreement of ideas and feelings."[13] She provided her husband with a refuge from the rigors of the world and also, stated Álvaro Bruno Cavalcanti de

Britto, taught him to become "accustomed to order, work and morality."[14] In order to ensure healthy children, the choice of a marriage partner was crucial: it should be made considering love and also the compatibilities of age, taste, morals, physiology, character, inclination, and the health of both partners. Consanguineous marriages were dangerous to children's health and should be avoided. The best age to get married, taking into consideration the Brazilian climate and average rate of development, was about twenty years old for women and twenty-five for men.[15] Clearly the young doctors were championing the notion of the "hygienic" nuclear family as opposed to the models of "degenerative" families that existed in Brazil.[16] They understood that the successful growth of medical authority lay in expanding into women's territory.[17]

Although the above prescriptions may first appear to be purely derivative of European ones, read in the Brazilian context they were an assault on the existing Brazilian family.[18] To forward-looking contemporary Brazilians, the traditional patriarchal upper-class family was seen as deficient for the purpose of "improving" the race. It was an institution bent more on cementing clan alliances, often through consanguineous marriage, in order to amass wealth and power, than on the production of biologically fit and morally sound Brazilian citizens.[19] In other words, it was an institution concerned with the transmission of precisely those traditional aspects of society being questioned by progressive, urban groups like doctors. Indeed, the manner in which the separation of gender was organized in this family presented grave dangers to a people's vigor, already threatened by tropical climate.[20] On one hand, the absolute authority exercised by the patriarch allowed men to frequent prostitutes, keep mistresses, and, sometimes, to run parallel households. On the other hand, women kept in seclusion, restricted by fathers and brothers, were forced into strategic marriages at too young an age to have healthy children.[21] This pattern of early, loveless marriage followed by men's immoral behavior was believed to lead to the production of dangerously unhealthy Brazilians. "What is certain," affirmed the medical graduate Silva Lisboa in 1870, "is that marriage must not take place too early [in life]. . . . The fruit of such a disastrous union almost always comes into the world as a victim of some terrible disease."[22] Moreover, the lack of a sound moral education, held Aprígio Ramos Proença, "has produced numerous disorders . . . [such as] syphilis, sodomy, onanism . . . which have [in turn] led to an infinite number of diseases rampant among us, [including] the terrible tuberculosis."[23] The disorders com-

mon to the progeny of consanguineous marriages, wrote Guarino Aloysio Ferreira Freire, were "epilepsy, deaf-muteness, idiocy, deformities, and,
often, general paralysis and various degeneracies."[24] The Brazilian patriarchal family, therefore, was not a suitable milieu within which to produce
the healthy and moral citizens a new nation like Brazil required.

At the other end of the class hierarchy, however, the unstructured family
of the populace was also seen as biologically and morally debilitating. The
sociologist Antônio Cândido, echoing the views of nineteenth-century
doctors, notes that "colonial society was divided into two parts, familial
and nonfamilial. . . . The nonfamilial portion consisted of a nameless mass
of the socially degraded. . . . They reproduced themselves haphazardly and
lived without regular norms of conduct."[25] More recently Dain Borges has
provided a more subtle description:

> Bahians had an offhand way of classifying crowds that suggests what
> the word "family" meant to them. Journalists describing a crowd would
> speak of as famílias e o povo. "Families" meant not just any family, but
> rather a properly organized establishment. Outside the "families," the
> rest of the Bahian society was disorganized, anonymous, the "popu-
> lace."[26]

There are several indications that such a "disorganized" family had long
existed in Bahia. In his study of the most serious slave revolt in Salvador
in 1835, the Bahian historian João Reis describes some of the patterns of
family life he discerned for urban slaves, and freedmen and women.[27] Because of the limitations of their freedom the slaves had few opportunities to
establish stable marital relationships; even when they did have long-term
relationships, these were played out in ways that differed markedly from
the model of the European, "hygienic" family.[28] Among the freedmen and
women there was a higher proportion of stable unions, although few legal
ones. Indeed, the norm among lower-class families in Salvador was not to
marry.[29] The unions produced few children. Sometimes, children from a
former union of one of the parents lived with their parent and his or her
new companion. But very often the household was composed of a mother
and her children without the permanent presence of the father.[30] Because of
the spatial relations of residence among different classes and races in Salvador, the lower-class models of unstructured households and families were
very much flaunted in the faces of the upper classes.[31] Until the turn of the
century there were few neighborhoods in Salvador exclusively inhabited

by the upper classes. Victoria and Pilar were two, the former pioneered by foreign merchants in the early nineteenth century. Only at the end of the century did more prosperous Bahian merchants and professionals begin to move out and build themselves palatial homes that advertised their wealth. Thus Salvador was a "residential melting pot" where all classes—rich, poor, free, and freedmen—lived alongside each other, often in the different levels of the same buildings.[32]

It was in opposition to the perceived morally and biologically insalubrious environments of the traditional patriarchal family and the unstructured popular family that the Bahian physicians posited a hygienic family. The context of such a family provided the possibility for the improvement of the Brazilian racial stock. Within its context the virtues of thrift, discipline, cleanliness, and morality could be instilled in the family members and the dangers of illicit and inconstant sexual relations contained. Above all, this sort of family followed the dictums of science and reason. Because the progeny of the hygienic family was seen as crucial, the doctor played an increasingly important role as the guardian of the mother's health, prescribing correct ways of living that would promote her own and her children's health. Indeed, in such a family the tyranny of the patriarch or slave owner, sometimes seconded by that of the priest, was replaced by the physician's guidance, wielded through the authority of science—often no less absolute than that of the patriarch.

The struggle to insert Western medicine into female and family life took place on several fronts. Doctors had to demonstrate to women and patriarchs that traditional ways of coping with the disorders of women, namely through the reliance of largely untrained midwives and healers, was no longer feasible. In other words, doctors had to demonstrate their efficacy in order to overcome competition from deeply entrenched traditional ways in healing, and women's reluctance to be physically examined by a male doctor. They were not altogether successful. In Bahia the modern-oriented, hygienic family remained largely an ideal despite doctors' concerted efforts to draw women into the territory of Western medicine and to extend their medical authority over women.[33]

The Tropicalistas were the Bahian physicians who made the most serious attempts in this direction. Their first battle was to wrest control of the sick woman's situation from female attendants and midwives. They tried to do this by challenging long-standing practices involving women's health and childbearing and counterpoising them with their superior knowledge of the great advances medicine had made over the course of the century, especially in the sphere of women's disorders.

The Tropicalistas' Modernity: Advances in the Treatment of Women's Disorders

Historians have mainly read the *Gazeta Médica da Bahia*, during the Empire years, as a journal of "tropical" medicine and have focused on the doctors' writings dealing with beriberi, filariasis, hookworm, and ainhum. However, an important subtheme of the journal was the story of the Tropicalistas' attempt to bring women in Bahia to accept the authority of scientific medicine, and to eclipse folk healing and the widespread use of officially untrained midwives. European doctors had already entered the realm of women's disorders and Brazilian doctors, the Tropicalistas believed, should follow suit. For the Tropicalistas, concerned as they were about the larger question of the intertwining of medicine and nation, the push into the female sphere was not mere imitation of Europeans but linked to the question of how to promote a fit population. Healing and preventing disease, reversing decline and decay meant combating defective and unsanitary practices—such as those used by ignorant midwives—and replacing them with the newest scientific medical techniques.[34] Women, the fulcrum of healthy reproduction, had to be directed away from the realm of backwardness into that of scientific medicine. In 1872 Silva Lima wrote wistfully of the day when every hospital in Brazil would have a well-attended maternity ward staffed by well-trained obstetricians who would write about the lessons they learned in their clinical practice.[35]

Advances in the treatment of women's disorders and childbirth had been going on apace throughout the nineteenth century in Europe and the United States.[36] Surgical techniques in gynecology were developed early in the nineteenth century and practiced, amid controversy, in both Europe and the United States. Ovariotomy (the extirpation of ovarian tumors or cysts) was first performed by the North American Ephraim McDowell in 1809. Successful surgery for the vesico-vaginal fistula was first performed by Marion Sims in the United States in 1849.[37] The removal of uterine fibroids, or tumors, was performed early in the nineteenth century by vaginal and abdominal hysterectomy in Europe and the United States.[38] Besides making advances in gynecological surgery, doctors began to decipher some of the processes involved in women's reproductive cycle. There was much debate, for example, about whether it was connected to ovulation and a healthy function of the body or whether menstruation was pathological and triggered by nervous excitement.[39] Much of the new knowledge remained shrouded by the attempt to use new discoveries about female biology as evidence for preconceived notions of female inferiority.[40] Nevertheless, Western medicine also made big strides in the case of childbirth and, through the use of better forceps, anesthesia, and antisepsis, made it safer and more comfortable.[41] All of these advances spurred the Tropicalistas to extend their practice into women's health.

Silva Lima called on Brazilian doctors to record and publish their cases on women's disorders in order to build up a body of local knowledge. He speculated that there were numerous techniques and therapies in use in Bahia for women's disorders that failed to become known to other doctors since they were never written about. As he noted, "Ours is a profession built mainly on facts and these, when faithfully recorded, always clarify our practice."[42] In 1868 he welcomed the publication of the first Brazilian book on obstetrics in Rio de Janeiro and also took the opportunity to reprimand local doctors:

> We are used to importing our books, our doctrine, our practice, and even the medical language we use in our professional lives. [These imported medical doctrines] almost dispense us of the trouble of thinking for ourselves . . . and prevent us from . . . contributing one iota to the universal patrimony of science.[43]

Just as the development of a knowledge of tropical medicine would help rescue Brazil from an association with inevitable backwardness, so, he believed, a medical profession fully conversant with the latest methods in women's medicine would be a sign of the nation's progress.

The Tropicalistas themselves practiced what they preached. In the *Gazeta Médica* they reviewed the writings of North American and European doctors in gynecology and obstetrics, and included an updated bibliographical section listing many publications concerning women's disorders. Indeed, they saw their journal as an important means of informing local doctors. In the introduction to an article on the current state of ovariotomy in Europe and the United States, the editor observed:

> What can be found here is a clear exposition on the advantages and disadvantages of [ovariotomy, a discussion] we believe is useful in order to

give the [operation] better exposure, and to inform our colleagues who have not yet had the chance to learn about this procedure.[44]

The Tropicalistas did not stop at reporting. They also pioneered the actual practice of gynecological surgery in Bahia. Such surgery started late in Bahia, retarded by most Bahian doctors' strict adherence to the French Academy of Medicine, which did not moderate its virulent opposition to ovariotomy until the 1860s.[45] By then, the Tropicalistas were already experimenting with the new surgical operations for women's disorders. In 1869, for example, Silva Lima carried out the first operation in Bahia for a vesicovaginal fistula.[46] John Paterson and later Pires Caldas followed his lead. In 1878 Paterson recorded a series of operations he performed for uterine fibroids with the help of Pires Caldas, Silva Lima, and his Anglo-Brazilian colleague Dr. Hall.[47] His were not the first operations on fibroids in that city but were the first to be written up in Salvador. The first ovariotomy performed in the city was carried out in the 1880s by Victorino Pereira. He was followed by Silva Lima and Pires Caldas.[48] Successful surgery moved into obstetrics in the 1880s when a number of cesarean sections were performed, although widespread use of this technique did not occur until after the turn of the century.[49] All of these procedures used by the Tropicalistas, successful or not, were described in detail in the *Gazeta Médica da Bahia,* thus ending the virtual silence in Brazilian medicine on clinical cases.

Like the unraveling of tropical disorders, understanding women's disorders, fertility, pregnancy, and birthing was important to sweep away false preconceptions about the meaning of living in a tropical country. As modern physicians bent on combating obstacles to progress, the Tropicalistas took as firm a stand against uninformed midwifery—which, they held, was rooted in ignorance and superstition, and a shameful sign of the country's backwardness—as they did against the idea of the inevitable backwardness of the tropics.

Tropicalistas and Midwives: Scientific Method or "Brutal Maneuvers"

As noted earlier, the Tropicalistas' greatest rivals in the sphere of women's disorders were female midwives. Known variously as *comadres, curiosas,* or *aparadeiras,* among other terms, midwives in Bahia, as in all of Brazil, were often mulattas or poor white women, who usually dressed in black, covered their heads with mantillas, and carried rosaries.[50] Midwives did more than simply deliver babies. After the birth they continued to visit the mother, giving advice on child care and nutrition for both mother and child. They helped mothers choose wet nurses. They were also healers, often applying their healing herbs and techniques with magic words and prayers, and treating women's "secret" ailments—which some doctors noted were abortions.[51] The exception to this sort of midwife was in Rio de Janeiro where, once the Portuguese court was installed in 1808, it became fashionable for the upper class to be attended by French midwives.[52] Madame Durocher was the most famous of the French midwives and was a member of the Academy of Medicine. These midwives who served in Brazil in the Empire years had mostly received formal training in obstetrics and were aware of the advances in instruments and techniques used by formal medicine. Madame Durocher, for example, wrote several tracts published by the Imperial Academy of Medicine. In Bahia, this sort of midwife was rare. In 1832, in an attempt to attract and train a higher class of woman into the profession, the medical schools created a one-year free course for midwives but the endeavor seems to have failed.[53] In 1871 Professor Elias Pedrosa reported in his "Memória histórica" that the course in obstetrics for women in Salvador was sinking into oblivion. He noted that since its creation, only two women had completed the course; the first had died soon after initiating her practice and the other had never exercised her skill. The failure is easily understandable because in order to be admitted, a woman had to know how to read and write and have "good manners."[54] Pedrosa did not think that the course had much to offer anyway, since the cornerstone of such a course—that is, practice in deliveries—was not offered.[55]

The Tropicalistas had several complaints against midwives. They noted that the women had no adequate training. In 1869 Silva Lima referred deprecatingly to the midwives and healers who "monopolize a good part of the practice of gynecology" and often mistreat their patients with their "brutal maneuvers."[56] In 1876 an editorial in the *Gazeta Médica* lamented that all over Brazil, even in the capital cities, healers and midwives exercised their callings ostentatiously, often employing powerful drugs illegally.[57] In general the Tropicalistas decried the fact that the profession was not strictly regulated by law. As things stood, they pointed out, the women were virtually unaccountable. How could they be tried for their botched actions if such actions were not criminalized? asked the *Gazeta Médica*. In day-to-day practice doctors often came into conflict with midwives. For example, physicians noted that midwives' attendance delayed entry of the doctor into a case jeopardizing the patient. Even when the doctor did enter a case, Silva Lima complained, midwives would not let the physician fully examine the patient, so he had to make do with the midwife's description of the situation in order to make a diagnosis.[58] Even worse, through pure ignorance, the Tropicalistas argued, midwives were often responsible for the spread of infection.

In March 1881 Silva Lima was called to examine a six-day-old infant who had been born easily but had developed a bad case of infection on the back of her head.[59] He treated the baby with a local application of phenic acid and very soon the baby recovered. By questioning the mother, he realized the baby had caught the infection from the attending midwife. On the day of delivery, he learned, the midwife, whom the woman had used before, had delivered the child easily, then bathed and dressed the infant, returning on subsequent days to keep a check on mother and child. The mother had noticed that the midwife's hands and clothes smelled badly, and when she asked the woman why this was so, the midwife explained that on the day of labor, as on all subsequent days, she had come straight from attending a patient suffering from "an ulcerated canker of the uterus." By the 1880s Silva Lima was very aware of the transmission of bacteria and the importance of asepsis. He quickly understood this was a case of infection passed on by the midwife to the infant. He decided to publish the case as a warning to other doctors about the dangers of midwives. Ironically, many contemporary doctors remained unsure of the implications of Pasteurian theories and often posed an even greater danger to their patients because Western medicine tended to be more interventionist with women's disorders than that of midwives.[60]

Not only did doctors blame midwives for the dissemination of disease through negligence, but they also derided midwives' lack of method and contrasted it to the methodicalness of physicians. We see this contrast in a case related by the Tropicalista Pires Caldas, a surgeon at the Santa Casa hospital.[61] In 1866 he was called to the Benedictine infirmary for slaves in Salvador to examine a twenty-five-year-old female slave. Two years before, the woman had had a stillborn baby after a very difficult labor. Ever since, urine leaked from her vagina. One day, suffering from greater discomfort than usual, she had passed a kidney stone and, alarmed, decided to consult a midwife. The midwife examined her internally and yanked at her organs believing she could rid her patient of any further stones but, instead, left her patient wracked by excruciating pains and wholly incontinent.[62] The slave woman despaired of anyone being able to help her, but her owner sent her into the city to consult a doctor. Pires Caldas, aided by Wucherer, found that she not only had a kidney stone but also was suffering from a vesico-vaginal fistula. They decided to treat the kidney stone first and then operate on her. After a discussion of various therapies, they chose one that seemed the most suitable to this case. After two months of treatment, the doctors agreed the woman was ready for the fistula operation. Pires Caldas was assisted in this operation, only the third of its kind performed in Bahia, by Wucherer, Silva Lima, and Paterson, and observed by faculty students. Pires Caldas gave a detailed description of the operation, the position of the patient, the use of the speculum, his method of sutures, making comparisons and comments on similar cases in the existing literature.[63] He documented the case on a day-by-day basis, describing the therapies administered in the postoperative period and the patient's response. By publishing the case, Pires Caldas juxtaposed the bungling ineptitude of the midwife to the theater of scientific endeavor provided by a team of physicians whose members not only discussed the case together, but had access to a whole body of medical literature, as well as to an arsenal of techniques and instruments that they sought to advance further by constructive comments and critiques.

The greatest chagrin for the Tropicalistas was that childbirth, the situation that most often led women to seek medical help, remained largely in the hands of untrained midwives. As normal births in Bahia were still seen as a natural and not a pathological event, doctors mainly attended women in cases of difficult labor and pregnancy-related disorders. They were usually called in after the presiding midwife admitted defeat and, often, once it was too late.[64] For example, in 1887 Deoclesiano Ramos was called to the bedside of a twenty-three-year-old black woman who lived at 44 Rua dos capitaes. She was experiencing severe birthing difficulties.[65] By the time he arrived, labor had been in progress for some forty-eight hours. Despite a smooth start, the fetus had not been expelled and the contractions had ceased. According to Ramos, the attending midwife did not know how to turn the fetus and ease it out and, therefore, had allowed the baby to die. She had then tried unsuccessfully to pull the dead fetus out by the protruding head but managed only to badly lacerate the scalp. Ramos was called only when the mother was close to death. Using forceps, he easily extracted the fetus but only just managed to save the mother's life. She remained in his care for a month, until she was fully recovered. Had he been called in time, Ramos asserted, he could have easily delivered the woman of a healthy child. Childbirth, Ramos seemed to be saying, should be redefined as an area for specialists, not amateurs.

Pacífico Pereira had similar experiences to relate concerning eclampsia during parturition. In 1874 he was called to see F., a robust Creole mother of four, whom he visited at her home on Rua do Bom Gosto.[66] She had had labor pains early the previous morning and by evening her water had broken but still labor had not commenced. Because of the poverty and ignorance of the people tending her, wrote Pereira, she had been left almost two days without adequate medical help. Only when she started to have convulsions had those in attendance become so frightened they had decided to call him. By that time the child was dead, although Pereira was able to revive the mother from her coma. Another of his eclampsia patients was a twenty-five-year-old black woman, S., who lived in Conceição da Praia and was having her first child.[67] After a long and difficult labor with no doctor in attendance, the child was born dead and the mother began to suffer convulsions alternating with states of coma. At this point Pereira was called. By the woman's swollen legs and face, her weak pulse, and the blood issuing from her mouth, he knew she was close to death and that he must take urgent action, but despite his attempts to save her, the patient died three hours later.

In another example that also underscored the ignorance of traditional midwives, Silva Lima told of a case he had in 1867. This concerned a pregnant young slave called Joanna who was many weeks overdue and very sick.[68] Because of her condition, Joanna had come in to the city from Camamu to consult local healers who proved to be of no help. Next she had turned to a Bahian male midwife who had also been unable to help. Finally, in desperation, she had sought out a doctor and ended up in Silva Lima's care. Although he had never seen such a case before, Silva Lima correctly diagnosed an ectopic pregnancy, a diagnosis seconded by Dr. Paterson. Joanna died, but Silva Lima, even though he had never seen such a case before, had the theoretical knowledge that enabled him to make a correct diagnosis. This was in contrast to the empirical knowledge of midwives and healers, who, having never or seldom seen such a case, did not know what they were dealing with.

Indeed, in all of these stories taken from the *Gazeta Médica* the doctors represented the choice of a professional doctor over that of an untrained midwife as one of reason over ignorance, caution over risk. What

Leavitt says about the nineteenth-century American perception of physicians saving women where midwives could not "because the doctors carried an image of expertise and knowledge along with the instruments and drugs in their medical bags" can also be said of Salvador.[69] According to the doctors' accounts, they arrived at their diagnostic and therapeutic decisions through deliberations with a team of doctors, and justified those decisions by appealing to the authority of science. Thus, Pacífico Pereira explained his heavy use of bleeding in the case of one of his eclampsia patients who then died by appealing to the debates in European medical literature and arguing that although he favored the shift in medicine against bleeding, there were some cases in which bleeding was indicated. Indeed, despite the deaths of two women and three babies in six of his birthing cases, Pereira presented these cases in support of "rational therapy." By this he meant deducing the correct medication for each case by relating observed clinical conditions to current debates in the medical literature. Framing his cases in this way made his article "scientific" and connected his discussion to larger debates within medicine.[70]

The Tropicalistas also had assorted drugs and instruments at their disposal. In the cases related above, they used forceps, speculums, and stethoscopes—tools the midwives did not have. Moreover, they not only used copious drugs, but pushed to gain exclusive access to these, lodging complaints with the authorities when they learned of midwives using the drugs.[71] Even though the drugs may not have made Western medicine any safer than traditional medicine, narcotics and anesthesia certainly made childbirth more comfortable and probably helped the doctors win over patients.[72] However, in several ways the contrasting images of doctor and midwife in the case of childbirth was ironic because not only did the doctors' patients die, but as we know today, many of the medications they administered probably did more harm than the midwives' less potent concoctions.

For example, in the cases described above, the doctors administered high dosages of chloral hydrate (a powerful and dangerous sleep-inducing drug), potassium bromide (a habit-forming sedative), ergot (a drug to tighten muscle tissue that when given in large amounts, causes dangerous muscular spasms), quinine, calomel (mercury), morphine, and ammonia, among other medications. In the case of S. related above, Pereira not only prescribed most of these medications together but he also bled his patient of five hundred grams of blood, explaining that he did so in order to stem an

imminent pulmonary or cerebral "congestion."[73] In the case of the overdue young slave, Joanna, suffering from an ectopic pregñancy, Silva Lima
decided, after several futile attempts to induce expulsion of the fetus with
hot poultices and castor oil, to operate on the woman with a team of his
colleagues. The patient was anesthetized with chloroform. No antiseptic
or aseptic precautions were taken, which is understandable given the date
(1867). As suspected, a fully developed dead fetus was extracted. After the
operation, the patient's wound festered badly. Her postoperative treatment
included castor oil, enemas, chlorine injections, soothing lotions, calomel,
opium, and belladonna (used to relax spasms, quicken heartbeat, and as a
purge). The patient also had poultices with laudanum applied to her wound
and was bled by leeches. She survived the operation by three weeks and
then died. When her autopsy was carried out, she was found to be riddled
with gangrene. Clearly, in the case of childbirth, medical science in Bahia
was less efficient than the image it projected.

Tropicalista contempt for midwives was not primarily because they believed women should not be allowed into the territory of healing. It had
more to do with the challenge that an area of healing outside the boundaries of formal medicine posed for these doctors. The Tropicalistas did not
deny that women had a role to play in certain areas of healing but believed
that they should be trained according to the canon of Western medicine in
order to perform this role adequately. When women like the French midwife Madame Durocher conformed to these rules, the men were willing
to accept and even praise their expertise. As long as women were not scientifically trained, the Tropicalistas rallied against them. The conflict between the Tropicalistas and the midwife can be seen, then, as a conflict
between a modern form of professional authority, largely a male preserve,
termed "scientific," and a traditional domain, largely controlled by lower-
class women, termed "ignorant."

Resisting the Tropicalista Embrace

For the Tropicalistas, the objective of a professionalized medicine implied
their hegemony in all realms of healing, including that of women's disorders. However, the extent to which they were successful in dislodging
the midwife and converting women into patients remained limited. This
becomes clear from the doctors' reports in this period on the prevalence of
midwives.[74] In the United States the shift away from midwives had started

as early as the eighteenth century, when upper-class women in Boston, Philadelphia, and New York began to accept the view that pregnancy and childbirth were medical problems to be dealt with by physicians. This view gained broader acceptance in the nineteenth century, when the traditional idea of childbirth as something that should take place in the community of other women vied with the new "scientific" notion of childbirth as a private event in which the kernel relationship became that between the woman and her physician. Once the importance of this relationship was recognized, and as anesthesia, asepsis, and surgery became more complex, so the woman patient was more and more extricated from her home milieu and placed under the increasing control of the physician—ultimately, as Leavitt has put it, "drugged and 'alone among strangers' in an impersonal hospital."[75] In Salvador, this shift—despite the Tropicalistas' efforts—was slow, and even well into the twentieth century the midwife remained an important figure in charge of normal childbirth and women's disorders.[76] Given the strong impetus from the Tropicalistas to draw in women as patients, why were they not more successful?

The first reason concerns the very weak tradition of Western medicine in Bahian, and indeed Brazilian, society.[77] During the colonial period, few Coimbra-trained physicians chose to serve in Brazil and, despite attempts by the Crown to exercise some sort of regulation on healing, the blend of several rich traditions in healing was hegemonic in Brazil and accepted and used by all classes.[78] Even where European-trained doctors were found, they shared business with barber surgeons, folk healers, and members of the religious orders. Moreover, the plantation, Brazil's formative institution, reinforced the use of a blend of African, Indian, and European folk healing, with occasional use of Western medicine.[79] Thus, unlike in Portugal and some areas in Spanish America, folk medicine in Brazil had never had to contend with an unrelenting barrage of criticism stemming from a jealous official medicine. This made it all the harder for Western-trained doctors to gain mainstream acceptance in a society where a simple dichotomy between Western and alternate healing was not common currency.[80]

A second factor that mitigated against the Tropicalistas' greater success was that most Brazilian doctors were very poorly trained in obstetrics and gynecology. Thus, in a way, the fact that women did not frequent doctors more can be seen as a very rational decision. This situation contrasted with that in the United States, where in the late–eighteenth and early–nineteenth centuries the appeal to discard tradition in women's medicine was strong because the formal teaching of physicians had provided them with a better understanding of female anatomy, making birthing with doctors safer than with traditional midwives.[81] In Bahia, for much of the nineteenth century, the only formal training in obstetrics, apart from a moribund course in midwifery, was a year-long course offered to male medical students. Until 1882 this course brought together a study of childbirth and the study of the disorders of pregnant women and infants. In that year two chairs were created: one in the disorders of infants and children, although no one was appointed to the chair until 1888, and another in obstetrics, to be complemented by a practical clinic in gynecology and obstetrics. However, no one was nominated to run the latter until 1886, and the Tropicalista Barão de Itapoan despaired that the medical school would ever introduce "demonstrative midwifery" so that young doctors could enter their professional lives at least having witnessed a delivery.[82] Thus, even though the Tropicalistas themselves claimed to be knowledgeable and successful in the treatment of women's disorders, it was difficult to overcome a general perception of the ineptitude of medicine in the area of women's disorders, a fact that worried some doctors at the medical school.[83]

A third factor working against the wider acceptance of physicians in women's disorders was that most women of all classes in Bahia, as in Brazil as a whole, were illiterate and thus had no knowledge of the changes taking place in women's health care. There was, therefore, no pressure from a well-informed group of women to introduce better birthing techniques as happened in the United States.[84] In her history of childbearing in North America, Leavitt argues that urban, privileged women were initially instrumental in bringing the male physician into the birthing process as they recognized that scientific medicine "held out promises for increased safety."[85] In Salvador the process was different. Literacy for the whole of Brazil remained low in the nineteenth century. The 1872 census noted Brazil's population as slightly more than 10 million, of which approximately 1 million men and half a million women were literate.[86] As June Hahner has noted, being literate provides for more than a technical skill. Rather, it makes possible exposure to ideas beyond the confines of an individual's world and enables a person to make choices and consider change. The lack of women's education, therefore, precluded pressures from women for change in the delivery of health care. Moreover, even when some people pushed to educate women in nineteenth-century Brazil, the content of education for women left much to be desired. The authorities viewed schools as places

to ensure that women might become better mothers and wives, not independent, critical, and self-assertive.[87] A handful of male physicians in
Bahia, particularly the Tropicalistas, moved to get innovative approaches
to women's health accepted. Women preferred the traditional midwife.

Women's preference was probably also related to the fact that given the
society's normative gender relations, fears about life cycles, problems and
questions about sexual relations and menstrual flows, unwanted pregnan-
cies, and abortions pertained to a woman's world and were not spoken
about with men. Even if some doctors were beginning to argue that they
too should be made the recipients of such confidences, it was not quite clear
that the men would respect the inviolability of the disclosures. One graduating doctor, Serafim Vieira de Almeida, who raised the issue of medical ethics, seemed to understand women's need for midwives, even if he
saw them as backward.[88] What should a doctor do, he asked, in the case
of a woman whose problem was a failed abortion attempt? The patient,
he noted, would have had accomplices who, by law, should be punished.
Many doctors would not hesitate to report such an incident to the authorities. However, reasoned Vieira de Almeida, it was not at all clear that
that was the right thing to do. A doctor should also consider his client's
reputation and her right to keep her secret. Sometimes, he stated, doctors
should even be prepared to provide an abortion. Doctors, it appeared, were
divided on how to behave in the face of abortion. Midwives were more
reliable.

A fourth factor impeding the acceptance of male physicians into the
sphere of female disorders in Salvador concerned women's reluctance to
be physically examined by, and reveal their genitals to, male doctors. This
situation was by no means peculiar to Bahia.[89] It has been well documented
in North American and European literature regarding the history of the
shift from female midwifery and the home to male physician and hospital.[90] But the pressures to adhere to tradition were particularly strong in
Bahia, a city less exposed than European and North American cities to
the forces of industrialization and urbanization. In Bahia, the seclusion of
upper-class women in their homes—a fact often remarked on in wonder by
foreign travelers, and bound up with the honor of the family—continued
until the turn of the century.[91] As the codes of behavior for women eased
in response to pressures from industrial capitalism for more active female
consumers and workers, so the strict seclusion of women came to be seen
as eccentric.[92] However, the separation of the spheres of gender in middle-

and upper-class families remained a centerpiece of Brazilian society until well into the twentieth century.

According to sociologist Emilio Willems, this fact followed from the asymmetrical roles ascribed to males and females in the family—an ascription he states can be traced back to previous centuries and remained remarkably resistant to change.[93] He argues that the female role centered around a cluster of values characterized as "virginity complex," which entailed a virtual separation of the sexes, chaperonage, and family-controlled courtship, before marriage, and a close tutelage by a jealous husband after marriage. Antithetical values were involved in the male "virility complex," whereby young men were expected to become actively interested in sex at puberty, to view frequent sexual intercourse as healthy and an essential attribute of their manhood, and to see marriage as in no way restrictive of their sexual activities and erotic adventures. Verena Martinez Alier has noted in her study of marriage and elopement in nineteenth-century Cuba that adherence to these kinds of social mores, with their strictly demarcated gender spheres, became even more complex in a slave society where, by definition, slaves had no honor.[94] According to her findings, in an attempt to differentiate itself from the slave community, the free mulatto community adopted the white codes of honor. From the evidence in the medical cases in my study, in which lower-class women showed great reluctance to expose themselves in front of male doctors, a similar situation existed in Salvador. Thus women of all classes felt that an examination of their genitals by a male doctor was an affront to their female modesty.

In 1877 twenty-two-year-old Maria Felippa de Conceição, a mulatta, married and bearing a second child with considerable difficulties, turned to several forms of futile "superstitious" healing and resisted calling a doctor because she was "constrained by her sense of chastity."[95] Only after six months of suffering, noted Dr. Aquello Leite, and when she lay at death's door, did her "instinct for preservation come over her" and she called in the doctor. Silva Lima came across the same problem with the mother who called him to attend to her infant suffering from an infection contracted from a midwife.[96] The woman told him she was suffering from the same problem as her baby, but when Silva Lima asked to examine her, she refused to allow him to do so.

If this attitude on the part of female patients interfered with the doctors' work, the physicians in Bahia understood the reticence and did not condemn it, for it was bound up with their own notion of a respectable woman. The doctors themselves identified with the cultural norms that made male and female spheres divergent from each other. Thus, it was not always the women who refused to be intimately examined. In 1879 Silva Lima told of a sixteen-year-old light mulatta who came to see him, complaining that her menstruation had stopped and that she was feeling sick.[97] Because he assumed she was a virgin, he examined her without giving her a vaginal examination. Only when it became clear to him that her problem was in fact pregnancy did he carry out a vaginal examination. In another case, Silva Lima attended a thirty-year-old Creole woman suffering from an intrapelvic abscess. He examined her and found she had a tumor; he explained that he had examined her by feeling her stomach and rectally but "as she was a virgin I did not attempt a vaginal exploration."[98] The physicians' scientific pursuit in the case of women's disorders was deflected not simply because women's ethical mores resisted it, but because the doctors, in part, accepted that resistance as valid. It is precisely in this area that the Tropicalistas showed they held attitudes concerning women remarkably similar to those recorded in the theses written by medical graduates—theses the Tropicalistas criticized because they confused morals with positive medical facts.[99]

A most instructive story in which we can observe the Tropicalista concern with the moral life of women is Silva Lima's case of the pregnant young woman who came to see him insisting she was a virgin.[100] Silva Lima recognized that his patient was a "decent" young woman: she was light brown in color, well constituted, with a wholesome appearance. She was poor but respectable and had a job as a seamstress. She lived with her family, and her mother had been concerned enough about her to bring her to the doctor. Silva Lima could see that although his patient had shown a momentary weakness, she identified with the "correct" canons on the sexuality of women and had a sense of modesty. Thus Silva Lima noted, when "I asked if she had partaken in lascivious acts with some man, she hesitated for a few moments before answering, and then, after a short silence, she lowered her eyes and said 'yes'."[101] She also presented him with extenuating circumstances: she explained that her boyfriend had promised to marry her and that they had engaged in "lascivious acts" only a few times. Moreover, these had always taken place standing up and fast for fear of being discovered by a member of her family. Upon inquiring about her boyfriend, Silva Lima learned he was an adult, of regular constitution, and single—all of which made him a good candidate for marriage. Silva Lima advised his patient that in order to rectify the mistake she had made, she should tell her family the truth and marry the young man. He was happy to report that the young woman had followed his counsel and that she later gave birth to a healthy child.[102]

Upon a first reading of this case, it is puzzling why Silva Lima should have bothered to publish it, for it seems full of trivial detail and was devoid of any medical or technical breakthroughs. Even more perplexing was that he should have included it in the prominent "Introduction" of the *Gazeta Médica,* a section usually reserved for a pressing issue. However, if we place the article within a broader context of the role of the physician in modern Bahian society, we can see that Silva Lima's message was that guiding patients in their lives was well within the boundaries of the physician's task—it was, in fact, an integral part of his job. Seen from this perspective, it becomes clear that the case was about the doctor's civilizing mission among the lower classes. In a society where the improvement of the race, and the "taming" of the restive lower classes into becoming orderly citizens, was an ever-present concern, Silva Lima was asserting that doctors in Brazil should be preoccupied with the "decency" of the popular class, and give guidance about the restrictions of place and the establishment of boundaries. The irony of Silva Lima's position was that the very principles he underscored as desirable for female conduct—modesty, delicacy, decorum—were also the ones that prevented male doctors from expanding their influence into the territory of female healing.

A final factor to consider in ascertaining the barriers to the Tropicalistas' influence over women concerns the affordability of Western medical treatment for the majority of Bahians. Was it in fact within reach for the popular classes? In his work on the family in Bahia, Borges argues that physicians attended the upper class directly, "through private visits," and attended the lower classes indirectly, "through appeals to the government for action" on hygiene and sanitation in the city.[103] However, the evidence from the Tropicalista medical cases indicates that they tended to all classes and, moreover, that they had vested interests in the poor as patients. Not only did attending such patients help them portray an image of the physician as a person with a keen sense of social responsibility, but the poor also provided the means to experiment with new techniques and therapies, as well as a population to use in the training of medical students. In 1881, for example, the *Gazeta Médica* noted enviously that a general polyclinic had recently been started in Rio de Janeiro.[104] The *Gazeta* stated that not only would such an institution provide organized medical charity to many needy people who at present relied on the personal charity of doctors, but it would also be a most fruitful place to train medical students. In 1876 the Barão de Itapoan was very disappointed when the promised birthing infirmary in the Santa Casa hospital, to which he had offered to render his services for free, failed to be set up. He had hoped that a large number of poor women would have access to superior treatment and that the infirmary would provide much-needed practical teaching for medical students.[105]

The mixture of self-interest and altruism was very evident in the case of female patients. The Tropicalistas tended to poor women in the charity infirmaries of the Santa Casa, they visited the poor in their own homes, and they even put them up in private infirmaries when necessary.[106] In 1859 Silva Lima became extremely interested in the case of Angelica, an African woman whom he suspected of having an advanced extrauterine pregnancy. Not only did he ask three of his colleagues to help him with the case, but he also placed her in a private infirmary. He noted:

> [My colleagues] advised me to closely observe the case and to place the patient in conditions where we could provide the professional services she might need. . . . That was why we placed her in an infirmary [*casa de saúde*], under the immediate vigilance of the director, who [had instructions] to inform me of any development which might require special attention.[107]

Even though the outcome of the case revealed that Silva Lima and his colleagues had made a mistaken diagnoses, Silva Lima decided to publish it because, as he put it, "I found this case to be . . . one of the most useful lessons that [clinical] practice has provided for me."[108] Clearly Silva Lima believed that whatever time and money had been spent on this poor patient had been well worth the learning experience. Indeed, it is no coincidence that there were more cases of lower-class female patients recorded in the *Gazeta Médica* than of upper- and middle-class women.[109] This does not necessarily prove that they treated more poor than rich but it does show that the cases that most interested the Tropicalistas, and which they found most worthy of reporting in a medical journal designed to professionalize medicine, were those dealing with the poor.

In Salvador, the gradual acceptance of the physician into well-off families to tend to the women was the result of the groundwork laid, to a large extent, by the Tropicalistas, often using the poorest patients. In this period, when the Tropicalistas were trying to extend their influence over women as patients, it cannot, therefore, be argued that affordability acted as a significant brake on the doctors' influence. What prevented physicians from making more formidable inroads with female patients had more to do with women's greater familiarity and trust of midwives than of male doctors. One solution to this problem was accepting the idea of women becoming doctors.

Despite an initial distrust, the Tropicalistas came to support the idea of women physicians for two reasons. One was that the tension created between advanced medical science and social mores between the sexes could be smoothed over by women doctors. That is, their gender allowed them to exercise the techniques of modern medical science without hurting their female patients' sensibilities. The second was that in more advanced countries, women were becoming doctors (often after a bitter struggle), and progressive doctors, like the Tropicalistas, came to see the existence of female doctors as yet another sign of Brazil's progress.[110]

The Carvalho educational reforms of 1879 allowed women to enter medical schools in Brazil.[111] The first woman to become a physician in Brazil was Rita Lobato, who graduated from medical school in Bahia in 1887.[112] She was a native of Rio Grande do Sul who had begun her studies at the Rio de Janeiro medical school but moved to Bahia for personal reasons. Between 1887 and 1900 another five women became doctors in Bahia, four of them native Bahians. The number of women physicians was small because the idea of "respectable" women earning their living came late in Brazil. Lobato's entry into the Bahian school caused a debate in Salvador about whether women's physical constitution, especially regarding brain size, might not be an obstacle to female intellectual prowess, and whether an upper-class woman's free perambulation in the streets would bring her purity into question.[113]

Rita Lobato was undoubtedly a pioneer in taking the earliest steps toward women's professional emancipation in Brazil. The travelers' stories we have about women managing their plantations and businesses are exceptional and nearly always refer to widows.[114] Poor women had, of course, always worked. Whether slaves, freedwomen, or free women, they served as domestic servants, laundresses, seamstresses, street-food vendors, nursemaids, ladies-in-waiting, and prostitutes. In the rural areas they also worked in agriculture.[115] The immediate obstacle to middle- and upper-

class women entering professions was their lack of access to a good education. The best schools, state or Catholic, were reserved for boys. Upper-
class girls who were educated received their instruction either at home with
a governess or at a Catholic school that emphasized the importance of
being good wives and mothers. State schools for women catered mainly to
poor girls, often orphans, whom the state wanted to get off its hands by
making sure that they were taught some sort of skill.[116]

In the second half of the nineteenth century women slowly began to
enter the ranks of teachers at elementary school, the role of teacher being
accepted as an extension of the nurturing role of a mother. It took longer
for women to enter into advanced education; the medical schools were
the first advanced schools to open their doors to women. In spite of a
few courageous women who demanded that Brazilian women be properly
educated, the 1879 educational reform allowing women into higher education, including medical schools, was not the result of a woman's movement
lobbying for change.[117] Rather, it was passed by men who made connections between the progress of the nation, the education of women, and the
modernization of motherhood, and who wanted to emulate the advanced
Western nations. The comment made by Joaquim Monteiro Caminhoá, the
medical professor who wrote the 1874 "Memória histórica" for the Rio de
Janeiro medical school, is a good illustration of this sort of thinking. After
noting that there were many worthy women doctors in the United States
and some in Switzerland, England, Scotland, and France, he went on to call
for immediate legislation in favor of training women doctors in Brazil. "It
is better to be in the vanguard of civilization," he wrote, "than to be pushed
by its waves. In the first case, there is awareness of the fact [of change], and
there is true progress; in the second, [change] acts on inert matter, which
does no more than react to an ousting force." [118]

Many men believed that, like the teacher, the female doctor had essential
nurturing qualities and natural kindness and tact, which many male doctors lacked. Furthermore, the question of moral ethics and women's modesty became almost redundant when women attended women. The areas of
study that women focused on were those that male doctors believed were
better suited to women. It is no coincidence that for their graduating dissertations, all the women wrote on obstetrical problems, except for one
who wrote on infant feeding.[119] Rita Lobato wanted to become a surgeon
but her adviser dissuaded her from doing so, whereupon she concentrated
on obstetrics.[120] Women were allowed into the medical profession but not

as equals; rather, they were allowed into a restricted area of medicine that male physicians found difficult to fully enter because of ingrained tradition.

How far did the Tropicalistas accept the idea of women as physicians? The evidence points to ambivalence and an evolution in their thinking. In 1868 the *Gazeta Médica* reproduced an article from a Portuguese journal about the horror of women becoming doctors and carrying out autopsies, and being called out late at night to attend to patients.[121] Women "were created to be wives and mothers. . . . Let her be instructed and educated in the most honorable functions of a good mother, an honest wife, and of an informed tutor. . . . [But] let us remember that women can be almost anything rather than doctors. If this is how she is emancipated, she will only fall."[122] A few years later, there was a report in the journal on the increase in numbers of women doctors in Zurich.[123] The tone was complimentary to the women, in particular for their good judgment in certain "delicate" situations so that embarrassments were avoided. In 1876 the *Gazeta Médica* seemed to further endorse such a view by publishing the graduation speech by Antônio Januário de Faria, director of the medical school and an early associate of the Tropicalistas, who listed what he believed were the great social questions of the day, among them the "elevation" of women in society.[124] Pacífico Pereira was more specific about one way of "elevating" women. He was particularly concerned with girls' physical development. He stressed that gymnastics were as important for them as for boys because exercise "prepares the young girl for her future role of motherhood, protecting her from the ill health that comes from a sedentary life."[125]

However, when the 1879 far-reaching educational reform allowed women to seek a university degree in Brazil, the *Gazeta Médica* was silent on that aspect of the reform—although it had a good deal to say about *ensino livre* (free teaching), another point in the new law.[126] The Tropicalistas' position was like that of José Alves de Mello, a professor at the medical school, who noted that the most important aspect of the 1879 reform was the question of ensino livre, which he worried about. Otherwise, he said, the reform contained many laudable points. He listed some of the latter, including the admission of women as just one more item alongside such seemingly noncontroversial changes concerning the creation of new chairs, making final examinations more exacting, and raising the standards of entry requirements.[127] Like Alves de Mello, the Tropicalistas seemed far more concerned with what they saw as lowering the standards of teaching than with women joining their ranks. The silence may have been because the Tropicalistas agreed with Alves de Mello, who saw the idea of educated women as uncontroversial and as an inevitable part of a grand sweep of changes "placing [Brazil] in the position of being able to accompany the progress of the era in which we live." Moreover, they must have known that it was likely that the number of women entering the schools would be too small to constitute a threat to male doctors.[128]

The evolution in Tropicalista thinking regarding women as professionals accompanied that of the intelligentsia more generally. From midcentury on, as the imprint of urban society became stronger and Brazilian society more complex, as the ranks of European immigration swelled and well-off Brazilians traveled abroad, read imported literature, and joined movements of abolition and reform, so material progress became associated, inevitably, with the opening up of new spaces for women in the society. The Tropicalistas, at the center of some of the key urban changes in nineteenth-century Brazil, slowly became inured to the shock of women's new roles, and even came to embrace the new female liberty.[129] Indeed, some of Rita Lobato's closest supporters in Salvador were Tropicalistas.[130] The Tropicalista support for women in higher education was not unlike that of the Recife positivist Tobias Barreto, who, in 1879, as a deputy of the Provincial Assembly in Pernambuco, argued forcefully in favor of women being allowed to participate in higher education. He saw the degree to which the Brazilian state held women back as a measure of Brazil's backwardness, the degree to which the state provided increasing opportunities as a measure of its advance.[131] Such views were simply reflections of the European debate over the education of women.

The definitions about the sorts of behavior expected from scientifically educated women was, again, similar to current European ideas. Thus, when Rita Lobato went to Bahia, she was particularly warmly received by the Tropicalistas Antônio Pacífico Pereira and the Barão de Itapoan, a reception made easy because of her understanding of the rules of decorum and the code of medical ethics for women, which still assigned "proper places" to women regardless of how far they might venture up the professional ladder.[132] She attended lectures accompanied by her father. She always dressed appropriately in dark, sober colors and limited her social life to members of her family and *gaúcho* friends known from her youth. One of the few exceptions to this was her attendance at the gatherings at Pereira's house, where she was taken in by his family and became a good friend of his wife. She did, for a moment, stray off the correct path by declaring she wanted to be a surgeon. However, she soon realized that this was not a wise choice and decided to specialize in obstetrics, one of the few areas of medicine deemed suitable to her gender.[133]

The Tropicalistas would, no doubt, have agreed with the woman's journal *A Mulher*, which in 1881 argued in favor of women entering medicine, because, in the paraphrasing of one historian, "gentle female doctors would inspire the necessary confidence in women patients who in Brazil were often reluctant to bare their bodies and their ills to male doctors."[134]

Conclusion

The Tropicalistas' interest in women's disorders must be understood within the context of their search for modernity and their desire to define Brazil as progressive. For the doctors, a modern medical corps had to strive vigorously to incorporate women within the sphere of officially accredited medicine and to combat the ignorance of charlatans, folk healers, and midwives. This is what the Tropicalistas worked for in Brazil. They saw the triumph of obstetrics and gynecology as important a sign of advancement as successfully unraveling the mysteries of tropical disorders. The management of women's fertility and health in the tropics was another means of neutralizing the dread of the tropics. Alternately, they viewed old-fashioned midwifery, with its stagnant, unchanging knowledge and its grip on Bahian women, as a metaphor of backwardness. They wanted to substitute such backwardness with their progressive and scientific enlightenment, an enlightenment that would entitle them not only to perform therapeutic and surgical interventions on the female body, but also to prescribe on all aspects of a woman's life.

The Tropicalistas' modernizing quest brought them into collision with untrained midwives who had long dominated the sphere of women's disorders and particularly birthing. Their struggle for control within this sphere, however, was not altogether successful. This can be attributed to the very poor training of young doctors in obstetrics, from whom women, wisely, kept away. There was little demand in Salvador, other than from a few doctors like the Tropicalistas, to improve the situation. Bahian women who stood to gain the most from improvements in obstetrics and gynecology did not know about the ongoing advances and thus never called for their implementation. Moreover, traditional mores regarding the separation of male and female in Bahia reinforced the popular practice of women seeking health care from women.

The Tropicalistas' activist endeavor to contribute to the knowledge about women's disorders represented a break with the passive Bahian approach to women's medical ailments. The Tropicalistas not only recorded, described, and published their cases with women, but they also performed operations that had never before been carried out in Bahia. In writing about their cases, they seldom used the prescriptive, moralistic language typical in Bahian medical writings on women. However, upon closer analysis of the cases they relate, it also becomes clear that although the Tropicalistas shed normative language, they retained many older ideas concerning women, ideas reinforced by unfolding European thinking on gender difference and the correct roles for women in a "civilized" nation. These notions were imported intact into Brazil and adhered to as much by the Tropicalistas as by other Brazilian doctors. This aspect of the Tropicalistas contrasts strongly with their refusal to accept, undiluted, European racial and climatological theories regarding medicine in the tropics. In the latter instance there was an obvious conflict between using science to further progress and, at the same time, being told by that very science that a nation like Brazil simply did not qualify for advanced civilization. The acceptance of such theories intact invalidated the enterprise of the Brazilian nation, that of the doctors' task in the tropics, and, on a more personal level, the civilized nature of the doctors themselves, many of them mulattoes and all of them denizens of the tropics. In order to break out of this deterministic trap presented to them by European scientific ideas, it was imperative that the Brazilian intelligentsia change these ideas. Doctors like the Tropicalistas made important contributions to enable Brazilians to arrive at a more hopeful concept of the nation.

By contrast, the Tropicalistas found European ideas on gender difference and the position of women in civilized nations relatively unproblematic. In fact, emerging ideas about the roles of women within the family, as well as new gender demarcations in a civilized, progressive nation, fit in well with the Tropicalista attempt to retain a malleable or "soft" hereditarian tradition within the damning context of hybridization in the tropics. They also served to establish new models of social control over women and their families in a society undergoing rapid urbanization and immense social change. European ideas about the roles of women and the relationship between women and doctors were retained intact by the Tropicalistas not because the doctors were purely imitative and unoriginal, but because these models suited them very well ideologically. Ultimately, both the notions about the improvement of the racial stock and the changing roles of women were parts of a larger canvas of images with which the Brazilian intelligentsia sought to portray Brazil's modernity.

CHAPTER FIVE

Moving into Mainstream

In the 1860s the Tropicalistas had been marginal men in several ways. The leaders of the Tropicalistas and many of their original followers had been outside the medical establishment in Bahia. The founders of the movement were foreigners and their early supporters associated with "foreign" ideas. Moreover, the group was geographically marginal within Brazil, developing, as it did, in Salvador rather than the more important city of Rio de Janeiro. Furthermore, many of the early Tropicalistas did not belong to traditional powerful families, but came from the ranks of the sons of immigrants and mulattoes seeking a way up in society.[1] Some, like the Pereira brothers, were still students and had not even set out on their lifelong careers. All of these factors reduced the men's impact as they assaulted the accepted paradigm that medical progress in Brazil should be measured by how closely Brazil followed medical practices in the leading European countries, especially France. It is ironic that these foreign-born doctors championed a Brazilian-oriented medicine whereas native doctors looked to Europe. But this irony runs through the history of Brazil and all of Latin America. It is something that the Tropicalistas were well aware of and often commented on.[2]

By the 1880s the Tropicalistas had become part of the mainstream. Their medical ideas had been endorsed. Their teachings had entered the medical school curriculum. Their ideas on how medical education should be organized had been accepted. And their demands for a focus on disorders common in Brazil, especially regional disorders, had been recognized. Indeed, by the fall of the Empire, the Tropicalistas had replaced their role of gadfly with one of accommodation.

Whereas in the early days their role of outside critics had promised the most in terms of recognition, prestige, and influence, by the 1880s accommodation and identification with the Bahian medical establishment was granting them most of these rewards.[3] It was not that the Tropicalistas were simply co-opted. Rather, when they had emerged as a critical force in the 1860s, they stood very much to the left of the political spectrum, particularly because they couched their criticism of medical practices in Bahia and Brazil within a broader criticism of a backward, "unscientific" social system generated by harmful governmental practices and neglect. But in the ensuing decades much of the political spectrum of Brazil shifted and what had been most radical about the Tropicalistas in the 1860s now seemed like common sense. Thus the Tropicalistas remained faithful to their original ideas but the political and social environment evolved around them. This was especially true in the urban settings and, in Bahia, even more so in the medical school and establishment. Thus, by the 1880s the Tropicalistas found a great deal with which to sympathize in the Bahian medical establishment. As the central government attempted to end what little autonomy the Bahian medical school had—an autonomy the Tropicalistas believed was a prerequisite to successful medical science—the Tropicalistas threw themselves wholeheartedly into the fray, supporting their local colleagues' struggle. The aims of the Tropicalistas and those of the local medical establishment had converged and so the separate identity of the movement was lost.

Through their defense of the medical school, the Tropicalistas were swept into the great political debates of the Empire's final decade, such as those concerning educational reform and provincial autonomy.[4] And as they mainstreamed, so their early creativity, such as when they made important contributions to parasitology, discovered a beriberi "epidemic" in their midst, and dared to speculate on Darwin's theories of evolution, all retreated into the past.[5] However, as I have tried to show throughout this book, although the Tropicalistas portrayed themselves as a group "above" politics, their agenda was always political.

Medical School and Tropicalistas

Although the Tropicalistas faced initial opposition at the medical school of Bahia, on the whole, and seen over several decades, the process of their acceptance went fairly smoothly. At first the very extramural quality of the group was viewed with distrust by nearly all of the school faculty. More-over, their assault on established theories of disease, and their preference for the new medicine emerging in Germany as opposed to France, was dis-turbing. Added to this was their critique of established topics and meth-ods of teaching in the school, all of which threatened to undermine en-trenched interests.[6] However, several factors helped the Tropicalistas. First, from 1871 to the fall of the Empire in 1889, the majority of the Bahian medi-cal school directors were sympathetic to the group. Second, in the 1870s, young Tropicalista followers began to enter the ranks of the faculty and to insert their ideas into the heart of the institution. Thus, the key decade for the acceptance of their ideas in the school took place in the 1870s. Third, in the increasingly bitter struggle between the Bahian medical school and the imperial government, the well-organized and internationally legitimated Tropicalistas became important allies of the school. And, finally, by the late 1870s and 1880s, what had been the novel ideas of the Tropicalistas in the early period had become the accepted ideas of the medical establishment. Thus, while Tropicalista ideas were being taken into the school through their disciples, the Tropicalista approach to medical practice was being re-inforced by the innovative trends in European medicine. At the same time, Tropicalista ideas meshed well with those of other rising urban groups who posed new political challenges for the Empire.

The Tropicalistas were fortunate that most of the school's directors after 1871 were sympathetic to them.[7] In 1871 João Baptista dos Anjos, director of the medical school in Bahia since 1857, died.[8] He had joined the fac-ulty as an adjunct in 1826 and by the time of his death had become an eminent figure of the Bahian medical establishment, representative of an early generation of Brazilian physicians who wished to Europeanize Bra-zilian medicine by replicating European, particularly French, medical insti-tutions in their own country. Thus, while he was in control, little headway could be made either in introducing new concepts of teaching, especially those coming from Germany, or in raising questions about the univer-sality or specificity of the disorders of Brazil. He was succeeded by Vicente Ferreira de Magalhães, who also belonged to the older generation of doc-tors, trained at Coimbra, and was professor at Bahia for forty years, but was sympathetic to the Tropicalistas.[9] Magalhães contributed several articles to the *Gazeta Médica* in its early years, and joined several core Tropicalistas to help found the Doctors' and Pharmacists' Mutual Aid Society in 1867.[10] He was elected president of the latter organization, serving with Almeida

Couto, Pacífico Pereira, Silva Lima (all core Tropicalistas), Goes Siqueira, and the pharmacist, Euclides E. Pires Caldas (early supporters).[11] Magalhães, in fact, was the first faculty member to praise the *Gazeta Médica* in an official document, citing admiringly several articles on physics, a subject he taught, that had appeared in the *Gazeta Médica*.[12] It was probably no coincidence that during his tenure the younger Tropicalistas began joining the faculty as adjuncts.

In 1874 the Tropicalistas gained an even stronger ally with the appointment of Antônio Januário de Faria as director of the medical school.[13] Faria was the first medical graduate from the Bahian medical school (1845) to become its director and remained in the post until 1881. As such, he represented a transition generation from the early European-trained physicians to home-trained doctors, some of whom were influenced by the Tropicalistas' emphasis on the development of a national agenda in medical inquiry.[14] He was primarily interested in French medicine, thus remaining true to the older generation, but Faria also wanted to open up new directions of medicine. Thus, he attended the meetings at Paterson's house in the mid-1860s and was one of the initial founders and editors of the *Gazeta Médica*. An early, albeit scant contributor to the journal, he participated in the Bahian debate on beriberi, a subject close to the Tropicalistas' heart.[15] He saw patients at the Santa Casa hospital and observed operations there, together with the core Tropicalistas Moura, Paterson, Wucherer, and Silva Lima. He was also, together with core Tropicalistas, among the early officers of the Doctors' and Pharmacists' Mutual Aid Society. Faria never became part of the core Tropicalistas, for by the first half of the 1870s, he devoted more time to his duties at the school, his considerable practice in Salvador, and his medical and autobiographical writings. He also traveled to Europe, including one trip made as a member of a government-appointed commission to look into developments in medical teaching in Europe.[16] But his relationship to the Tropicalistas remained good, and upon his death an editorial in the *Gazeta Médica* remembered him in the glowing terms reserved for only a handful of physicians.[17]

In 1881 Francisco Rodrigues da Silva became director of the school. A graduate of the Bahian medical school (1853), he was not a Tropicalista supporter: he never contributed to their journal, he was not a member of the Doctors' and Pharmacists' Mutual Aid Society, he did not attend the meetings at Paterson's house, and although he was appointed to head the Santa Casa hospital, he seems never to have worked with the Tropicalis-

tas on any of the many cases the latter attended. In 1870 he bitterly opposed the Tropicalista Virgílio Clímaco Damázio's joining the faculty at
the Lyceu, the city's most prestigious high school. Formed in the mold
of an older generation of Brazilian physician, Silva was renowned for his
classical erudition, and was probably opposed to the new teachings in natural history, particularly those stemming from Darwin's work. This would
certainly have pitted him against the Tropicalistas, for in Salvador, it was
Wucherer, writing in the *Gazeta Médica,* who had first made admiring references to Darwin's ideas in the medical press.[18] However, Rodrigues da
Silva's active tenure was brief, for he fell seriously ill and traveled to Paris for
treatment, where he later died. During his official tenure there were a number of acting-directors, including the Tropicalistas Antônio Pacífico Pereira
(1883–84) and Ramiro Affonso Monteiro de Carvalho (1884–86).

The clinching of the relationship between the Tropicalistas and the medical school occurred during Pacífico Pereira's interim tenure. By then, Pacífico Pereira had been active for more than a decade as a core Tropicalista. He
had carried out research on beriberi, he had been a director of the *Gazeta
Médica* since 1869, and in his clinical practice at the Santa Casa hospital, he
had worked with other Tropicalista doctors observing, investigating, and
experimenting on beriberi and other disorders central to Tropicalista interests. He called for an epidemiological approach to medicine that would
involve record-keeping, statistics, and greater sanitation awareness. Like
other Tropicalistas, he was especially eager to develop an understanding of
Brazilian nosology and thus of exploring the notion of tropical disorders.
In order to do this, he believed it was crucial to train doctors in a more
positivistic approach to medicine; that is, he wanted medical students to
focus on the research of the disorders of Brazil and write dissertations on
subjects relevant to Brazilian health problems, and he wanted a practical
approach to teaching, in which knowledge of experimental science, learned
through the laboratory, was made central to the curriculum.

By 1881 Pacífico Pereira's dedication had earned him admiration from
some members of the school. Thus in his 1881 "Memória histórica," Claudemiro Augusto de Morais Caldas noted that the faculty considered Pacífico
Pereira to be one of its most distinguished professors and he was especially
commended for having provided his students with microscopes at his own
expense.[19] Because he was so well respected within the medical school, Pacífico Pereira was able to exercise considerable influence in gaining acceptance of his Tropicalista ideas on medical practice and education, an influ-

ence that proved particularly significant because the years when he headed the school coincided with the most far-reaching educational changes in the Empire.

Whatever acceptance Tropicalista ideas had gained under the leadership of Pacífico Pereira was consolidated under that of his successor, Ramiro Affonso Monteiro de Carvalho, full director between 1886 and 1891. Monteiro graduated from the Bahia medical school in 1865, a year before Pacífico Pereira, and joined the medical school faculty in 1871 as an adjunct in medical sciences. In 1883 he was appointed to one of the two chairs in clinical medicine, which meant he spent a good deal of time at the Santa Casa hospital, the forum for his practical teaching and also alongside some of the leading Tropicalistas. He was an official of the Doctors' and Pharmacists' Mutual Aid Society, contributed to the beriberi debate, and in 1886, coincident with his appointment to the faculty directorship, joined the editorial board of the *Gazeta Médica*.[20] Thus, after the long stewardship of Baptista dos Anjos ended in 1871, the medical school was, for the most part, directed by men who sympathized or were actively engaged with the Tropicalistas' modern outlook. They therefore took seriously the Tropicalistas' criticism of local medical education and practice.

Among the rank-and-file faculty members it is also possible to trace the Tropicalistas' increasing influence. Of the fourteen men Silva Lima recalled at the meetings held in the early 1860s at Paterson's house, only two were on the medical school faculty, namely Antônio José Alves and Antônio Januário de Faria. By the end of the Empire, however, sixteen Tropicalistas had served on the medical faculty.[21] Moreover, in the 1870s, the bulk of Tropicalista sympathizers on the faculty were to be found among the adjunct professors (called variously *opositores* and *sustitutos*).[22] By 1883 all of the adjuncts identified with the Tropicalistas had moved up the faculty hierarchy to become full professors.

For example, in 1871 Luís Alvares dos Santos, Demétrio C. Tourinho, and José Affonso Paraíso de Moura, adjuncts closely identified with the Tropicalistas, moved into the ranks of full professors. The promotion of the three men indicated a receptivity of their viewpoints from at least an important sector of the congregation, for until 1876 it was the faculty congregation, made up by full professors, who proposed adjuncts for the posts of professors, after which a competition was held to choose the final candidate.[23] Monteiro and Antônio Pacífico Pereira also entered the faculty as adjuncts in 1871.[24] José Luís De'Almeida Couto, also editor of the *Gazeta*

Médica, was appointed adjunct in 1873, as was Manoel Victorino Pereira in 1878. Between 1876 and 1883 Monteiro, Virgílio Clímaco Damázio (an adjunct since 1863 and editor of the *Gazeta Médica*), Pacífico Pereira, and Victorino Pereira all became full professors. By the mid-1880s there were approximately fifteen Tropicalista supporters, including a number of core members, on the medical school staff.[25] Not only had the number of Tropicalista supporters on the faculty become weightier, but more significantly, as they moved up the faculty ladder, they had a stronger voice in the faculty congregation, the highest decision-making body within the school.[26]

Even if men favorable to Tropicalista ideas about medicine and science were entering the ranks of teachers at the medical school, this did not necessarily mean they were able to initiate real intellectual innovation or debate. Pacífico Pereira may have made his students more aware of the importance of microscopes for clinical pathology, and new disorders, like beriberi and filariasis, became objects of study. But fundamental engagement with the new materialist forms of thinking such as Darwinism, Spencerism, "Germanism"—ideas already being discussed and argued outside the medical school—did not take place within it.[27] The congregation remained adamant about this. The extent to which this was so can be gleaned from the debates among the faculty congregation dealing with the "Memória histórica" presented by Luís Alvares dos Santos in 1876, which the congregation rejected.

Dos Santos cannot be considered a core Tropicalista. His energies were dispersed in too many directions to merit this label, but he was always a firm supporter of the Tropicalistas and appreciated their desire to change the mold of medicine in Bahia. The son of an important Bahian family, he held many civil service appointments in the true Bahian fashion of the well connected.[28] He served as inspector of health from 1874, taught at the Lyceu da Bahia, and was appointed to the medical school faculty in 1861, becoming full professor, as noted earlier, in 1871. He represented Brazil at two international exhibitions, the first in Argentina (1872) and the second in Austria (1873). He was also a writer and a poet, and in his last decade he entered politics, becoming a deputy in the Provincial Assembly and joining the campaign for the abolition of slavery.[29] As a close sympathizer of the Tropicalistas, dos Santos attended their early meetings in the 1860s, and served on the editorial board of the *Gazeta Médica* in 1876. He shared Wucherer's interest in Darwinism and natural history, the latter a subject he taught at the Lyceu da Bahia.[30] He sided with Silva Lima on the debate over beriberi, and one of his first actions on becoming health inspector was to declare a beriberi epidemic in the province. When he died in 1886, the *Gazeta Médica* dedicated its opening editorial article to Luís Alvares, recalling his life in laudatory terms. The editorial remarked that if "a slight excess sometimes led him to become enraptured by the latest ideas which over excited this fervent apostle of progress, this was [because of] a noble passion."[31]

This "excess" seems to have nettled some of the conservative spirits on the congregation. In March 1876 dos Santos read his "Memória histórica" to the congregation as part of the routine procedure for the approval and dispatch of the report to the imperial government. However, on this occasion a series of acrimonious debates followed the reading, culminating in the September 1876 rejection of the "Memória."[32] The report offended for two reasons. First, dos Santos defended the 1875 graduating dissertation presented by Domingos Guedes Cabral titled "Funções do cérebro," in which the student promoted Darwinist ideas. The congregation had rejected the dissertation the previous year, a decision that dos Santos, an advocate of Darwinism, challenged.[33] Second, dos Santos criticized the government's 1875 law suppressing competitions for professorships. According to this law, competitions were to be held only for adjunct positions, while professors were to be appointed by the government from among the adjuncts, with special weight given to seniority.

Dr. Manoel Joaquim Saraiva launched the attack on the "Memória."[34] Saraiva held that in his critique of the 1875 law, dos Santos was being contemptuous of the high capacity and standards found among the adjuncts of the medical faculty who did not need to be subjected to further competition to show their worth. Saraiva also objected to dos Santos's proposal that foreign doctors be asked to teach at the faculty and put in charge of practical instruction, and that the school faculty do more practical teaching in the military hospitals, again implying that the Bahian medical establishment was in some way deficient.[35] Both these suggestions had upset the sensibilities of many professors. The mention of "foreign" doctors in Bahia was synonymous at this time with the leaders of the Tropicalistas, a group that, with its controversies over beriberi, hookworm, and its repeated calls for innovation in medical teaching, was unsettling to the Bahian status quo. Moreover, military hospital doctors and surgeons were traditionally considered of low status.[36] Thus dos Santos was asking the faculty to turn to two sources they were most loath to use—one, because of their nationalistic pride; the other, because it was beneath their dignity to do so.[37] Dr. Domingos Carlos da Silva stated that dos Santos was offending "the dignity of the faculty." He proposed that only those parts of the "Memória" that referred specifically to the events in the faculty be accepted, and all the rest expunged.[38] Dr. Claudemiro A. Morais Caldas noted that, in contrast to what dos Santos believed, "Darwinism [is] a heretical doctrine, a scientific fad, ominous to religion."[39] Despite some compromise suggestions proposed by Jerônymo Sodré Pereira and Almeida Couto, both dos Santos and the congregation refused to change their positions and the "Memória" was rejected.[40]

Two fundamental issues were really being debated in the exchange over dos Santos's report. One concerned the kind of knowledge that the medical school accepted and approved of and that "foreigners" (like leading Tropicalistas) criticized as being outdated; the other concerned the limits of the imperial government's right to dictate terms to the provinces. On both these issues dos Santos emerged wholeheartedly on the side of change, thus showing himself to be within the camp of the Tropicalistas. The timing of the "Memória histórica" is also crucial in understanding the fate of the report, for the 1870s revived vigorous debates dormant since the Conciliação (the period from 1852 to the mid-1860s when liberals and conservatives agreed to share power) about the role of slavery in modern and progressive nations, the benefits of federalism as opposed to centralism, and the anachronism of monarchy in a continent of republics. All events became politicized and all issues polemical.

Although no physician at the medical school would have disagreed with dos Santos and the Tropicalistas about the importance of the advances in medicine as a result of French clinical advances and pathological anatomy and more recent German advances in microscopy, physiology, and biochemistry, there were conservative physicians who distrusted the philosophical underpinnings of scientific and positivistic trends. They believed that the new trends in medicine, as in other intellectual fields, went too far and too fast, particularly when the advances, such as those in Germany, were linked to an interest in materialist philosophies and sometimes radical political activism that undermined long-held philosophical and religious positions.[41] Thus when Saraiva argued that the school did not need the intervention of foreigners to supplement its practical teaching, he was suggesting that the Bahian medical school was as good as any top European school but—even more—he was suggesting that change would come to the

Bahian school in an orderly manner according to the rhythms of change fostered by the traditional authority of French medicine, working its way, like much else in the Brazilian Empire, from the top down. It was anathema to such conservative physicians to contemplate change in the Bahian medical school because of some upstart foreigners living in Salvador who had managed to canvas a local following for their ideas.

The threat the "foreign" doctors represented to the old-guard physicians can best be appreciated by recalling that the Tropicalistas were among the first men in Bahia to show an interest in Darwin's evolutionary ideas. In 1866, under the guise of reporting and reviewing a talk given by Benjamin E. Cotting to the Massachusetts Medical Society, Wucherer indicated his approval of and familiarity with Darwin's ideas. In the article, Wucherer betrayed a Darwinian-like view of a world in constant flux, where some species died and others transformed into new ones, one group living off and destroying another.[42] As early as 1801, Wucherer wrote, Lamarck had talked of the transformation of species. However, the theory had never had many followers until Darwin, who was its best expounder. Wucherer continued:

> "Darwinism," like all doctrines that question prejudices and traditional myths, is still strongly opposed. However, it is being taken up, openly or covertly, by a growing number of investigators. . . . The work of Carpenter (on foraminifera), of Bates (on Amazon butterflies), of Wallace (on India's butterflies and birds), of the tireless Fritz Müller in the [Brazilian] wilderness, and of many other famous naturalists, both zoologists and botanists . . . , are gradually solidifying the basis of this interesting doctrine.[43]

Moderate as this statement may seem today, the fact that Wucherer dared to argue publicly in favor of a doctrine that was alarming European conservatives in many countries indicated to die-hard conservatives that foreigners living in Bahia could be dangerously subversive, introducing ideas that assaulted long-held religious beliefs already undermined by anticlericalism and positivism.

Such discussions of Darwin's ideas became even more dangerous to the conservative elite in the 1870s when Brazilians began importing French evolutionary debates. The debates surged in France after the shock of defeat by Germany and the rise of the Paris Commune, and as Darwin's evolutionary theories became common currency among the French, so they were introduced into Brazil by the progressive intelligentsia.[44] In 1875 a series of well-attended seminars on Darwin's ideas were held in Rio de Janeiro.[45] That same year the Bahian medical student Guedes Cabral wrote his dissertation following Darwin's evolutionary ideas.[46] That Darwin's *transformisme* drew strong opposition among some medical circles can be seen in the medical school's rejection of Guedes Cabral's dissertation. The following year another student, whose work was accepted, wrote his dissertation attacking the Darwinian ideas expounded by Guedes Cabral.[47]

More familiar with the ruckus that Darwin's ideas had caused than with his work, conservative groups in Bahia, as in Brazil, tended to reject the Englishman's theory as an assault on religion.[48] Although the Brazilian upper class was very far from devout, as Richard Graham has noted, it did care a great deal about the "religious orthodoxy of social institutions which . . . was to prove the chief weapon used by the defenders of the old order against the attacks of the modernizers and rationalists."[49] Thus the French debate of the 1870s that pitted defenders of the Catholic Church together with the "spiritualists" (both of whom stressed the functional structure of the universe) against the unmitigated struggle approach of some Darwinian transformists found its counterpart in Brazil in the 1870s and 1880s. This was not a mere imitation of what was going on in the metropolis but was a debate about the role traditional institutions should play in an increasingly troubled Brazilian nation, and, if the institutions were to be changed, what the pace of that change was to be. Were the nation's problems to be solved by rationally applying scientific ideas, or by revitalizing the authority of old institutions like the Church, the monarchy, and slavery?[50] In the specific case of dos Santos's report, the conservative group was trying to check a Darwinian cancer from developing in the midst of the medical school, a cancer they had already detected the previous year with Cabral's dissertation. Not only did they therefore disavow dos Santos's more radical theoretical ideas, such as his Darwinism, but they also opposed the idea of "foreigners" telling them what to teach and how best to do it.[51] The debate over dos Santos's report was not about narrow medical matters but about contrasting forms of knowledge and, thus, differing positions on how far to dismantle the old in bringing about the new.

The second issue Luís Alvares dos Santos raised in his "Memória histórica" concerned the extent of power the imperial government should exercise over the provinces. As a liberal and a federalist, dos Santos opposed the newly instituted system of government appointment of full professors to their chairs, instead of competitive examinations. The new system, he believed, would enable the government to dispense patronage with ever greater impunity and thus give it greater control over the medical school's affairs.[52] The conservatives challenged dos Santos, for even if they were not averse to progress, they wished to slow the pace of change and were therefore far more respectful of the decisions originating from the central government. Domingos Carlos da Silva, for example, did not stop at taking a stand in favor of the government over the promotion of adjuncts by appointment. He also supported the imperial government in its proposal to create a centralized university, an anathema to the liberal federalists who feared the autonomy of provincial faculties would be completely eclipsed by such a development.[53]

By the 1880s the conservatives were forced to change their position. The central government's blatant favoritism toward the Rio de Janeiro school made their position untenable and they closed ranks with the liberals they had formerly vilified. For example, the much heralded educational reforms of 1878–79 and 1884 promised a great deal in terms of modernizing medical teaching in Brazil, and bringing the faculties of Bahia and Rio de Janeiro more in line with each other. Initially, nearly all groups hailed the proposed changes. But the Bahian school's raised expectations were dashed when the monies needed to enact the reforms were not forthcoming. The Bahian faculty was further irritated when the imperial government managed to get wealthy sponsors to underwrite many of the changes in Rio de Janeiro but never bothered to resolve the Bahian school's money shortage.[54] By 1887 Saraiva, who had formerly defended the imperial government, had changed his position. In fact, he joined eleven faculty members, including seven Tropicalistas, in publicly disobeying a ruling of Prime Minister Barão de Mamoré concerning competitions.[55] Thus, although at the time of the discussion about dos Santos's "Memória" the dividing line had been between the innovative faculty members, closer to the Tropicalistas' modernity, and the conservative members who opposed change unless sanctioned from above, by the early 1880s the perception of government high-handedness had forced the two groups together.

While the imperial government was proving to be a dissatisfying Maecenas and a capricious meddler in medical school affairs in Bahia, the Tropicalistas' status had become established. Even the most recalcitrant among the Bahian faculty found the Tropicalistas, with their journal, their international prestige, their clear agenda for change, and their willingness to take up the battle on behalf of the faculty, a natural and formidable ally. By then, too, some very influential core Tropicalistas had become regular faculty and were successfully pressing from inside to make the Tropicalistas' agenda that of the medical school. Also, as more Tropicalistas joined the medical school faculty, so the school's preoccupations became the concerns of the Tropicalistas. If the 1870s saw the Tropicalistas enter the ranks of the faculty, the 1880s were when the medical school's demands for its autonomy and the Tropicalistas' demands for modernizing medical teaching intertwined. Now Tropicalista demands for change and innovation and those of the medical school faculty were indistinguishable; the Tropicalistas were no longer outsiders.

Tropicalistas, Students, and the Critique of Medical Teaching

The pages of the *Gazeta Médica* are full of examples of the Tropicalistas as critical reviewers of the teaching and facilities at the medical school.[56] At first sight their demands do not seem unlike those reiterated year after year in the annual medical school reports.[57] However, there were subtle but far-reaching differences. To elucidate these, it is instructive to look at two articles published in the *Gazeta Médica* in 1884. The first was by Louis Couty, a French industrial biologist who was one of a handful of foreign scientists appointed to the National Museum in Rio de Janeiro in 1876.[58] In his article on the state of higher learning in Brazil, Couty wrote that in terms of money invested in laboratory equipment for teaching and research, Brazil compared favorably to what many well-known European scientists had to work with. However, he continued:

> with each new step [in the research] one is obliged to enter into paperwork, and to make special petitions for the purchase of an animal, a small instrument, a reagent, [all of which] are needed urgently and, if the money to be spent exceeds a certain amount, then the petition must be submitted to the congregation. Often a professor, in the face of so many obstacles, becomes discouraged and follows the easiest path: a lecture. . . . In Europe things are very different. A laboratory may have fewer resources, but the resources it has belong to it exclusively: every professor disposes of the resources as he sees fit, he must only justify his expenses. Then every laboratory becomes a real working center where

the cabinets are probably not as tidy as they might be, and the books and administrative paper are paltry but where disciples can be formed who are useful to their country.[59]

As a solution, Couty called for decentralization of the medical laboratories in the schools and for professors and researchers to be released from continual government accountability. As long as the organization of education was not changed, no amount of equipment and new laboratories would make the least difference. Moreover, argued Couty in a passage reminiscent of Tropicalista writings, Brazilian doctors and researchers failed to stress Brazilian themes. He went on:

> When the research carried out in a laboratory is on yellow fever, beriberi, tuberculosis; when attempts are made to determine the properties of various medicinal plants, some of which, like ipecacuanha and jaborandi, are already being exported; when the properties of animal poisons are probed, . . . then [researchers] work for the good of all.[60]

It is significant that the Tropicalistas published this article in their journal. They believed, with Couty, that a part of the failure of medical education was the government's heavy control over education but, even more, they believed the problem also involved an erroneous approach by medical professors themselves. As Silva Araújo put it:

> we are blinded by the brilliancy of [European achievements]. . . . For too long we have been a mere extension of European science . . . producing inadequate [science] because of a lack of autonomy and [failing] to live up to the mettle of an advanced, independent nation.[61]

Thus the Tropicalistas blamed an attitude prevalent in the school itself. They asked that the school not wait for changes initiated by the government, but that the professors themselves begin to adapt to a changing medical world.

The second article that illustrates Tropicalista thought regarding medical education in Brazil was by Pacífico Pereira. In an extensive review of the flaws of Brazilian education and the recent attempts to overhaul it, he added a further critique to Couty's assessment.[62] Quoting from the Bahian legislator and educator, Rui Barbosa, he wrote, "The central problem of . . . education among us is that, until today, it has been almost exclusively literary. . . . We enter our academies . . . with a baggage of useless teach-

ings, without even minimum requirements to understand science and life."
Pereira lamented that "the men who are to form the intellectual cream of
our nation do not have a complete . . . education, do not know the principal languages of today [i.e., German as opposed to Latin], or do not know
the explanation of some of the most common phenomena in the natural
sciences, and do not appreciate the value of these sciences."[63]

Developing a scientific approach to medicine did not only entail new
equipment and experimentally based teaching. It required a new mind-set.
As an editorial in the *Gazeta Médica* noted,

> In this era of positivism . . . there can be no place for abstract ques-
> tions. Clinical observation, investigations with the microscope, chemi-
> cal analysis, animal experimentation, these are the bases on which to-
> day's medicine builds; [theories developed] without these [foundations]
> may be ingenious but they only satisfy and nourish dreamers.[64]

This meant that the language of medical instruction must change; it
must be oriented toward positivistic science, shed of moralistic, literary,
and polemical tones. A good place to observe the change in scientific language as well as the choice of subject for investigation is in the graduating
dissertations written by medical students. As a requirement to receive the
medical degree, students had to write a dissertation in their final year that
they defended orally in front of members of the faculty congregation and
the public. They could choose the topics from a list of possible subjects
drawn up by the congregation, most of them replicas of French graduate
dissertation topics.[65] There was, however, some flexibility, as was evident
when Domingos Pedro dos Santos approached his adviser, the Tropicalista
Ramiro Affonso Monteiro, for help in choosing a topic and together they
came up with beriberi, a subject they felt was particularly relevant to Brazilian medicine.[66]

It is instructive to contrast the older French-oriented dissertations with
those the Tropicalistas chose to publish in their journal. In the traditional
dissertation written in Bahia, it was common for students to discuss questions drawn from European dissertations and wholly irrelevant to Brazil, such as the dangers during pregnancy for women living in the Vosges
mountains or the cold in Copenhagen.[67] The language used in these dissertations was erudite, flowery, vague, and moralistic. The authors moved
easily from references to religion and God, ancient civilizations, the won-
ders of history, and the medical subject in hand.[68] These dissertations con-

trasted sharply with the few the Tropicalistas published in their journal, all of which concentrated on common local disorders and on Brazilian pharmacopoeia. For example, one thesis dealt with hookworm; two were on beriberi; another investigated the therapeutic properties of araroba, a Brazilian medication; another treated leprosy in the Brazilian Northeast; another was a Brazilian medical bibliography.[69] All the dissertations were based on original research and contributed to ongoing debates rather than recycling old ones, and were written mainly in factual, descriptive language that avoided prescription.

Another way the Tropicalistas encouraged students to learn a more scientific-oriented language was by directing them to new sources of medical discovery. Thus they recommended students to familiarize themselves with medical developments in Germany and Austria. There, medicine was becoming a more exact and scientific science, and the Tropicalistas approved of the way it was taught in small classes with a hands-on experimental approach instead of the literary and lecturing approach still in use in much of France and in Brazil. Wucherer's old teacher and correspondent Wilhelm Griesinger noted that the new German teaching was designed to provide "a personal familiarity with the objects of research, the sharpening of the senses and the actual handling of instruments."[70] This is what the Tropicalistas, with limited resources, equipment, and facilities, tried to do with interested students who worked alongside them at the Santa Casa hospital, helped in autopsies, and attended informal sessions of instruction on the use of the microscope and chemical tests. Through the *Gazeta Médica,* too, students read about the work of Ludwig Traube and Rudolf Virchow in pathology; Ernst Felix Hoppe-Seyler and Carl von Voit in biochemistry; Max von Pettenkofer in physiological chemistry; Theodor Billroth in surgery; Carl Wunderlich and Ernst von Leyden in medicine; and Griesinger and Leuckart in parasitology. The Tropicalistas called for a knowledge of German as a prerequisite for entry into medical school (a suggestion that was not accepted), and following the advice of their mentors, several of the younger Tropicalistas not only learned German but also spent time in Germany and Vienna.[71]

That the Tropicalistas exercised considerable influence on students in the 1870s and 1880s is also evident from the number of dissertations that were prefaced by acknowledgments of the Tropicalistas or included references to their example in the text. Through their journal, their meetings to discuss Brazilian disorders, their unofficial teaching at the Santa

Casa hospital, and the official teaching of their members who joined the medical school faculty, the Tropicalistas became a central force in Bahian medicine.[72] What made them a more formidable influence than they might otherwise have been was that in the politically charged atmosphere of the late 1870s and 1880s, they became central to the debates over ensino livre and over the relationship of the central government to the Bahian medical school.

The Tropicalistas and the Reform of Medical Education

If a salient feature of Brazilian education during the Empire years had been its centralization, a characteristic of education in the Old Republic that followed was decentralization. As Simon Schwartzman has noted, important efforts were made toward geographical and geological research, toward the creation of medical institutes for research and practical applications, and toward the setting up of new secondary schools and universities.[73] This activity was mainly the result of state, not central, governments, and although most of it was unleashed after the fall of the Empire, the loosening of central control began with the the liberal prime minister Leôncio de Carvalho in 1878–79. His educational reforms affected the primary school system all the way up to the institutions of higher education, such as medical schools.[74] The ensino livre policy became the single most controversial issue in the new law.

There were three different aspects to ensino livre. First was the right to set up schools or universities separate from the umbrella of the state, a policy that private educational enterprises, including the Catholic Church, homeopathic centers, and a few Protestant schools, greatly favored. Second was the liberty of qualified outsiders and faculty to teach specialized courses in schools of higher education, additional to the official program of studies—a liberty given in order to end the uniformity of the official syllabi and introduce the possibility of real academic debate within the schools. Third was the noncompulsory class attendance of students in the higher education institutions that, liberal legislators argued, would lead to the creation of more responsible and motivated students, as well as force professors, who now had to compete for student attendance, to improve their teaching.[75]

Overall, the stipulations concerning the medical schools were designed to update medical teaching in Brazil. Thus, for example, practical teaching was to be carried out in properly equipped and staffed laboratories, entry requirements to the schools were raised, new chairs were created in recognition of new medical fields, clinical teaching was extended, and women were allowed entry into the schools. Although all sectors of the intelligentsia agreed on the need for a fundamental reappraisal of the educational system, including that of the medical schools, there was also a good deal of political jockeying for power between the conservatives and the liberals, the latter recently returned to power after a ten-year conservative stint and anxious to reduce conservative hold over patronage and diffuse centralized power. With an unstable cabinet and a divided Chamber of Deputies, the various aspects of the law were often more the result of opportunistic policies and, as Fernando de Azevedo has put it, "the transitory influence of the cabinets of ministers" rather than a coherent program for reform and renovation.[76]

Indeed, much of the seeming incoherence of the educational policies in this era had to do with the elite's recognition that although progress must come to Brazil, they wanted to somehow fit it into existing social and power relations. One of the conservatives' accusations was that Carvalho's ensino livre policy was the liberal answer to the conservative demand for a centralized university. The debate over the formation of a centralized university was an old one in Brazil. José Bonifácio de Andrada e Silva, a founding father of independent Brazil, had recommended the creation of a university in the instructions he drafted for the São Paulo delegates to the Constituent Assembly of 1823 but had failed to get the measure accepted. Two more attempts failed in 1870 and 1880. If the earlier endeavors to create a centralized university system floundered on the anachronism of creating a literate public in a slavocratic and agrarian nation, the latter endeavors failed primarily because they ran contrary to the decentralizing trends gathering force from the 1870s on. In fact, there were liberals who believed that the creation of one or more universities was a prerequisite for progress in Brazil and they looked to Germany and Austria as their model. However, in the atmosphere of growing distrust of the grasping tentacles of the imperial government, the liberals resisted the creation of a university, fearing the government would see this as an excuse to create a "Napoleonic" university with tight central control. Thus although in theory there was no contradiction between the demand for a university system and the demand for ensino livre, at this point the liberals waved the flag of ensino livre (and opposed a central university), for this was useful to the liberals' objective of reducing the government's central control over higher education.[77]

Carvalho, who was adamant that an educational reform had to be carried out and fearful that an acrimonious debate would result in the bill's being thrown out, resorted to the high-handed method of governmental decree in order to pass some of the most polemical aspects of the bill, such as free attendance, free courses, and a stipulation that there be competitions for all medical and law school posts.[78] In 1879 ensino livre became a fact in Brazil and liberal politicians hailed the law as breaking imperial government's stranglehold on education. Carvalho's reform laid the basis for far-reaching changes in medical education. However, the reform was also general rather than specific and led to a great deal of confusion, opposition, and criticism, including from his own party. Moreover, it quickly became clear that noncompulsory attendance, particularly in the medical profession where laboratory training and practical teaching were crucial, was a failure.[79] In Salvador, Pacífico Pereira, writing in the *Gazeta Médica,* became central to the liberal discussion about ensino livre, a policy he had initially favored but later came to reject.

In October 1880 Pacífico Pereira wrote the lead article in the *Gazeta Médica* on the reform of the medical schools that he said was "agitating all enlightened people of the nation."[80] The intent of Carvalho's reforms was to be highly commended, he wrote; however, the actual stipulations had gone too far in some aspects and not far enough in others. For example, the notion of "free teaching" had been misunderstood. Although the decentralization of higher education was a laudable aspect of the new laws, Pereira did not believe that Brazil was ready for the proliferation of degree-granting private universities, and in its present stage of development, he warned, the nation might end up with the sort of devalued medical schools that existed under the proprietorial medical school system in the United States. There, the sale of medical diplomas by some so-called accredited medical schools in the United States was a notorious fact.[81] Moreover, the "mania of diplomas" that existed in Brazil would make many vulnerable to the sort of hoaxes and lowering of standards common in the United States. "How can we permit the creation of free universities in [Brazil]," an editorial in the *Gazeta Médica* asked, "where charlatanism is encouraged by the negligence of the authorities, where medical responsibility is not [clearly] defined, where there is no regularly organized sanitary police force?" A more desirable form of freedom was that which existed in German, Austrian, and British medical schools, which were autonomous in their right to set syllabi, choose their directors, and allocate their resources, but still had to conform to certain nationally required standards for their degrees.[82]

Freedom of attendance, for Pacífico Pereira, was another great mistake in the Brazilian context. Such freedom, which existed in some advanced countries, assumed that the responsibility required to wield the freedom had been inculcated into people from preparatory school. This was not the case in Brazil and no law could simply legislate responsibility into creation. The reform of education in Brazil, therefore, argued Pacífico Pereira, had to be tackled on a much more fundamental level and would take considerably more time and effort than the mere passage of a law. Moreover, while the entry requirements in the German and British universities were valid exercises in choosing the best students, in Brazil such examinations were a farce the well-connected could easily circumvent, thus obtaining admission and gaining degrees through favoritism rather than merit.[83] If freedom for individual students had gone too far, however, argued Pereira, the new law still failed to clearly define those areas in which the medical schools must have autonomy. For example, the faculty congregation should be allowed to elect its director rather than have him appointed; the role of the director should be that of mediator between the minister of the Empire and the school; and all of the latter's concerns, whether scientific, regulatory, or administrative, should be the prerogative of the director.

On one level, Pacífico Pereira's critique of Carvalho's reform provides yet another example of the way in which the Tropicalistas believed European ideas were to be adapted to conform to the Brazilian context, rather than merely imitated. Indeed, the heart of his critique was that, much as traditional Brazilian doctors were content to imitate European medicine rather than develop a national medicine, Carvalho's reforms simply replicated a European policy created for a very different social context. On another level, Pereira was arguing in favor of granting increased power to local doctors. Pereira wanted to see the decentralization of teaching insofar as it involved the end of the imperial government's interference in the provinces. But this did not mean that he advocated its complete liberalization. In his thinking, Salvador should replace imperial government control and become the metropolis of medical teaching in the north. The regulation of teaching would come from modern-minded Bahians like himself, men who saw the advantages of progressive government regulation, and who understood the importance of having experts within government.

As a rejoinder to the flaws in the reform laws, Pacífico Pereira outlined a detailed plan of an ideal general educational reform (*plano*) that would free the Bahian medical school of restrictive government regulations, lay the base for the pursuit of high standards in medical teaching, and enable the school to become a center of "investigations that could one day develop a medical science and therapy suitable to our own climate."[84] The plan included recommendations that the directors to the school be elected by the congregation for two years at a time, that they have ample powers, that students attend both theoretical and practical classes, and that entry requirements include German.

Pereira's *plano* became the basis of the petition for reforms that the Bahian faculty presented to the Chamber of Deputies in 1880. Pacífico Pereira, Ramiro Affonso Monteiro, and Claudemiro A. Morais Caldas were chosen to take the document in person to the chamber.[85] This "notable petition" was a key influence on the compromise educational reform passed by the prime minister, Felipe Franco de Sá, on October 25, 1884.[86] The amended reform pulled together the educational reforms of the previous decade, particularly those from 1878–79 on, into a coherent package, pruning and discarding the most unpopular and unworkable stipulations, while keeping the spirit of innovation of Carvalho's law. Thus, for example, more teaching laboratories were set up, bringing the total to fourteen, the number of personnel to help in the practical teaching increased, and the policy of free attendance was severely restricted. Above all, the government promised to provide the money needed to implement the changes. Pereira, who had fought hard for this more balanced change, was optimistic. Sabóia's educational policy was a step forward; it seemed to Pereira that the medical schools might finally get on with the real business of producing well-trained medical students in Brazil.[87]

Besides entering the debates of ensino livre, the Tropicalistas defended the medical school from an often arbitrary imperial government. In particular they waged a campaign in their journal against the government's failure to finance its reforms, and they challenged the government's right to override the school congregation on such issues as faculty appointments and promotion. From the late 1870s on, the faculty of the Bahian medical school became far less tolerant of government meddling in its affairs than it had been in former times.

This increasing politicization on the part of the school faculty was directly related to the great political struggles that swept through Brazil in the 1870s and 1880s and, ultimately, led to the fall of the monarchy in 1889. Groups from all ends of the political spectrum began pointing an accusing finger at the central government as the cause for their grievances and this one point of agreement made for some unlikely political alliances. Dissatisfied sectors of the army fueled by the ideas of positivism and republicanism forged alliances with ultramontane sections of the Catholic Church that disputed the emperor's right to become involved in Church decisions.[88] Urban middle-class groups—such as university professionals—and lower-middle-class groups—swelled by European immigration—questioned the power and influence of the rural aristocracy. Gaining momentum in the political effervescence was the movement for the abolition of slavery that emerged as the first truly national movement cutting across geographical, class, racial, and political groupings.

In Bahia, the medical school became one of the main centers in the debate about Brazil's future and the place where the Republican Party found its staunchest support in a city that remained largely loyal to the monarchy. Indeed, the founder of the Republican Party in Bahia, Virgílio Clímaco Damázio, was both a Tropicalista and a medical school faculty member. It is within this context that we must place the medical school's criticisms and challenges to the central government, all diligently reported by the *Gazeta Médica*. In particular, the journal supported Pacífico Pereira, who, as interim director of the school (1883–84), struggled over finances with the central government. For example, renovations in the medical school for new laboratories in compliance with the law started in June 1883, but by December the work had to be suspended for lack of money.[89] An annoyed Pereira complained that this was in contrast to Rio de Janeiro, where the promised innovations had been successfully carried out. When the Chamber of Deputies discussed Pereira's complaints in a session on government spending, the *Gazeta Médica* noted bitterly:

> Without allowing ourselves to care that [the money provided for the Rio de Janeiro school] is evidence of the special relationship the government has with the [Rio] school, whose faculty is enticed with favors and titles; . . . without comparing the two schools because we are not moved by jealousy (but certainly by sadness for the way we are abandoned), we will show that . . . the government did have the means to finance the new laboratories and new chairs.[90]

When informing its readers about a pedagogical conference organized by the central government to be held in June 1883, the journal warned that the conference was simply a diversionary tactic:

> Questions on . . . the autonomy of the schools in the three [northern] provinces, which have fought for so many years against an atrophying centralization . . . are going to be decided by a congress in which there are six votes to represent the three provincial schools and fifty votes to represent the court faculty.[91]

And after receiving the decrees that were formally announced in the conference, the *Gazeta Médica* proclaimed, "We were right not to believe that the conference would be an occasion for pushing through the needed reforms in the schools."[92]

Even when competitions in faculty positions, as demanded by the Tropicalistas, replaced the practice of government appointments from 1883 on, the more radical members of the Bahian faculty, seconded by the Tropicalistas' journal, refused to tone down their criticisms. The progressive liberal Victorino Pereira, one of the first to benefit from the reformed law and earn an appointment to a newly created chair (clinical surgery), assailed the government in his acceptance speech:

> This government has enslaved everything. . . . Today we have a new reform as a result of a long struggle in which we members of the Bahian school played a primary role. . . . For science to live, it needs talent which nature provides, and resources which [a government] provides. [This government] wants to make us unequal in a manner no law did: [it] is miserly, giving little and late from [a fund] which provided plenty to our sister school.[93]

The belief that the government had no real intentions of giving up its central control in spite of the educational reforms of the previous decade was confirmed yet again in 1887 when the prime minister, Barão de Mamoré, invalidated the outcome of a competition in the Bahian medical school on the grounds that there was insufficient evidence to prove the candidate's competence. He ordered a new competition to be held to select another candidate.[94] The *Gazeta Médica* immediately took up the school's cause, writing that the government's action was "arbitrary and illegal" and assaulted the school's rightful prerogative to decide who was most fit, according to scientific criteria, for faculty posts.[95] The journal applauded the faculty congregation's move to reject the minister's order to hold a new competition.[96] The *Gazeta* placed the incident within a broader pattern of recurring ignominies, reminding its readers of several similar incidents.[97] The journal also published the full letter of complaint forwarded by the congregation to the government. Eleven members of the congregation signed the letter, seven of whom were core Tropicalistas or supporters.[98]

Where once they had been outsiders looking in and criticizing, now the Tropicalistas were a part of the Bahian medical establishment. Their minute attention to debates in the Chamber of Deputies, their account of the interchanges between representatives, their publications of correspondence passing between the medical school and the government are all evidence of this shift. Whereas before the late 1870s, the articles published in the *Gazeta Médica* focused on clinical practice and original pieces, with medical news relegated to the "Notices" section, now an increasing number of key articles focused on the question of medical education. Such a shift in the content of the journal was, of course, partly in response to the big educational changes that were being nationally debated, but it was also a result of the closer association of the Tropicalistas and the medical school, and a coalescing of aims.

Conclusion

From the very start the *Gazeta Médica* had been a political journal, but it had sought to develop a "new" physician-politician. That is, the Tropicalistas had wanted entry into the great national debates as a result of their scientific expertise and merit, and not through playing the established political game of ascendancy through patronage and connections. They represented themselves as a group somehow above the fray of politics. But in the political ferment of the late 1870s and 1880s, in which all issues and government actions came to be interpreted in highly charged terms, the true political nature of the Tropicalistas became ever more evident. As the allies of faculty members, they wholeheartedly took on the fight against what they saw as arbitrary and high-handed actions from the central government, using their journal as an overtly political publication. At the same time, individual Tropicalistas entered politics, lobbying for political posts and influence.[99] By the 1880s the Tropicalistas had also largely shed their image of "foreignness." Not only had some of the original foreign leaders died, but there were sufficient numbers of Brazilian-born followers for the movement to be seen as a Bahian one. There were also enough Tropicalistas within the medical school faculty for the movement to be seen as having started within the medical school, and while much of what the Tropicalistas had preached in the 1860s had seemed new and unsettling, by the 1880s it become accepted within mainstream medicine. By the time of the fall of the Empire in 1889 the Tropicalistas had shed their outsider status.

Silva Lima's plaintive comment that his son-in-law Victorino Pereira should never have entered politics because in so doing he sacrificed his early promise of excellence in science is typical of the Tropicalistas' representation of themselves.[100] According to this portrayal, they had started out with the disinterested ideal of pursuing pure scientific knowledge that, when applied to medicine in Brazil, would have far-reaching implications for medical practice in the tropics and for Brazil by developing tropical medicine, or *pathologia intertropical*. The success of their ideal would professionalize medicine in Brazil and redefine doctors as crucial agents of national improvement.

However, this portrayal of altruistic doctor-scientist is simplistic. In fact, the Tropicalistas had always been an inherently political group. Like other new professional groups with a clear technical orientation, such as engineers, the Tropicalistas tried to use their privileged knowledge within the political arena to advance their professional and political interests. In so doing, they became increasingly caught up in the political struggles of the Empire and focused less on original research.

Silva Lima's complaint probably had more to do with the fact that in the end, the Tropicalistas, for all their apparent successes, made less of a sustained impact to eradicate the "literary" tradition in medical teaching and practice than they would have liked. It is indicative that one of the most prestigious centers for "high" culture in Bahia in the 1890s became the Bahian Geographic and Historical Institute (Instituto Geográfico e Histórico da Bahia), founded in 1894, a literary and philosophical center for general, rather than specialized, "scientific" culture. In its early lists of members, there were many doctors, including eleven members more or less closely associated with the Tropicalistas.[101] In Bahia, as in France, the "ideal of general culture remained the final crowning of life."[102] The Tropicalistas were successful in many ways, but in the final analysis, they were not successful in converting a creative scientific moment into a sustained scientific enterprise.

CONCLUSION

The Tropicalistas can be viewed as a success in many ways. By the 1880s they had gained some of the acceptance beyond Bahia that they had sought. The original leaders moved from being obscure clinicians in a tropical back-water to participants in an international debate and the founders of a pres-tigious journal. The movement helped modernize the medical school and medical establishment in Bahia. Brazilian doctors's interests expanded from purely European concerns in medicine to Brazilian ones. The group was an important influence on some of the most far-reaching educational reforms in the Empire. When later innovating doctors started their own medical journals, even in Rio de Janeiro, they emulated the *Gazeta Médica da Bahia*. After the turn of the century, however, as the last of the Tropicalistas died, little was left of the group other than the nostalgic memory of a time when medical science in Bahia had achieved international recognition. Even if the Tropicalistas can be considered an example of "scientific excellence under adversity" in the sense of creating knowledge recognized by international peers, they cannot be so considered in the sense of organizing stable insti-tutions that made a sustained contribution to medical science and trained disciples to carry on their work.[1] Thus their investigations may have been an inspiration, but they provided no foundation on which later researchers like Oswaldo Cruz could build. Why did the Tropicalistas fail to establish a lasting tradition in Brazilian tropical medicine that could be built on by future generations of doctors?

The first part of the answer lies in the Tropicalistas' marginal status within Brazil. One of the greatest obstacles the Tropicalistas faced in order to gain recognition was the marginal nature of Bahia. As a result of its being close to the seat of power and center of patronage, the Rio medical community had many advantages over its sister medical community. Not only was there an unbalanced granting of noble titles to doctors from the capital city, but the government took a series of steps to benefit its local community. Thus in the early 1880s the imperial government financed the building and setting up of fully equipped laboratories in the Rio de Janeiro medical school, but not the Bahian one. It provided resources to set up a polyclinic in Rio de Janeiro to be used for training students but ignored demands for a similar polyclinic in Salvador. It set up a medical research center at the National Museum but did little to upgrade the facilities in the Bahian medical museum. It underwrote the costs of the Imperial Academy of Medicine and its journal but did not replicate the academy in Salvador.[2] The justification given for this state of affairs was that Rio de Janeiro attracted the more brilliant minds. This relationship explains why Tropicalista discoveries, like Wucherer's discovery of the hookworm parasite, were received in the capital city, on the whole, with skepticism.

Only once the Tropicalistas' work gained recognition in European journals did the Rio community start to take notice of the Bahian doctors. Even then, however, the Tropicalistas lamented that the journal of the Imperial Academy of Medicine, the *Anais Brasilienses de Medicina*, seldom acknowledged the work of the *Gazeta Médica da Bahia*. Despite all the Tropicalistas' demands for domestic support, official medical circles in the capital city largely ignored them. As a result, they never received any financial or other official backing for their efforts. For this reason, the Bahian doctors were unable to truly institutionalize their early ideal of medical research in the tropics so as to train a school of disciples and leave behind a scientific legacy on which others could build.

A second reason for the Tropicalistas' failure to establish a lasting tradition was the timing of their enterprise. As one historian of Brazilian science has noted, "in the few instances of research work being carried out in Brazil before 1900 such work was sporadic, isolated, . . . or incapable of being self-sustaining."[3] The Tropicalistas set out on their journey of medical discovery in the 1860s, when it was still possible for individual doctor-scientists to hope for recognition, even fame, from their activities as freelance clinicians and researchers. It was also a period when the unspecialized nature of the biomedical sciences made it easy to move from one subject to another in an interdisciplinary manner, an approach that began to change radically by the 1870s.[4]

Then the increasingly specialized character of the biomedical sciences led to a few, well-financed, and mainly European centers emerging at the forefront of medical advances.[5] Moreover, the development of parasitology and bacteriology in the laboratory, and later "the alliance between field-work and laboratory," required funding, most coming from governments now willing to reconceptualize health as a national question worthy of investment.[6] The change in thinking was directly linked to the coincidence of growing international economic competition and the triumphs of the germ theory, especially regarding the disorders of the tropics. Not only were colonial powers ready to take on tropical disease that they saw as a major obstacle to colonial development by funding research on such disorders, but the governments of independent tropical countries, like Brazil, also began to invest money to solve the problems of tropical disease.[7]

In addition, by the 1890s Brazil's new republican government was forced to confront the issue of health as part of its efforts to replenish the labor force in a postslavery society. International capitalism presented huge new opportunities for Brazil to become one of the leading agro-export countries in Latin America. To provide the labor to attain that progress, the Brazilian elite looked both to encouraging more European immigrants and to improving the miserable living conditions of Brazilians in the backlands.[8] By the time of this heightened concern for "national efficiency," many of the Tropicalistas had died, others were old men, and although they had attracted younger doctors into their ranks, they had never trained up a cadre of disciples single-mindedly pursuing a research agenda. The impulse for research moved south to Rio de Janeiro and São Paulo.[9]

A final reason for the eclipse of the Tropicalistas was the amazing success of Western European medical science, which, from the 1880s on, swamped homebred traditions, such as that begun by the Tropicalistas.[10] In addition, from the 1870s on, materialist philosophies such as positivism, social Darwinism, and "Germanism" had begun to take hold in Brazil. Brazilian social thought was growing increasingly complex, raiding foreign models for elements that could provide answers to Brazil's particular national problems and yoking them in a variety of ways to Brazilian nationalism.[11]

The Tropicalistas themselves were eclectic in the way they bundled new European medical ideas with older ones that had taken root locally. After the 1880s, however, one of the key problems in medicine—namely, the yawning gap between the increased understanding of disease and the lack of therapeutic advances to cure disease—appeared to be shrinking, as an unprecedented series of discoveries concerning bacteriology and vector-borne parasites made disease eradication and prevention seem possible.[12] Unlike the multifaceted etiological framework of the Tropicalistas that included biting social critiques and broad demands for environmental improvements to accelerate the melioration of the Brazilian people, a highly practical model of tropical medicine now emerged. By the turn of the century, the Brazilian government could target helminths, germs, and vectors and leave virtually untouched the underlying social relations of inequality, the source of much ill health in the tropics.[13]

Along with the triumphant germ theory that dislocated nascent local traditions came other Western medical theories, such as those of innate criminality, proposed by the Italian psychiatrist Cesare Lombroso, and inheritance, proposed by the British scientist and eugenicist Francis Galton, theories that bolstered the story of European superiority to the detriment of other peoples.[14] Brazilian doctors increasingly adopted these theories, for it was difficult to reject the immense authority of European medical science, with its unfolding cluster of brilliant discoveries. As Thomas Skidmore has noted for the Brazilian intelligentsia more broadly, "Brazilians were ill equipped intellectually to refute the supposedly scientific theories of race pouring out of Europe and North America" because their intellectual tradition was recent, insecure, and characterized by a sense of cultural inferiority.[15] By the turn of the century, in order to impose "civilization" on Brazilians, the country was importing racial determinism, criminal anthropology, and legal medicine—artifacts disguised as neutral, scientific, and universal, and developed by colonial nations for their own needs. By then, the Tropicalistas' attempt to define the idea of the tropics and of tropical disorders had been eclipsed by a tropical medicine and a racial determinism constructed by the colonial nations of the more developed world.

Nevertheless, the Tropicalista episode of science under adversity is impressive and revises the long-standing image of nineteenth-century Latin American physicians faithfully (and passively) reproducing European science in their mainly tropical countries. The Tropicalista school of medicine in Bahia offers a clear example of doctors in Brazil attempting to rethink the idea of disease in the tropics. In so doing, they began a shift from thinking of the tropics as a region of physical and mental degeneration to the assertive view that through medical improvements, Brazil and its people could participate in the long march toward civilization. If for some European nations "the study of tropical diseases [was] a means of promoting imperial policy," in Brazil the reframing of tropical disease and the pursuit of tropical medicine were primarily nationalistic ventures intended to redefine Brazil's place in the world.[16]

The study of the Tropicalistas corrects another depiction of nineteenth-century doctors in Brazil—namely, that they were a more or less homogeneous group throughout the century, adhering to medical ideas emanating from Rio de Janeiro and of minor historical interest. This view has led to a long neglect of a study of the doctors except for the period around the turn of the century, when individual doctors are catapulted as heroes into history with little sense of whether they represent continuity with a tradition or a break with it. The Tropicalistas, an example of an independent strand in the tradition of medical science in Brazil, show how simplistic such an image is. Similar to the way the positivist Tobias Barreto in Recife was able to become a source of considerable influence on intellectual thought in the south, so, for a while, the newest and most controversial thinking in nineteenth-century medical science and practice came from the Tropicalistas in Bahia and moved south. Among the reasons they were able to develop as a new school was their positioning on the periphery of the imperial power and official medicine, which gave them the necessary latitude to develop their ideas unimpeded. From the 1880s on, as the laboratory became a central tool in medical science and the rise of bacteriology marked the "real point of disjuncture with the past," the Tropicalistas' medical discourse became "typical."[17] This study has shown that the group was an early precursor of the shift in medical paradigm that made the discourse typical.

Finally, this study of the Tropicalistas also casts doubt on the wisdom of using only a European colonial framework to try to understand the history of the rise of tropical medicine. Indeed, one of the remarkable aspects about recent studies on the history of tropical medicine has been the relative absence of Latin America from the story.[18] Once Latin America is included, it becomes evident that the push to develop tropical medicine came not only from the colonial powers like Britain and France, but also from new nations like Brazil. This work has shown how a study of the tradition of Western medicine in tropical Latin America can provide rich insights into the diverse ways in which Western medicine, including tropical medicine, was taken up in regions linked to, yet far from, metropolitan sources.

APPENDIX 1

Table 1. Numbers of Students at the Bahian Medical School 1861–89

Year	Matriculated (doctors only)	Medical graduates	Pharmacy graduates	From Bahia (prov./ city)
1861	104	11	4	98
1867	170	8	4	157
1868	199	10	14	188
1869	212	29	6	217
1870[a]	242	40	29	265
1871	215	53	17	217
1872	193	23	26	197
1873	243	34	19	—
1874	260	32	—	—
1875	299	30	26	273
1876	369	25	10	—
1877	402	35	18	348
1878	405	40	15	336
1879	411[b]	53	14	323
1880	406	68	20	—
1881	425	41	7	315
1882	428	64	15	271
1883	383	60	12	—
1884	390	36	6	314
1885	—	104	26	—
1886	612	95	21	43[c]
1887	398	—	—	—
1888	—	62	17	—
1889	—	54	10	—

Total Graduated: 1,007

Source: "Memórias históricas dos acontecimentos mais notáveis ocorridos na Faculdade de Medicina da Bahia, 1868–1884," in Brazil, Ministério do Império, *Relatórios ministeriais,*

Época do Império (1832–88); reels 1–21; *Gazeta Médica da Bahia* (1866–90). There are small discrepancies in figures given in the two sources.

[a] Includes those returning from Paraguayan War.

[b] Does not include 78 students from Rio de Janeiro who transferred to Bahia after a conflict with the Rio Medical School.

[c] This figure is for graduate doctors only.

Table 2. Numbers of Students at the Rio De Janeiro Medical School 1867–89

Year	Matriculated	Medical graduates	Pharmacy graduates
1867	272	19	11
1868	358	16	19
1869	305	31	30
1870	435	44	—
1871	467	56	33
1872	470	50	18
1873	503	93	23
1874	502	53	30
1875	492	70	27
1876	481	75	15
1877	519	63	15
1878	530	67	20
1879	497	104	20
1880	587	86	19
1881	626	66	39
1882	911	62	35
1883	1,012	78	25
1884	1,145	101	31
1885	306	106	40
1886	783	91	25
1887	560	126	26
1888	437	77	52
1889	—	—	—

Total Graduated: 1,534

Total in Brazil: 2,541

Source: "Memórias históricas dos acontecimentos mais notáveis ocorridos na Faculdade de Medicina do Rio de Janeiro," in Brazil, Ministério do Império, *Relatórios ministeriais,* Época do Império (1832–88), reels 1–21.

Table 3. Movement of Patients at the Santa Casa da Misericórdia Hospital 1843–78

Year	Entry		Died		Cured		Remained	
1843	1,669		316		1,148		161	
1846–47	1,642		329					
1852–53	1,561		400		1,195		191	
1853–54	1,916		349		1,335		232	
1856–57	1,605		307		1,113		185	
1866–67	1,973		410		1,352		210	
[1860–68	15,051[a]		3,425[b]]					
1873–74	2,648	1,768[m] 880[f]	600	335[m] 265[f]	2,044	1,423[m] 621[f]	218	130[m] 88[f]
1874–75	2,442		480		1,940		272	
1875–76	2,761		607		2,205		221	
1876–77	2,691	2,000[m] 691[f]	533	319[m] 214[f]	2,099	1,640[m] 459[f]	280	172[m] 108[f]
1877–78	3,058		619		2,419		300	

Source: Brazil, *Relatórios da Província da Bahia*, Época do Império (1832–88); reels 1–18; *Gazeta Médica da Bahia* (1866–90).
[a] Annual average for 1860–68: 1881.
[b] Annual average deaths for 1860–68: 428.
m = male; f = female

The Making of the Tropicalistas:
Institutional Base

Core Tropicalistas

Antônio José Pereira da Silva Araújo (1853–1900)

Manoel Maria Pires Caldas (b. 1818)

Ramiro Affonso Monteiro de Carvalho (1839–1902)

Paulino Peres da Costa Chastinet (d. 1887)

José Luís D'Almeida Couto (1833–1895)

Virgílio Clímaco Damázio (1838–1913)

José Francisco da Silva Lima (1826–1910)

Joaquim dos Remédios Monteiro (1827–1901)

John L. Paterson (1820–1882)

Antônio Pacífico Pereira (1846–1922)

Manoel Victorino Pereira (1853–1902)

Demétrio Ciríaco Tourinho (1826–1888)

Otto H. Wucherer (1820–1875)

Second-Generation Tropicalistas

Braz H. do Amaral (1861–1949)

Alfredo Tomé de Britto (1863–1909)

Ezequiel Cândido de Souza Britto (1860–1922)

Antônio Pacheco Mendes (1856–1941)

Deoclesiano Ramos (n.d.)

Raimundo Nina Rodrigues (1862–1906)

Domingos Pedro dos Santos (n.d.)

---

* These are second-generation Tropicalistas; most of their articles were written after 1889.

** Not from Bahia but published in the *Gazeta Médica da Bahia*.

Tropicalista Supporters

Antônio José Alves (1818–1866)
Augusto Freire Maia Bittencourt (1847–1890)
Antônio Mariano do Bonfim (1825–1875)
Antônio Januário de Faria (also called Farias) (1822–1883)
Ludgero Ferreira (d. 1867)
José Antônio de Freitas (1825–1894)
Luís Adriano Alves de Lima Gordilho, Barão de Itapoan (1830–1892)
Thomas Wright Hall (1831–1911)
Pedro Severiano de Magalhães (1850–1927)
João Baptista Bueno de Mamoré (n.d.) **
José Affonso Paraíso de Moura (1822–1898)
Júlio Rodrigues de Moura (1839–1892) **
Alexander Paterson (nephew of John) (n.d.)
Francisco dos Santos Pereira (1844–1912)
Jerônymo Sodré Pereira (1840–1900)
Luís Álvares dos Santos (1825–1886)

*Physicians Who Participated in Meetings That Led to Founding
of the* Gazeta Médica *and the School*

Jonattas Abbot (1796–1868)
Antônio José Alves
Antônio José Pereira da Silva Araújo
Augusto Freire Maia Bittencourt
Antônio Mariano do Bonfim
Manoel Maria Pires Caldas
Ramiro Affonso Monteiro
José Luís D'Almeida Couto
Antônio Januário de Faria
Ludgero Ferreira
A. Garcia (n.d.)
Thomas Wright Hall
José Francisco da Silva Lima
A. Almeida Marques (n.d.)
Santos Paiva (n.d.)
John L. Paterson
Antônio Pacífico Pereira
Manoel Victorino Pereira
Otto H. Wucherer

Editors of Gazeta Médica

Antônio José Pereira da Silva Araújo
Ezequiel Cândido de Souza Britto
Manoel Maria Pires Caldas
Ramiro Affonso Monteiro de Carvalho
Paulino Pires da Costa Chastinet
José Luís D'Almeida Couto
Virgílio Clímaco Damázio
Antônio Januário de Faria
José Francisco da Silva Lima
Antônio Pacheco Mendes
Joaquim dos Remédios Monteiro
Antônio Pacífico Pereira
Manoel Victorino Pereira
Luís Álvares dos Santos
Demétrio Ciríaco Tourinho
Raimundo Nina Rodrigues

Doctors Publishing Two or More Articles in Gazeta Médica *up to 1889*

J. M. Aguiar 2 (n.d.)
Braz H. do Amaral 3 *
Antônio José Pereira da Silva Araújo 16
Antônio Mariano do Bonfim 5
Alfredo Tomé de Britto 1 *
Manoel Maria Pires Caldas 27
José Luís D'Almeida Couto 3
Antônio Januário de Faria 2
José Antônio de Freitas 9 (1825–1894)
Rosendo Aprígio Pereira de Guimarães (1826–1907) 5
Thomas Wright Hall 2
José Francisco da Silva Lima 53
José Lourenço Magalhães 8 (b. 1831)
Pedro Severiano de Magalhães 12
João Baptista Bueno de Mamoré 7 **
Antônio Pacheco Mendes 3 *
Joaquim dos Remédios Monteiro 15
Affonso José Paraíso de Moura 6
Júlio Rodrigues de Moura 10 **
Alexander Paterson 3
John L. Paterson 19

Antônio Pacífico Pereira 38
Francisco dos Santos Pereira 2
Jerônymo Sodré Pereira 2
Manoel Victorino Pereira 7
Deoclesiano Ramos 3 *
Raimundo Nina Rodrigues 4 *
Domingos Pedro dos Santos 5 *
José Goes Siqueira (1817–1874) 3
Demétrio Ciríaco Tourinho 5
Otto H. Wucherer 10

Doctors Who Worked at the Santa Casa Hospital

Antônio José Alves
C. de Andrade (n.d.)
Antônio José Pereira da Silva Araújo
Augusto Freire Maia Bittencourt
Alfredo Tomé de Britto
Ezequiel Cândido de Souza Britto
Manoel Maria Pires Caldas
Ramiro Affonso Monteiro
H. César (n.d.)
Paulino Pires da Costa Chastinet
José Luís D'Almeida Couto
Antônio Januârio de Faria
E. M. Ferreira (n.d.)
José Antônio de Freitas
Luís Adriano Alves de Lima Gordilho, Barão de Itapoan
José Francisco da Silva Lima
Affonso José Paraíso de Moura
Ignácio d'Oliveira (n.d.)
Alexander Paterson
John L. Paterson
Antônio Pacífico Pereira
Francisco dos Santos Pereira
Manoel Victorino Pereira
Raimundo Nina Rodrigues
Francisco Rodrigues Silva (1831–1886)
Otto H. Wucherer

Doctors Who Observed or Cooperated with Each Other
on Cases at the Santa Casa

Antônio José Alves
Braz H. do Amaral
Augusto Freire Maia Bittencourt
Manoel Maria Pires Caldas
Ramiro Affonso Monteiro de Carvalho
E. M. Ferreira
José Antônio de Freitas
Luís Adriano Alves de Lima Gordilho, Barão de Itapoan
José Francisco da Silva Lima
Domingos Alves de Mello (n.d.)
Joaquim dos Remédios Monteiro
Affonso José Paraíso de Moura
Ignácio d'Oliveira
Alexander Paterson
John L. Paterson
Antônio Pacífico Pereira
Francisco Santos Pereira
Manoel Victorino Pereira
José Goes Siqueira
José Teixeira (n.d.)
Affonso Vianna (n.d.)
Otto H. Wucherer

Members of the Doctors' and Pharmacists' Mutual Aid Society

Alves de Abreu (pharmacist) (n.d.)
J. M. Aguiar
Augusto Freire Maia Bittencourt
Antônio Mariano do Bonfim
Euclides E. Pires Caldas (n.d.)
Anísio Circundes de Carvalho (b. 1855)
Ramiro Affonso Monteiro de Carvalho
Paulino Pires da Costa Chastinet
José Luís D'Almeida Couto
J. Cunha (pharmacist) (n.d.)
Virgílio Clímaco Damázio
M. Devoto (n.d.)
Sátiro Oliveira Dias (1844–1913)
A. Diniz (n.d.)

Antônio Januário de Faria
Luís Adriano Alves de Lima Gordilho, Barão de Itapoan
José Francisco da Silva Lima
C. Machado (n.d.)
Vicente Ferreira de Magalhães (1799–1877)
Souza Marques (n.d.)
Domingos Alves de Mello
Affonso José Paraíso de Moura
Ignácio d'Oliveira
John L. Paterson
Antônio Pacífico Pereira
Francisco dos Santos Pereira
A. Cerqueira Pinto (1820–1895)
J. J. Ribeiro (n.d.)
C. Ferreira Santos (n.d.)
Cardoso Silva (n.d.)
M. D'Assis Souza (n.d.)
Otto H. Wucherer

*Tropicalista (Core or Supporters) Bahian Medical School
Faculty Between 1868 and 1889*

Ramiro Affonso Monteiro de Carvalho
José Luís D'Almeida Couto
Virgílio Clímaco Damázio
Antônio Januário de Faria
José Antônio de Freitas (1825–1894)
Luís Adriano Alves de Lima Gordilho, Barão de Itapoan
José Affonso Paraíso de Moura
Antônio Pacífico Pereira
Jerônymo Sodré Pereira
Manoel Victorino Pereira
Luís Álvares dos Santos
Demétrio Ciríaco Tourinho

Sources: *Gazeta Médica da Bahia;* Ordival Cassiano Gomes, *Manoel Victorino Pereira: Médico e cirurgião* (Rio de Janeiro: Agir, 1957), 53. Lycurgo Santos Filho, *História geral da medicina brasileira,* 2 vols. São Paulo: Hucitec, 1991.

Numbers of Practicing Doctors in Bahia

How many practicing doctors were there in Bahia in the second half of the nineteenth century? This question is difficult to answer with certainty because, although we have annual figures for the numbers of graduating doctors, many doctors used their degree to enter careers in the civil service, journalism, or politics. Other medical graduates returned to their provincial places of origin to practice. However, it is possible to arrive at some estimates.

The *Gazeta Médica* noted in the 1880s that France, Germany, Austria, Norway, and England had doctor/population ratios varying between 1,350 and 1,500 people for every one doctor.[1] According to the journal, the United States had a far higher doctor/patient ratio, of 1 doctor for every 600 inhabitants; Russia was at the other extreme, with 1 doctor per 6,200.[2] In the nineteenth century Russia was clearly not a model of progress and it is likely that the low number of doctors in that country was seen as a sign of its backwardness. Yet, the *Gazeta Médica* did not view the United States's high number of doctors as a sign of that country's advancement but of U.S. laxity in the accreditation of medical schools that led to a proliferation of bogus or unqualified doctors. This complaint was raised many times in the journal, accompanied by warnings against U.S. men posing as doctors in Brazil.[3] It is also probable that the Western European ratio was comparable to what existed in the main Brazilian cities. Certainly the doctors never voiced a desire that fewer men be trained as doctors. Even during the debates over ensino livre that led to a sharp increase in the production of doctors, few voices were raised against the increase. Rather, doctors demanded that Brazilians turn

[1] For some doctor/population ratios, see *Gazeta Médica* 8 (1876): 44; 16 (1885): 506; 18 (1886): 426.
[2] *Gazeta Médica* 18 (1886): 426.
[3] For critique of U.S. medical schools, see *Gazeta Médica*, 11 (1879): 260–261.

more to "allopathic" medicine instead of various folk medicines and homeopathic remedies (which the emperor favored) and that more doctors be willing to practice in the countryside. They also asked that statistics be compiled in order to know exactly what the doctor/patient ratio was in Brazil.

Taking the country as a whole, Brazil's doctor/population ratio was much closer to the Russian than the Western European one throughout most of the nineteenth century. In 1888, even if all the doctors who had graduated between 1866 and 1888 had actually practiced, the doctor/population ratio would have been approximately 1 to 5,600. However, in the cities, the doctor/population ratio was much lower because so many professionals wanted to remain in the urban areas.[4] A ratio closer to the European one would give the following figures for practicing physicians in Bahia:

Year	Population	Doctors	
		Ratio of 1:1,500	Ratio of 1:1,000
1872	129,000 [a]	86	129
1890	174,000 [a]	116	174
	144,000 [b]	96	144

[a] Emília Viotti da Costa, *The Brazilian Empire: Myths and Histories* (Chicago: University of Chicago Press, 1985).
[b] Kátia M. de Queirós Mattoso, *Bahia: A Cidade do Salvador e seu mercado no século XIX* (São Paulo: Hucitee, 1977).

It is likely that the doctor/population ratio in Bahia remained relatively stable between 1860 and 1890, for even as more doctors were graduating, the population of Bahia increased through natural growth and provincial migration into the city. However, competition among the doctors must have become harsher for there is no reason to suppose that the number of people turning to Western medicine increased proportionally to the rise in population. Moreover, the increase in population was occurring among the poorer people. This offered the doctors a greater pool of patients to "experiment" on but there was probably more competition for the paying patient. The pool of paying patients was relatively inelastic and this would account for the growing numbers of complaints in the *Gazeta Médica* about the unethical practices of some doctors in Bahia and for demands that standard fees be charged by all doctors.

4 See, for example, the complaint to this effect by the Bahian health inspector Goes Siqueira in Brazil, *Relatórios da Província da Bahia,* Época do Império, reel 9, annex (1869), 8–9; and reel 10 (1870), 17–18.

NOTES

Introduction

1   "Western" medicine, a shorthand term used by historians of medicine, refers to the tradition that emerged over centuries, through the work mainly of literate men, in Western Europe, Germany, Austria, and Italy. In this book it refers especially to nineteenth-century French, British, German, and Austrian medicine and surgery. I use "school" loosely. This school did not have official backing and thus it did not have the sort of institutional base of the first European tropical schools founded at the turn of the century. It did, however, create its own institutional base, from whence its members carried out their research and taught. On the school, see Antônio Caldas Coni, *A Escola Tropicalista Bahiana: Paterson, Wucherer, Silva Lima* (Salvador: Typ. Beneditina, 1952); Edgard de Cerqueira Falção, *As contribuições originais da "Escola Tropicalista Bahiana* (Centro de Estudos Bahianos, Universidade Federal da Bahia, 1976); Carlos Roberto Oliveira, "Medicina e estado: Origem e desenvolvimento da medicina social no Brasil, Bahia, 1866–1896" (master's thesis, Universidade do Estado do Rio de Janeiro, 1982); Julyan G. Peard, "Tropical Medicine in Nineteenth-Century Brazil: The Case of the 'Escola Tropicalista Bahiana,' 1860–1890," in *Warm Climates and Western Medicine: The Emergence of Tropical Medicine, 1500–1900,* ed. David Arnold (Amsterdam: Rodopi, 1996), 108–32; Peard, "Tropical Disorders and the Forging of a Brazilian Medical Identity, 1860–1890," *Hispanic American Historical Review* 77 (1997); 1–44; Madel T. Luz, *Medicina e ordem política brasileira: Políticas e instituições de saúde, 1850–1930* (Rio de Janeiro: Graal, 1982), 139–164; Pedro Motta de Barros, "Alvorecer de uma nova ciência: A medicina tropicalista bahiana," *História, Ciências, Saúde Manguinhos* 4, no. 3 (1997): 411–59.

2   By institutionalized tropical medicine I mean "a discipline with its own journals, institutions, qualifications, and an exclusive discourse [that] did not emerge until the last decade of the nineteenth century, and partly in response to metropolitan

imperatives." Mark Harrison, "Tropical Medicine in Nineteenth-Century India," *British Journal for the History of Science* 25 (1992): 299.

3   For discussion on the recent shift in the history of medicine and public health in Latin America, see Marcos Cueto, "Introducción," in *Salud, cultura y sociedad en América Latina: Nuevas perspectivas históricas,* ed. Cueto (Lima: Instituto de Estudios Peruanos, 1996), 13–30; Nancy Leys Stepan, "Tropical Medicine and Public Health in Latin America," *Medical History* 42 (1998): 104–112.

4   I use "metropolitan" medicine as synonymous with European, Western, and, after 1910, U.S. medicine. For the purposes of this book I justify this very general label because Brazilians, like other Latin Americans, imported ideas eclectically, often interweaving strands of theories that may originally have come from opposing sides of a debate. For a discussion on how to define Western medicine, see Arthur Kleinman, "What Is Specific to Western Medicine?" in *Companion Encyclopedia of the History of Medicine,* ed. W. F. Bynum and Roy Porter (London: Routledge, 1994), 15–23.

5   Recent works on the history of medicine and public health for Latin America in the national period include Jaime L. Benchimol, "Domingos José Freire e os primórdios da bacteriologia no Brasil," *História, Ciências, Saúde, Manguinhos* 2, 1 (1995): 67–98; Jaime L. Benchimol and Luiz Antônio Teixeira, *Cobras, lagartos e outros bichos: Uma história comparada dos Institutos Oswaldo Cruz e Butantan* (Rio de Janeiro: Universidade Federal do Rio de Janeiro, 1993); Benchimol, *Manguinhos do sonho à vida: A ciência na belle époque* (Rio de Janeiro: FIOCRUZ, 1990); Benchimol, "Do Pasteur dos micróbios ao Pasteur dos mosquitos: Febre amarela no Rio de Janeiro, 1880–1903" (Ph.D. dissertation, Universidade Federal Fluminense, 1996); Sidney Chalhoub, *Cidade febril: Cortiços e epidemias na corte imperial* (São Paulo: Companhia das Letras, 1996); Nancy Leys Stepan, *Beginnings of Brazilian Science: Oswaldo Cruz, Medical Research, and Policy, 1890–1920* (New York: Science History Publications, 1981); Stepan, *"The Hour of Eugenics": Race, Gender, and Nation in Latin America* (Ithaca: Cornell University Press, 1991); Stepan, "Initiation and Survival of Medical Research in a Developing Country: The Oswaldo Cruz Institute of Brazil, 1900–1920," *Journal of the History of Medicine and Allied Sciences* 30 (1975): 303–325; Stepan, "The Interplay between Socio-Economic Factors and Medical Science: Yellow Fever Research, Cuba, and the United States," *Social Studies of Science* 8 (1978): 397–423; Marcos Cueto, "Excellence in the Periphery: Scientific Activities and Biomedical Sciences in Peru" (Ph.D. dissertation, Columbia University, 1988); Cueto, "The Rockefeller Foundation's Medical Policy and Scientific Research in Latin America: The Case of Physiology," *Social Studies of Science* 20 (1990): 229–254; Cueto, ed., *Missionaries of Science: The Rockefeller Foundation and Latin America* (Bloomington: Indiana University Press, 1994); Cueto, "Sanitation from Above: Yellow Fever and Foreign Intervention in Peru, 1919–1922," *Hispanic American Historical Review* 72 (1992): 1–22; Cueto, "Science under Adversity: Latin Ameri-

can Medical Research and American Private Philanthropy, 1920–1960," *Minerva* 35 (1997); 233–245; Luiz Antônio de Castro Santos, "Power, Ideology, and Public Health in Brazil, 1889–1930" (Ph.D. dissertation, Harvard University, 1987); Santos, "A reforma sanitária pelo alto: O pionerismo paulista no início do século XX," *Dados* 36 (1993): 361–392; Santos, "O pensamento sanitarista na Primeira República: Uma ideologia de construcção da nacionalidade," *Dados* 28 (1985): 193–210; Nara Britto, *Oswaldo Cruz: A construção de um mito na ciência brasileira* (Rio de Janeiro: FIOCRUZ, 1995); Nísia Trinidade Lima and Gilberto Hochman, "Descobrindo a nação, construindo o estado: O movimento pela reforma de saúde pública no Brasil da Primeira República" (paper presented at the 1995 meeting of the Latin American Studies Association, Washington, D.C., September 28–30); Robin L. Anderson, "Public Health and Public Healthiness, São Paulo, Brazil, 1876–1893," *Journal of the History of Medicine* 41, 3 (July 1986): 293–307; Sam C. Adamo, "The Broken Promise: Race, Health, and Justice in Rio de Janeiro, 1890–1940" (Ph.D. dissertation, University of New Mexico, 1983); Ilana Lowry, "Yellow Fever in Rio de Janeiro and the Pasteur Institute Mission (1901–1905): The Transfer of Science to the Periphery," *Medical History* 34 (1990): 144–163; Donald B. Cooper, "Brazil's Long Fight against Epidemic Disease, 1849–1917, with Special Emphasis on Yellow Fever," *Bulletin of the New York Academy of Medicine* 51, 5 (1975): 672–696; D. Cooper, "The New 'Black Death': Cholera in Brazil, 1855–56," *Social Science History* 10 (winter 1986): 467–488; Teresa Meade and Mark Walker, eds., *Science, Medicine, and Cultural Imperialism* (New York: St. Martin's, 1991); Kenneth F. Kiple, "Cholera and Race in the Caribbean," *Journal of Latin American Studies* 17 (1985); 157–177; Jeffrey D. Needell, "The *Revolta Contra Vacina* of 1904: The Revolt against Modernization in 'Belle Époque' Rio de Janeiro," *Hispanic American Historical Review* 67, (1987): 233–270; James D. Goodyear, "Agents of Empire: Portuguese Doctors in Colonial Brazil and the Idea of Tropical Disease" (Ph.D. dissertation, Johns Hopkins University, 1982).

6 Some important recent contributions include Warwick Anderson, "Immunities of Empire: Race, Disease, and the New Tropical Medicine, 1900–1920," *Bulletin of the History of Medicine* 70 (1996): 94–118; Mark Harrison, " 'The Tender Frame of Man': Disease, Climate, and Racial Difference in India and the West Indies, 1760–1860," *Bulletin of the History of Medicine* 70 (1996): 68–93; Michael Worboys, "The Emergence of Tropical Medicine: A Study of the Establishment of a Scientific Speciality," in *Perspectives on the Emergence of Scientific Disciplines,* ed. G. Lemaine et al. (The Hague: Mouton, 1976), 75–98; Worboys, "The Emergence and Early Development of Parasitology," *Parasitology: A Global Perspective,* ed. Kenneth S. Warren and John Z. Bowers (New York: Springer-Verlag, 1983), 1–18; Worboys, "Tropical Diseases," in *Companion Encyclopedia of the History of Medicine* 1 ed. Bynum and Porter, 512–536; David Arnold, ed., *Imperial Medicine and Indigenous Societies* (Manchester: Manchester University Press, 1987);

Arnold, *Colonizing the Body: State Medicine and Epidemic Disease in Nineteenth-Century India* (Berkeley: University of California Press, 1993); R. MacLeod and M. Lewis, eds., *Disease, Medicine, and Empire* (London: Routledge, 1988); John Farley, *Bilharzia: A History of Imperial Tropical Medicine* (Cambridge: Cambridge University Press, 1991); Maryinez Lyons, *The Colonial Disease: A Social History of Sleeping Sickness in Northern Zaire, 1900–1940* (Cambridge: Cambridge University Press, 1992); Mark Harrison, *Public Health in British India: Anglo-Indian Preventive Medicine, 1859–1914* (Cambridge: Cambridge University Press, 1994); Philip D. Curtin, *Death by Migration: Europe's Encounter with the Tropical World in the Nineteenth Century* (Cambridge: Cambridge University Press, 1989), and his older but still important *Image of Africa: British Ideas and Actions, 1780–1850* (Madison: University of Wisconsin Press, 1964); Martin F. Shapiro, "Medicine in the Service of Colonialism: Medical Care in Portuguese Africa, 1885–1974" (Ph.D. dissertation, University of California at Los Angeles, 1983).

7   Patrick Manson, "Tropical Medicine and Hygiene," *British Medical Journal* 2 (July 1917): 103.

8   On defining tropical medicine, see David J. Bradley, "Tropical Medicine," in *The Oxford Companion to Medicine,* ed. John Walton, Paul B. Beeson, and Ronald Bodley Scott (Oxford: Oxford University Press, 1986), 1393.

9   Some have called this "pre-Mansonian" tropical medicine.

10   M. Yoeli calls the period from 1890 to 1912 the "Age of Discovery." See "The Evolution of Tropical Medicine: A Historical Perspective," *Bulletin of the New York Academy of Medicine* 48 (1972): 1237–1238.

11   H. Harold Scott, *A History of Tropical Medicine,* 2 vols. (Baltimore: Williams and Wilkins, 1939); M. Gelfand, *Tropical Victory: An Account of the Influence of Medicine on the History of Southern Rhodesia, 1890–1923* (Cape Town: Juto, 1953); Yoeli, "Evolution of Tropical Medicine," 1231–1246. Many, of course, stayed home and investigated in their laboratories, but all recognized that the advancement of tropical medicine depended on investigators in the field.

12   For some cogent statements on this approach, see Elizabeth Fee and Daniel M. Fox, "Introduction: AIDS, Public Policy, and Historical Inquiry," and Charles E. Rosenberg, "Disease and Social Order in America: Perceptions and Expectations," in *AIDS: The Burdens of History,* ed. Fee and Fox, (Berkeley: University of California Press, 1988) 1–11, 12–32; Judith Walzer Leavitt, "Medicine in Context: A Review Essay on the History of Medicine," *American Historical Review* 95 (1990): 1471–1484; Karl Figlio, "The Historiography of Scientific Medicine: An Invitation to the Human Sciences," *Comparative Studies in Society and History* 19 (1977), 262–86; Everett Mendelsohn, "The Social Construction of Scientific Knowledge," in *The Social Production of Scientific Knowledge,* ed. Everett Mendelsohn, Peter Weingart, and Richard Whitley (Dordrecht: D. Reidel, 1977), 1:3–26: For recent assessments of the social construction approach to the history of medicine, see Charles E. Rosenberg, "Disease in History: Frames and Framers,"

Millbank Quarterly 67 (1989): 1–15; Ludmilla J. Jordanova, "The Social Construction of Medical Knowledge," *Social History of Medicine* 7, 3 (1995): 361–381.

13 For example, Sheldon Watts, *Epidemics and History: Disease, Power, and Imperialism* (London: Yale University Press, 1997); Maynard W. Swanson, "The Sanitation Syndrome: Bubonic Plague and Urnad Policy in the Cape Colony, 1900–1909," *Journal of African History* 13, 3 (1977): 387–410; John W. Cell, "Anglo-Indian Medical Theory and the Origins of Segregation in West Africa," *American Historical Review* 91 (1986): 307–335; Philip D. Curtin, "Medical Knowledge and Urban Planning in Tropical Africa," *American Historical Review* 90 (1985): 594–613; Vicente Navarro, ed., *Imperialism, Health, and Medicine* (Farmingdale: Baywood, 1981).

14 See, for example, Maryinez Lyons, "Sleeping Sickness Epidemics and Public Health in Belgian Congo," in *Imperial Medicine and Indigenous Societies,* ed. Arnold 105–124; Farley, *Bilharzia,* 298–302.

15 See, for example, Harrison, *Public Health in British India;* and Arnold, *Colonizing the Body.*

16 There is a large literature on the subject. Seminal works include Edward Said's *Orientalism* (New York: Vintage, 1979), and the essays in Ranajit Guha and Gayatri Chakravorty Spivak, eds., *Selected Subaltern Studies* (New York, 1988). See also Gyan Prakash, *After Colonialism: Imperial Histories and Postcolonial Displacements* (Princeton: Princeton University Press, 1995) and Prakash, "AHR Forum: Subaltern Studies as Postcolonial Criticism," *American Historical Review* 99, no. 5 (1994): 1475–1490; Gayatri Chakravorty Spivak, *In Other Worlds: Essays in Cultural Politics* (New York: Methuen, 1987); Anne McClintock, *Imperial Leather: Race, Gender, and Sexuality in the Colonial Contest* (New York: Routledge, 1995); Inderpal Grewal, *Home and Harem: Nation, Gender, Empire, and the Cultures of Travel* (Durham: Duke University Press, 1996). For Latin American works following this approach, see the next note. On nations and nationalism, see E. J. Hobsbawm, *Nations and Nationalism since 1870: Programme, Myth, Reality* (Cambridge: Cambridge University Press, 1990); E. J. Hobsbawm and Terence Ranger, *The Invention of Tradition* (Cambridge: Cambridge University Press, 1983); Benedict Anderson, *Imagined Communities: Reflections on the Origin and Spread of Nationalism* (London: Verso, 1990).

17 For such writings on Latin America, see Mary Louise Pratt, *Imperial Eyes: Travel Writing and Transculturation* (London: Routledge, 1992); Patricia Seed, "Colonial and Postcolonial Discourse," *Latin American Research Review* 26 (1991): 181–200; Michael Taussig, *Shamanism, Colonialism, and the Wild Man: A Study in Terror and Healing* (Chicago: University of Chicago Press, 1987); Jean Franco, *Plotting Women: Gender and Representation in Mexico* (New York: Columbia University Press, 1989); Florencia Mallon, "AHR Forum: The Promise and Dilemma of Subaltern Studies: Perspectives from Latin American History," *American Historical Review* 99, no. 5 (1994): 1491–1515, and n. 1, where Mallon gives

a small bibliography of Latin American scholars associated with the subaltern studies approach; Mallon, *Peasant and Nation: The Making of Postcolonial Mexico and Peru* (Berkeley: University of California Press, 1994); Frederick Cooper et al., *Confronting Historical Paradigms: Peasants, Labor, and the Capitalist World System in Africa and Latin America* (Madison: University of Wisconsin Press, 1993). Recent studies in colonial Latin America have focused on understanding the "interior architecture" of the perceived meanings and understandings resulting from unequal conquest and colonial relationships.

18   The nineteenth-century Brazilian elite's sense of wanting to be both like Europeans and different from them has been much analyzed by Brazilian scholars. See, for example, Thomas E. Skidmore, *Black into White: Race and Nationality in Brazilian Thought* (New York: Oxford University Press, 1974), 3–77; and chap. 3 n. 21. Less looked at is what doctors had to say on these issues.

19   There are, of course, classic attempts in Latin American literature to draw such cleavages. For example, Domingo Faustino Sarmiento, *La civilización o la barbarie;* see also E. Bradford Burns, *The Poverty of Progress: Latin America in the Nineteenth Century* (Berkeley: University of California Press, 1980). But equally strong was the more malleable approach that Stepan discusses in "*The Hour of Eugenics.*"

20   John Lynch, *The Spanish-American Revolutions, 1808–1826* (New York: Norton, 1973); Leslie Bethell, "The Independence of Brazil," in *Brazil: Empire and Republic, 1822–1930,* ed. Bethell (Cambridge: Cambridge University Press, 1989), 3–44; Emília Viotti da Costa, *The Brazilian Empire: Myths and Histories* (Chicago: University of Chicago Press, 1985), esp. the essay "Independence: The Building of a Nation" 1–23. Brazil, in contrast to all the other Latin American countries (with the brief exception of Mexico), retained the monarchy, calling itself an empire. The institution remained until 1889, when a military coup abolished the monarchy and set up the First Republic.

21   In Spanish America the equivalent of *mazombo* (the child of Iberians born in America) was Creole.

22   The Spanish American countries that retained slavery were Cuba and Puerto Rico, which remained Spanish colonies. By the 1820s most of the Spanish American mainland nations had initiated a process of freeing slaves through the "free-womb" laws. Thus slavery dwindled, ending for many of these nations by the 1850s, by which time the numbers of slaves were small. See Herbert S. Klein, *African Slavery in Latin America and the Caribbean* (New York: Oxford University Press, 1986), 250–252.

23   Actually, the question of whether the United States was an appropriate model for slavery and progress was debated with much vigor. See, for example, the texts in the Congresso Agrícola, *Collecção de documentos* (Rio de Janeiro: Typ. Nacional, 1878).

24 Chap. 3 deals with ideas on whitening and the improvement of the racial stock in some detail.

25 I use B. Anderson's phrase, *Imagined Communities* 70.

26 By then not only doctors asserted this but all sectors of the elite believed—and debated—it. See, for example, Afonso Celso's "Porque me ufano do meu país" (Why I Am Proud of my Country). Skidmore, *Black into White*, 100, discusses this poem. Another, more complex example of an "optimistic" position is Sílvio Romero's "História da literatura brasileira" (1888), in Skidmore, *Black into White*, 32–37, 55–56.

27 For examples of the new work, see the bibliographies in the articles by Cueto and Stepan cited in n. 3.

28 See Thomas E. Skidmore, "Studying the History of Latin America: A Case of Hemispheric Convergence," *Latin American Research Review* 33 (1998): 105–127; Charles Gibson, "Latin America and the Americas," in *The Past before Us,* ed. Michael Kammen, (Ithaca: Cornell Univeristy Press, 1982), 187–204; William Taylor, "Between Global Process and Local Knowledge: An Inquiry into Early Latin American Social History, 1500–1900," in *Reliving the Past: The Worlds of Social History,* ed. Oliver Zunz (Chapel Hill: University of North Carolina Press, 1985), 115–190; Tulio Halperin Donghi, "The State of Latin American History," in *Changing Perspectives in Latin American Studies: Insights from Six Disciplines,* ed. Christopher Mitchell, 13–62 (Stanford: Stanford University Press, 1988).

29 Steve J. Stern, "Feudalism, Capitalism and the World System in the Perspective of Latin America and the Caribbean," *American Historical Review* 93 (1988): 829–872; Tulio Halperin Donghi, "'Dependency Theory' and Latin American Historiography," *Latin American Research Review* 17 (1982): 115–132.

30 Stuart B. Schwartz, "Somebodies and Nobodies in the Body Politic: Mentalities and Social Structures in Colonial Brazil," *Latin American Research Review* 31 (1996): 114; Brooke Larson, "Shifting Views of Colonialism and Resistance," *Radical History Review* 27 (1983): 3–20. Both refer specifically to scholarship on colonial Latin America but their remarks can be extrapolated for later periods. See also Skidmore, "Studying the History of Latin America."

Chapter One The Escola Tropicalista Bahiana: A Creative Response in Adversity

1 For colonial education and cultural and educational reforms introduced during the Portuguese Crown's stay in Brazil, see Fernando de Azevedo, *Brazilian Culture: An Introduction to the Study of Culture in Brazil,* trans. William Rex Crawford (New York: MacMillan, 1950), 165–178, 370–374; Robert J. Havighurst and J. Roberto Moreira, *Society and Education in Brazil* (Pittsburgh: University of Pittsburgh Press, 1965), 36–66; Maria do Carmo Tavares de Miranda, *Educação no Brasil: Esboço de estudo histórico* (Recife: Imprensa Universitária, 1966), 13–44; Sérgio Buarque de Holanda and Boris Fausto, eds. *História da civilização brasi-*

leira: O Brasil monárquico (São Paulo: Difusão Européia do Livro, 1971), Part 3: 467–489, Part 4: 366–384; Octávio Torres, *Esboço histórico dos acontecimentos mais importantes da vida da Faculdade de Medicina da Bahia, 1808–1946* (Salvador: Vitória, 1952), 10–12; Eduardo de S. Oliveira, *Memória histórica da Faculdade de Medicina da Bahia* (Bahia: EDUFBA, 1982); Lycurgo Santos Filho, *História geral da medicina brasileira,* 2 vols. (São Paulo: Hucitec, 1991). For an introduction to medical education in Latin America, see John Z. Bowers and Elizabeth F. Purcell, eds., *Aspects of the History of Medicine in Latin America* (New York: Josiah Macy Jr. Foundation, 1979), 124–131; and Agueda María Rodríguez Cruz, *Historia de las universidades hispanoamericanas: Período hispánico,* 2 vols. (Bogotá: Instituto Caro y Cuervo, 1973). See also Ronald L. Numbers, ed., *Medicine in the New World: New Spain, New France, and New England* (Knoxville: University of Tennessee Press, 1987).

2   Before that time, Brazil had no community of doctors trained in Western medicine in that country. In more than three centuries of colonial history only about one hundred European-trained physicians had served in Brazil, either as personal physicians to high-ranking civil servants or as part of the imperial bureaucracy. Most of the health care in colonial society, therefore, was provided by religious orders, low-ranking barber-surgeons, apothecaries, midwives, and faith healers. Even after the creation of the medical schools, the colonial tradition of health care remained paramount so that, for the vast majority of Brazilians, there was no great improvement in health care. James D. Goodyear, "Agents of Empire: Portuguese Doctors in Colonial Brazil and the Idea of Tropical Disease" (Ph.D. dissertation, Johns Hopkins University, 1982), esp. chap. 4, "Portuguese Physicians and Colonial Curers"; Santos Filho, *História geral,* 2: 432–444; Dain Edward Borges, *The Family in Bahia, Brazil, 1870–1945* (Stanford: Stanford University Press, 1992), 94.

3   "Empiricism" was the term used to refer to folk healing learned directly through practice rather than formally in medical schools.

4   The Paris medical school, the most influential in Western medicine in the first half of the nineteenth century, was where "the clinical approach based on bedside observations and postmortem findings" first emerged. See Günter B. Risse, "History of Western Medicine from Hippocrates to Germ Theory," in *The Cambridge World History of Human Disease,* ed., Kenneth F. Kiple (Cambridge: Cambridge University Press, 1993), 17. However, more Brazilians studied at Montpellier than at the Paris school. See Santos Filho, *História geral,* 2: 164–167, 168–171. On Brazilian independence, see Emília Viotti da Costa, *The Brazilian Empire: Myths and Histories* (Chicago: University of Chicago Press, 1985), esp. the essays "Independence: The Building of a Nation," 1–23, and "José Bonifácio de Andrada e Silva: A Brazilian Founding Father," 24–52; A. J. R. Russell-Wood, ed., *From Colony to Nation: Essays on the Independence of Brazil* (Baltimore: Johns Hopkins University Press, 1975); Francisco Adolfo de Varnahagen, *História da indepen-*

dência do Brasil (Rio de Janeiro: Imprensa Nacional, 1940); Roderick J. Barman, *Brazil: The Forging of a Nation, 1798–1852* (Stanford: Stanford University Press, 1988); Alan K. Manchester, "The Growth of Bureaucracy in Brazil, 1808–1821," *Journal of Latin American Studies* 4, (1972): 77–83. For independence in Salvador, Luís Henrique Dias Tavares, *A independência do Brasil na Bahia* (Salvador: Civilização Brasileira, 1982).

5   The Regency was the period between Pedro I's abdication in 1831 and the crowning of his son as Emperor Pedro II at age fourteen in 1840.

6   For medical education under the Empire, see Primitivo Moacyr, *A instrucção e o Império: Subsídios para a história da educação no Império, 1854–1889,* 3 vols. (São Paulo: Companhia Editora Nacional, 1938), 2: 145–212; Lycurgo Santos Filho, *História da medicina no Brasil: Do século XIV as século XIX* 2 vols. (São Paulo: Brasiliense, 1947), 1: 167–291; Nancy Leys Stepan, *Beginnings of Brazilian Science: Oswaldo Cruz, Medical Research, and Policy, 1890–1920* (New York: Science History Publications, 1981), 47–65; Simon Schwartzman, *Formação da comunidade científica no Brasil* (São Paulo: Companhia Editora Nacional, 1979); Roque Spencer Maciel de Barros, *A ilustração brasileira e a idéia de universidade* (São Paulo: Universidad de São Paulo, 1959); Gilberto Freyre, *Order and Progress: Brazil from Monarchy to Republic,* trans. Rod W. Horton (Berkeley: University of California Press, 1986), 103–165; see also various sections of F. Azevedo, *Brazilian Culture,* and Havioghurst and Moreira, *Society and Education.* For contemporary writings, see Manoel José de Araújo, "Breve notícia sobre a fundação e marcha do ensino médico na Bahia," *Gazeta médica da Bahia* 10 (1877): 506–514; Braz H. do Amaral, "O centenario do Ensino Médico no Brasil," *Gazeta Médica* 14 (1882): 146–147; Luiz Couty, "O ensino superior no Brasil," *Gazeta Médica* 15 (1884): 521–532; "O ensino médico no Brasil," *Revista do Instituto Geográfico e Histórico da Bahia* 15, 34 (1908): 47–51; Antônio Pacífico Pereira, *Memória sobre a medicina na Bahia* (Salvador: Imprensa Oficial do Estado, 1923).

7   For example, in 1857 Antônio José Alves, one of the early Tropicalista supporters, noted ironically: "The 1854 reform, instead of improving [medical] teaching, has, for the most part, brought us promises that four years later, have still not been fulfilled. It promised us practical teaching and it has given us theoretical professors; instead of laboratories, it has provided us with employees; instead of instruments and appliances, it has provided us with notebooks to keep a record of students' punctuation errors." Quoted by Ordival Cassiano Gomes, *Manuel Vitorino Pereira: Médico e cirurgião* (Rio de Janeiro: Agir, 1957), 35. For a fuller account of the reform, see Flávio Coelho Edler, "As reformas do ensino médico e a profissionalização da medicina na corte do Rio de Janeiro, 1854–1884" (master's thesis, Universidade de São Paulo, 1992).

8   In 1887 the minister of the Empire invalidated the outcome of a competition for a faculty post in the Bahian medical school on the grounds that it was insufficient to prove the candidate's competence. He ordered a new competition

to select another candidate. See S. R. "A Faculdade de Medicina da Bahia e o Ministrado Imperio," *Gazeta médica* 18 (1887): 529–532. The first issue of the *Gazeta Médica* came out on July 10, 1866. The journal appeared every fortnight and was numbered consecutively until it reached volume 7, issue number 168, in July 1874. The journal suffered some interruptions in publication, but the longest break came between 1874 and 1876 when it closed for eighteen months. It started up again in January 1876 and then it appeared once a month. This was volume 8, issue number 1. In 1880 there was another break and then it recommenced publication in July 1880 with volume 12, issue number 1. This is why volume numbers often span two years. There were also errors made in the numbering of the journal. For example, volume 12 (August 1880) is issue number 2. But the following issue, volume 12, number 3, is also dated August 1880; volume 14 runs for only six months, from July to December, issues 1–6. Volume 15 runs for eighteen months: from January 1883 to June 1883 with issues 7 through 12; and then from July 1883 to June 1884 with issues 1 through 12. Because this numbering was confusing I decided to use only volume number, year, and page numbers.

For an example of the central government's intervention on minute matters in the organization of the medical schools, see the decree issued in 1883 on the exact time a competition should take a candidate and what steps to take if the candidate took more or less time; "Noticiário," *Gazeta médica* 15 (1883): 424; Moacyr, *Instrução*, 145–212, has a long section on some of the many decrees passed.

9   Araújo, "Breve notícia," 510.

10 Joseph-F.-X. Sigaud, *Du climat et des maladies du Bresil; ou statistique medicale de cet empire* (Paris: Fortin, Masson, 1844).

11 See tables 1 and 2.

12 Robert Dundas, *Sketches of Brazil; Including New Views on Tropical and European Fever* (London: John Churchill, 1852), 389. Emphasis in the original. For other contemporary accounts of Brazilian medicine, see L. Papillaud, "Etat de la médecine du Brésil; condition des médecins," *Gazette Médicale de Paris* 3, 2 (1847): 215–223; J. McF. Gaston, "Brazil in Its Relation to Medicine," *Gaillard's Medical Journal of New York* 32 (1881): 289–294.

13 In 1881 another foreign observer, Dr. Gaston, noted, "The personal and professional relations of Brazilian doctors are often bad and they display their animosities in the press." See "Brazil in Its Relation to Medicine," 291. Barman, *Brazil,* 238, discusses competition in relation to law graduates. On the importance of patronage in nineteenth-century Brazil for success in almost any field, see E. Costa, *Brazilian Empire,* 188–190, 196–197, 243, and 277 n. 21, where she gives a small bibliography on the subject. See also Richard Graham, *Patronage and Politics in Nineteenth-Century Brazil* (Stanford: Stanford University Press, 1990).

14 R. de G. Daunt, "On the Status of the Physician in Brazil," *Medical Times and Gazette* 1 (1871): 439.

15 Santos Filho, *História da medicina*, 2: 376–378. The one physician who became a baron in Salvador was Lima Gordilho, named Barão de Itapoan in 1872. A good example of the sort of frustration Bahian doctors felt is given by a rather bitter obituary notice that appeared in the *Gazeta Médica* in 1885: noting the death of a Dr. Luiz Carlos da Fonseca in Rio de Janeiro and giving his biographical details, the obituary commented, "[In accounting for] his election as a senator, it is perhaps not irrelevant that he was also a member of the Emperor's council of doctors, because there was nothing in his political life that made him in any way more exceptional than [the others] who made up the electoral list. . . . Bereft of talent, but greatly favored by partisan politics, Dr. Luiz Carlos da Fonseca managed to accede to a position that many other men, recognized for their talent and services, have not been able to achieve in this country of nepotism [*filhotismo*] and godparenthood [*compadrismo*]." *Gazeta Médica* 18 (1885): 574.

16 For example, one of Dundas's close associates in Salvador, Dr. José Lino Coutinho, "who sprung from the humblest origin," was in 1819 "a simple physician absorbed in the duties of his profession." After independence he was elected deputy to the general legislative assembly in Rio de Janeiro, later nominated to the Senate. Dundas, *Sketches*, 392.

17 Barman observes, "Because of the superior economic, social, and cultural opportunities it offered, Rio de Janeiro city acted as a magnet, attracting from the provinces anyone of talent, thus reinforcing its hegemony over the nation." *Brazil*, 219. On a visit to the Bahian medical school in 1859, Pedro II made scathing remarks about some of the professors. Of the professor of general and anatomical pathology, he noted, "What I heard was really bad." Of the physiology professor, "Less than mediocre." Of the hygiene professor, "Seemed to have learned his talk off by heart." Of the botany professor, "Diffuse and verbose." The emperor did praise some of the faculty. Santos Filho, *História geral*, 2: 147–148. See also Santos Filho, *História da medicina*, 1: 272–273; Schwartzman, *Formação da comunidade*, 79–80. Among the doctors who were Tropicalistas or close to them and who moved to Rio de Janeiro between 1866 and 1889 were Silva Araújo, member of a very wealth family, and Pedro S. de Magalhães, who came from a more humble background.

18 On the importance of law graduates for supplying the pool of civil servants and politicians, see Roderick J. Barman and Jean Barman, "The Role of the Law Graduate in the Political Elite of Imperial Brazil," *Journal of Inter-American Studies and World Affairs* 18, 4 (November 1976): 423–450; José Murilo de Carvalho, *A construção da ordem: A elite política imperial* (Rio de Janeiro: Campus, 1980); Carvalho, "Political Elites and State Building: The Case of Nineteenth-Century Brazil," *Comparative Studies in Society and History* 24 (1982): 378–399.

19 Gomes, *M. V. Pereira*, 29. Richard Graham, in *Britain and the Onset of Modernization in Brazil, 1850–1914* (Cambridge: Cambridge University Press, 1968), 16, notes how the sons of Portuguese immigrants sought to difference themselves

from their fathers' humble background by entering one of the institutions of higher learning.

20   Manoel Victorino Pereira is better known for his political activities than his medical ones. He became vice president of the Republic in the 1890s in the administration of Prudente José de Morais (1891–94), against whom he later conspired. In pre-Republic days he was one of the leaders of the Liberal Party in Salvador and an active abolitionist. See Gomes, *M. V. Pereira*, 179–250; Luís Henrique Dias Tavares, *História da Bahia* (São Paulo: Ática, 1973), 164–166; June E. Hahner, *Civilian-Military Relations in Brazil, 1889–1898* (Columbia: University of South Carolina Press, 1969), 149–182. On Magalhães, see Renato Clark Bacellar, *Brazil's Contribution to Tropical Medicine and Malaria: Personalities and Institutions* (Rio de Janeiro: Olímpica, 1963), 74. After the three founders of the Tropicalista school, Antônio Pacífico Pereira was undoubtedly its most important and influential member, becoming head of the medical school (1895–98) and director of public health after the fall of the Empire. Santos Filho, *História geral*, 152–153, vol. 2; Luiz Anselmo de Fonseca, *Gazeta Médica* 30 (1898): 215–227, 251–260, 300–312, 346–353.

21   Gilberto Freyre, *The Mansions and the Shanties: The Making of Modern Brazil*, trans. Harriet de Onis (Berkeley: University of California Press, 1986), 355–358, 367–368.

22   Thomas E. Skidmore, *Black into White: Race and Nationality in Brazilian Thought* (New York: Oxford University Press, 1974), 23; Freyre, *Order and Progress*, 166–197.

23   The situation was repeated in Rio de Janeiro, where, for example, Torres Homem, the most renowned physician in the capital in the 1870s and 1880s, was mulatto. Some have questioned whether Nina Rodrigues was indeed mulatto. See chap. 3 n. 111.

24   Freyre, *Order and Progress*, 121. Despite the conservative tradition regarding medical education, politically there were always radical voices among Bahian doctors, as can be seen in the rebellions of the 1820s and 1830s when some of the most radical participants were doctors.

25   According to Torres, *Esboço histórico*, Antônio José Alves was the first professor to introduce the microscope to his students; see the caption under his picture, no page number. Alves was one of the early Tropicalista supporters who died soon after the group formed. The systematic use of the microscope was certainly a result of Wucherer's efforts.

26   German medicine did, of course, become influential in Rio de Janeiro too. Thus by the 1880s, Billroth (who practiced mainly in Austria) is listed as an honorary member of the Imperial Academy of Medicine in Rio de Janeiro. But the Tropicalistas' interest in German medicine developed earlier. One of the reasons for the longer influence of French medicine in the capital city was that there were many more French doctors practicing there.

27   On the epidemics, see Sidney Chalhoub, *Cidade febril: Cortiços e epidemias na corte imperial* (São Paulo: Companhia das Letras, 1996); Chalhoub, "The Politics of Disease Control: Yellow Fever and Race in Nineteenth-Century Rio de Janeiro," *Journal of Latin American Studies* 25 (1993): 441–463; Donald B. Cooper, "Brazil's Long Fight against Epidemic Disease, 1849–1917, with Special Emphasis on Yellow Fever," *Bulletin of the New York Academy of Medicine* 51, 5 (1975): 672–696; D. Cooper; "The New 'Black Death': Cholera in Brazil, 1855–56," *Social Science History* (winter 1986): 467–488. Cooper includes Silva Lima as one of the foreign doctors who opposed local ones. I have found no evidence that he was involved in the episode and it seems unlikely for he graduated only in 1851. For Salvador specifically, see David Onildo Reis, "O inimigo invisível: A epidemia do cólera na Bahia, (1855–1856)" (master's thesis, Universidade Federal da Bahia, 1994); Anna Amélia Vieira Nascimento, "A 'cholera morbus' como fator de involução populacional da cidade de Salvador," *Anais do Arquivo do Estado da Bahia* 45 (1981): 263–289; Kátia M. de Queirós Mattoso and M. Johildo de Athayde, "Epidemias e fluctuações de preços na Bahia no século XIX," In *Collóque international sur l'histoire quantitative du Brésil de 1800 a 1930,* ed. Frederic Mauro, Colloques Internationaux du Centre Nacional de la Recherche Scientifique, no. 543 (Paris: Editions du Centre Nationalde la Recherche Scientifique, 1973), 185 n. 3; and for contemporary reports, José Francisco da Silva Lima, "O Dr. Paterson, sua vida e sua morte: Esboço biográphico," *Gazeta Médica* 18 (1887): 337–344, 385–394, 433–439, 481–492; "Falla ao Presidente da Província da Bahia, Álvaro Tibério de Moncorvo e Lima," in Brazil, *Relatórios da Província da Bahia,* reel 3 (May 1856), 5–15, and appendix relating to health by Malaquias Álvares dos Santos.

28   Antônio Caldas Coni, *A Escola Tropicalista Bahiana: Paterson, Wucherer, Silva Lima* (Salvador: Progresso, 1952), 43, says: "Paterson and Wucherer . . . held . . . that the disorder was produced by a virus (Fracastorian concept) whose mechanism of transmission was still unknown. Rejecting the doctrine of atmospheric effluvia, they forecast, as contagionists, that the epidemic 'would follow the most frequent and rapid trade routes and not the winds.'" See also Erwin H. Ackerknecht, "Anticontagionism between 1821 and 1867," *Bulletin of the History of Medicine* 22 (1948): 574. The Council of Health is a good example of the way in which the early generation of doctors in Brazil sought to replicate French medical institutions in Brazil. As in France, the council, founded in 1838, was a public health advisory board. Twelve men sat on the council, most of them physicians. For a list of the men on the council, see *Gazeta Médica,* 10 (1878): 480. For an analysis of the Parisian council, see Ann F. La Berge, "The Paris Health Council, 1802–1848," *Bulletin of the History of Medicine* 49 (1975): 339–352.

29   Coni, *Escola Tropicalista,* 42.

30   Appendix on health in Brazil, *Relatórios da Província da Bahia,* reel 3 (May 1856), 2.

31   Nascimento, "'Cholera morbus,'" 265–266; D. Cooper, "New 'Black Death,'"

471. Although there is no direct evidence that the issue of contagionism was raised on this occasion, it is very probable that it was one of the points of contention. According to Ackerknecht, the belief in anticontagionism and cholera began to lose its hold in the third great cholera pandemic of 1852–55 and generally dropped in the fourth pandemic of 1865–67. See his "Anticontagionism," 581–582. However, in the health report presented after the cholera epidemic in Salvador, it is clear that the source of the disease was viewed not as a result of contagion but as a result of a "miasma" from overcrowding, filth, dampness, and faulty drainage.

32 "A nova organisação do serviço sanitário," *Gazeta Médica* 17 (1886): 392. For the 1882 reforms to the sanitation system, see "Hygiene pública," *Gazeta Médica* 13 (1882): 436–439, 477–485. Some members of the council were impressed by the acuity of the foreign doctors and later supported the Tropicalistas; among these were Luís Álvares dos Santos, Virgílio Clímaco Damázio, Antônio Januário de Faria, and Vicente Ferreira de Magalhães.

33 For example, they served on commissions for the inspection of ships regarding beriberi (see "Beriberi no esquadrilla de evoluções," *Gazeta Médica* 15 (1883): 1); and on another to find out about beriberi in the province of Salvador (1878); "Commissoes medicas para o estudo do beriberi," *Gazeta Médica* 11 [1879]: 526. Silva Lima also served on a commission formed in 1873 because of a yellow fever epidemic (Brazil, *Relatórios da Província da Bahia,* reel 12 [1873], 16), and on another for smallpox vaccination in 1883 (reel 17 [1883–85], 11). In 1892 Silva Lima became president of a newly created council of public health in Bahia.

34 This was true, too, for many local doctors who stayed in the city to help with the crises. See Nascimento, "'Cholera morbus,'" 275. Santos Filho, *História da medicina,* 1:278, gives the names of some local doctors; Santos Filho, *História geral,* 2: 210, refers to Antônio José Alves turning his home into a hospital.

35 Chalhoub, "Politics of Disease Control," 443–446, shows how strong the arguments in favor of miasmatic approaches were. For medical theories of a later period, see Jaime L. Benchimol, *Manguinhos do sonho à vida: A ciência na belle époque* (Rio de Janeiro: FIOCRUZ, 1990), 5–22; Jaime L. Benchimol and Luiz Antônio Teixeira, *Cobras, lagartos e outros bichos: Uma história comparada dos Institutos Oswaldo Cruz e Butantan* (Rio de Janeiro: Universidade Federal do Rio de Janeiro, 1993); Benchimol, "Domingos José Freire y los comienzos de la bacteriología en Brasil," in *Salud, Cultura y Sociedad en América Latina,* ed. Marcos Cueto, Lima: Instituto Estudios Peruanos, 1996, 53–86. Dr. D. Rodrigues de Seixas, one of the leaders in the 1855 effort to combat the cholera epidemic, wrote about it in 1860 and stated that his experience with the disorder had convinced him that it was not contagious. See Nascimento, "'Cholera morbus,'" 272. For a different view, see D. Cooper, "New 'Black Death,'" 484, who holds that anticontagionist beliefs were dropped by doctors in Brazil as a result of the two epidemics. For changing ideas regarding etiology, see Erwin H. Ackerknecht,

"Hygiene in France, 1815–1848," *Bulletin of the History of Medicine* 22 (1948): 117–155; Ann F. La Berge, *Mission and Method: The Early-Nineteenth-Century French Public Health Movement* (Cambridge: Cambridge University Press, 1992). On miasma, see Caroline Hannaway, "Environment and Miasmata," in *Companion Encyclopedia of the History of Medicine*, ed. W. F. Bynum and Roy Porter (London: Routledge, 1994), 292–308.

36 On Wucherer's bibliography, see Antônio Pacífico Pereira, "Esboço biográfico do Dr. Wucherer," *Gazeta Médica* 6 (1873): 305–309; Julio de Moura, "Dr. Otto Wucherer," *União Médica* 1 (1881): 178–179, 226–228.

37 Erwin H. Ackerknecht, *A Short History of Medicine* (New York: Ronald, 1955), 157. For changes in clinical medicine around midcentury, see Kenneth D. Keele, "Clinical Medicine in the 1860s," in *Medicine and Science in the 1860s*, ed. F. N. L. Poynter (London: Wellcome Institute for the History of Medicine, 1968), 1–11; for a discussion of German medical schools and ideas from this period, see Thomas Neville Bonner, *Becoming a Physician: Medical Education in Britain, France, Germany, and the United States, 1750–1945* (New York: Oxford University Press, 1995); Timoth Lenoir, *Laboratories, Medicine, and Public Life in Germany, 1830–1849: Ideological Roots of the Institutional Revolution* (Cambridge: Cambridge University Press, 1992); Erwin H. Ackerknecht, *Rudolf Virchow: Doctor, Statesman, Anthropologist* (Madison: University of Wisconsin Press, 1953).

38 Ackerknecht, *Virchow*, 46. In a sense the Tropicalistas' "hygienism," like that of the Germans, continued the older French and British medicine and its insistence on the relationship between poverty and disease, but like the Germans, who tried to work out exactly how poverty led to disease, the Tropicalistas investigated how poverty and conditions *in the tropics* led to disease. Wucherer's links to German circles can be seen in the articles he published in Germany. He was published or cited in *Archiv für pathologische Anatomie und Physiologie und für klinische Medecin* (also known as *Virchow's Archives*), *Deutsches Archiv für Klinische Medicin, Zeitschr. für Parasitenkunde,* and August Hirsch's *Handbook of Geographical and Historical Pathology* (1883). See also Carlos Roberto Oliveira, "Medicina e estado: Origem e desenvolvimento da medicina social no Brasil, Bahia, 1866–1896" (master's thesis, Universidade do Estado do Rio de Janeiro, 1982), 192–202.

39 Bacellar, *Brazil's Contribution,* 61–73; for a slightly different version of Wucherer's early life, see the bibliographical article on Wucherer in Julio de Moura, "Dr. Otto Wucherer," *União Médica* 1 (1881): 178–179, 226–228. Despite a steady economic decline from mid–nineteenth century on, the city of Salvador remained a thriving commercial city throughout the Empire era and was home to several communities of foreign merchants, the most important of whom were the British, the German, and the Portuguese, with their own hospitals and cemeteries. The estimates for the numbers of foreigners living in Salvador vary greatly but since there is no definition of whether the figures include Africans and Portuguese, they are not very helpful. See Moema Parente Augel, *Visitantes estrangeiros*

na Bahia oitocentista (São Paulo: Cultrix, 1980), 196 n. 80. For the importance of the German community in Salvador, which was prominent in several economic enterprises, especially tobacco, see Frederico G. Edelweiss, "A secular presença da Alemanha na Bahia," *Anais do Arquivo do Estado da Bahia* 39 (1970): 223–242; and Otto Quelle, "A Actuação germânica no Estado da Bahia," *Revista do Instituto Geográphico e Histórico da Bahia* 59 (1933). On German influence in northern Brazil and mainly in Pernambuco, see Gilberto Freyre, *Nós e a Europa germânica: Em torno de alguns aspectos das relacões do Brasil com a cultura germânica no decorrer do século XIX* (Rio de Janeiro: Grifo, 1971).

40   For Wucherer's herpetology, see O. Wucherer, "Sobre a mordedura das cobras venenosas e seu tratamento," *Gazeta Médica* I (1867): 229–232, 241–243; and "Sobre o modo de conhecer as cobras venenosas do Brasil," *Gazeta Médica* I (1867): 193–196. For his work on hookworm and filariasis, see chap. 2.

41   This was, of course, an axiom in the rise of public health, for which there is a large literature. George Rosen, *A History of Public Health,* expanded ed., introduction by Elizabeth Fee (Baltimore: Johns Hopkins University Press, 1993), remains a classic. See also Ackerknecht, "Hygiene in France," and M. W. Flinn, ed., *Report on the Sanitary Condition of the Laboring Population of Great Britain* by Edwin Chadwick, 1842 (Edinburgh: University of Edinburgh Press, 1965), esp. Flinn's "Introduction."

42   For my account of Paterson's life and work, as well as the secondary sources cited above for the history of the Tropicalistas, I have drawn mainly on an article by Paterson's friend and colleague Silva Lima, "O Dr. Paterson."

43   When he was buried, a mass of poor people insisted on carrying his coffin, thus paying a Bahian homage to the doctor. *Gazeta Médica,* 14 (1882): 245.

44   Some earlier medical and literary journals launched by the members of the medical school in Salvador were *O Ateneu* (1849), *O Acadêmico* (1853), *O Prisma* (1853), and *Revista Acadêmica* (1864). They all lasted between one and two years. Attempts to found privately financed journals from the 1870s on were not any more successful. See Santos Filho, *História da medicina* 1: 264–270.

45   Just how much of a turning point can be gauged by an article Paterson wrote in 1867 before his meeting with Lister and while still in Salvador. He described an operation he had performed during which the patient had died of septic fever. He wrote that the fact that his patient had contracted septic fever at the same time he had been operated on was pure coincidence. The fever, Paterson asserted, had been caught from the "miasm" of a slaughterhouse near the patient's home. In 1869, before his trip to Scotland, Paterson helped his nephew, Alexander, who had recently graduated from the University of Edinburgh, to perform an operation during which they used carbolic acid according to a new theory of antisepsis, a theory that the young physician had learned about in Scotland. John Paterson was therefore aware of the method, if not yet of its momentous implications,

before he made Lister's acquaintance. "Caso de febre séptica rapidamente fatal," *Gazeta Médica* 2 (1867): 17–18.

46 "A medicina no Brasil," *Quarto Congresso Médico Latino Americano* (Rio de Janeiro: Imprensa Nacional, 1909), 66. Silva Lima was profoundly affected by his encounter with Wucherer and Paterson. This can be seen from the fact that his graduating dissertation of 1851 followed the line of French vitalism, exactly the sort of medical approach the Tropicalistas later gave as an example of what was outdated about Bahian medicine. See Coni, *Escola Tropicalista*, 36.

47 Kenneth Kiple, ed., *Cambridge World History of Human Disease* (Cambridge: Cambridge University Press, 1993), 561.

48 See "O Dr. Silva Lima," *Gazeta Médica* 41 (1910): 337–357; "O jubileo do Dr. Silva Lima," *Gazeta Médica* 33 (1901): 247–252. For the Doctors' and Pharmacists' Mutual Aid Society, see, for example, "Sociedade Médico-Pharmacêutica de Beneficência mútua," *Gazeta Médica* 17 (1885): 193–196; for the Bahian Medical Society, see "Sociedade Médica de Salvador," *Gazeta Médica,* 19 (1888): 433–438; *Gázeta Médica* 25 (1894): 186–187; Madel T. Luz, *Medicina e ordem política brasileira: Políticas e instituições de saúde, 1850–1930* (Rio de Janeiro: Graal, 1982), 152; C. Oliveira, "Medicina e estado," 175–259.

49 In his work on the Tropicalistas, Caldas Coni dwells mainly on the contributions of Wucherer, Paterson, and Silva Lima, though he also mentions some of their most prominent followers, such as Antônio Pacífico Pereira, Demétrio Ciríaco Tourinho, José Luís D'Almeida Couto, and Manoel Victorino Pereira. But Coni gives little indication of the size of the school.

50 Silva Lima, "O Dr. Paterson," 389.

51 See appendix 1 for the lists of names.

52 Hall graduated from the University of Edinburgh in 1853, after which he worked for a time in Salvador as well as in Pará and his native Maranhão. After Paterson's death, he became the main doctor to the British community, according to Silva Lima. "O Dr. Paterson," 341. See Santos Filho, *História Geral* 2: 167. On the usefulness of prosopographical analyses for the history of science, see Lewis Pyenson, "'Who the Guys Were': Prosopography in the History of Science," *History of Science* 15 (1977): 155–188.

53 The following core or supporter Tropicalistas made trips to Europe, although there may well have been more: Faria (1873), Moura (1873), Silva Lima (1854, 1858, 1870, 1875, 1881), Damázio (1875), Luís Alvares dos Santos (1873), Sodré Pereira (1873), Victorino Pereira (1879–81), Pacífico Pereira (1871, 1877), Carvalho (1889), Mendes (1880).

54 This is a tentative figure. See appendix 2.

55 One of the two men was Antônio José Alves, father of the poet Castro Alves, who held a chair in external clinical medicine. He was one of the best-known surgeons in Salvador and held an appointment at the Santa Casa charity hospital.

The other was Antônio Januário de Faria, who held a chair in internal clinical medicine and was also on the staff at the Santa Casa. The relationship between the Tropicalistas and the medical school is the subject of chap. 5.

56   On the Santa Casa de Misericórdia Brotherhood, see A. J. R. Russell-Wood, *Fidalgos and Philanthropists: The Santa Casa de Misericórdia of Bahia, 1550–1755* (Berkeley: University of California Press, 1968); Carlos Ott, *A Santa Casa de Misericórdia da cidade do Salvador* (Rio de Janeiro: *Diretoria do Patrimônio Histórico e Artístico Nacional* 1960); Joaquim dos Remédios Monteiro, "A Santa Casa de Misericórdia," *Gazeta Médica* 11 (1879): 474–482. The *Relatórios da Província da Bahia*, reels 1–18 (1823–1888), also include an annual report on the Santa Casa and its business.

57   Remédios Monteiro, "a Santa Casa," 478.

58   The other charity hospitals were the Santa Casa of Cachoeira, of S. Amaro, of Maragogipe, of Nazareth, and of S. Pedro in the village of Barra. The numbers of patients they had, respectively, in 1853 were 324, 617, 19, 106, and 79.

59   This had been the site of the military hospital installed in 1759 after the expulsion of the Jesuits. The Santa Casa's finances must also have been impacted by a law passed in 1860 authorizing the chartering of associations and mutual aid societies. Many former sponsors of brotherhoods like the Santa Casa de Misericórdia now turned to these secular groups. See Borges, *Family*, 161.

60   Brazil, *Relatórios da Província da Bahia*, reel 2 (March 1853), 17–21.

61   On the rise of the hospital in the nineteenth century, see Charles Rosenberg, *The Care of Strangers: The Rise of America's Hospital System* (New York: Basic, 1987); Judith Walzer Leavitt and Ronald L. Numbers, eds., *Sickness and Health: Readings in the History of Medicine and Public Health* (Madison: University of Wisconsin Press, 1985), esp. articles in "Institutions" section, 273–312; Michel Foucault, *The Birth of the Clinic* (New York: Vintage, 1975); Paul Starr, *The Social Transformation of American Medicine* (New York: Basic, 1982), 145–179; Lindsay Granshaw, "The Hospital," *Companion Encyclopedia of the History of Medicine* ed. Bynum and Porter, 1180–1203.

62   Brazil, *Relatórios da Província da Bahia*, reel 9 (March 1868), 73–74.

63   The space for women in labor was still inadequate and in 1877 a new ward was under construction. See Brazil, *Relatórios da Província da Bahia*, reel 14 (1877), 28. The insane asylum was called Asylo dos Alienados de São João de Deos and was headed by Demétrio Ciríaco Tourinho. In 1877 the asylum had 145 patients. *Gazeta Médica* 9 (1877): 82; Joaquim dos Remédios Monteiro, "Asylo dos Alienados de São João de Deus," *Gazeta Médica* 12 (1880): 205–214, 262–271; Pedro Salles, *História da medicina no Brasil* (Belo Horizonte: G. Holman, 1971), 128–130. See also Robert M. Levine, "The Singular Brazilian City of Salvador," *Luso-Brazilian Review* 30, 2 (1993): 60.

64   E. Costa states that the population of Salvador at the end of the eighteenth century was close to 45,000. In 1872 the population was 129,109 and by 1890 had

grown to 205,813; *Brazilian Empire,* 173, 199. Kátia M. de Queirós Mattoso's figures are 45,600 for 1805; 108,138 for 1872; and 144,959 for 1890; *Bahia: A cidade do Salvador e seu mercado no século XIX* (São Paulo: Hucitec, 1977), 135–137. Borges gives 130,000 for the population of the city of Salvador in 1772. From the 1840s to the end of the 1860s the average number of patients entering the hospital per year was in the order of 1,700 patients, but from the 1870s through the following decade the average jumped to 2,600. See table 3 on the breakdown of the annual entries. Two reasons for the increase in numbers, given by Dr. Remédios Monteiro, were the rise in the city's population and its growing poverty. See "Santa Casa," 474–482. Another reason must certainly have been the repeated droughts in the arid *serão,* which sent many people sick through malnutrition into the city of Salvador and the Misericórdia Hospital. On the drought, see Gerald Michael Greenfield, "The Great Drought and Elite Discourse in Imperial Brazil," *Hispanic American Historical Review* 72 (1992): 375–400.

65 See "Os beribericos do hospital de caridade," *Gazeta Médica* 11 (1879): 91; "O novo hospital da Misericórdia," *Gazeta Médica* 17 (1886): 337–341. In 1882 a commission was appointed to reform the regulations of the Santa Casa; it included Victorino Pereira, Almeida Couto, Pacífico Pereira, and Pires Caldas. See "Santa Casa," *Gazeta Médica* 13 (1882): 136.

66 *Relatórios da Província da Bahia,* reel 13 (May 1876), 60. In 1879 Monteiro, "Santa Casa," 481, had a less positive assessment of the hospital, noting that there was a severe space problem, especially since poverty had increased and there were more people going to the Santa Casa for help.

67 In 1872 a news item stated that the appointees would receive no remuneration. See *Gazeta Médica* 5 (1872): 80. In 1879 they were to receive the paltry sum of 50$000 mil-réis per month; *Gazeta Médica* 11 (1879): 476. As a point of comparison, in 1886 a provincial inspector of hygiene received 2,400$000, and the inspector general in Rio de Janeiro 6,000$000. See *Gazeta Médica* 18 (1886): 279. Arnold Thackray has some suggestive remarks on the importance of the infirmary in eighteenth-century provincial Manchester for the advancement of careers and status of physicians. See "Natural Knowledge in Cultural Context: The Manchester Model," *American Historical Review* 79 (1974): 672–709; Jack Morrell and Arnold Thackray, *Gentlemen of Science: Early Years of the British Association for the Advancement of Science* (Oxford: Clarendon, 1981).

68 In 1879 the intern was Dr. Ignácio d'Oliveira, and the Tropicalistas with appointments were Silva Lima, Almeida Couto, Pires Caldas, Faria, Bittencourt, Affonso José P. de Moura, and the Barão de Itapoan. For a description of the Rio de Janeiro Santa Casa hospital, see Thomas B. Peacock, "Brief Notes on a Voyage to Brazil," *Lancet* (July 17, 1880): 88–89.

69 The chairs that included practical instruction at the Santa Casa hospital were external clinical medicine, internal clinical medicine, and childbirth and the disorders of pregnant women and children. In 1883 seven new chairs in clinical medi-

cine were created to carry out practical instruction in the hospitals and infirmaries of Salvador. The imperial government, however, took a long time to implement these reforms and to actually fill the new posts. See "Os últimos decretos para as faculdades de medicina," *Gazeta Médica* 15 (1883): 302–304.

70   All Santa Casa hospitals traditionally made use of the physicians in the vicinity. The situation in Salvador was somewhat different from those of other towns and cities where there was no medical school and thus fewer doctors available. In Salvador being well connected either through patronage or to doctors already appointed was indispensable.

71   See appendix 1.

72   However, even charity patients exercised quite a lot of control: they often decided whether to allow operations on themselves, and often checked out against the doctor's wishes.

73   For an example of the sort of dilemma progressive doctors found themselves in, see the case of the Tropicalista supporter Pedro S. Magalhães, who was experimenting with glycerin as a cure for the disorders that filariasis caused, and noted that he had been unable to ascertain whether the results obtained from many of the patients in his private practice had been due to glycerin, for "great as the desire of a doctor to see through the action of a medication, he cannot forget his responsibility toward the health of his fellow-being and, *especially in private practice,* he is forced to use several methods at the same time in order to get the fastest cure possible." See "Aplicações da glicerina contra esta helmintiasi," *Gazeta Médica* 13 (1881): 111. My emphasis.

74   Of thirty-eight cases involving surgery reported by Pires Caldas, Silva Lima, Pacífico Pereira, Paterson, and Victorino Pereira in the *Gazeta Médica* between 1866 and 1888, thirty dealt with patients from the lower classes; four were from the middle or upper classes; four were unclear. I have defined the lower classes according to color, occupation, and place attended. Although in Salvador there were members of the upper class who were mulatto, because of the code of silence on race (a theme E. Costa explores in her "Myth of Racial Democracy," *Brazilian Empire,* 234–246) it is unlikely any doctor would have recorded this for the upper class. On the use of poor patients for experimentation, see João Baptista Bueno de Mamoré, "Novas tentativas para a cura da elefantíase dos gregos: Ensaios sobre o tratamento do Dr. Beauperthuy no Hospício de Tucunduba (Pará)," *Gazeta Médica* 8 (1876): 411–417.

75   This theme is further explored in chap. 4.

76   Antônio Pacífico Pereira, "Aos médicos deputados," *Gazeta Médica* 9 (1877): 437. Also Pacífico Pereira, "Memória histórica dos acontecimentos mais notáveis na Faculdade de Medicina da Bahia no anno 1882," in Brazil, Ministério do Império, *Relatórios ministeriais,* Época do Império, reel 19 (1832–88), 43–44.

77   See A. Pacifico Pereira, "Estudo sobre a etiologia e natureza do beriberi," *Gazeta Médica* 12 (1881): 455.

78 *Gazeta Médica* 1 (1866): 27.
79 For an account of Wucherer's ideas on tuberculosis in Brazil, see chap. 3. Subsequent articles on these disorders by other Tropicalistas include Antônio Pacífico Pereira, "Contágio da lepra: Investigações histológicas e bacteriológicas que demonstram sua natureza parasitária," *Gazeta Médica* 19 (1887): 527–541; 20 (1888): 1–10, 51–60, 99–104, 149–156, 245–253; see also his "Colônias agrícolas para morféticos," *Gazeta Médica* (1885): 1–6; Raimundo Nina Rodrigues, "Contribuição para o estudo da lepra na província do Maranhão, "*Gazeta Médica* 20 (1888): 105–113, 205–211, 301–314, 358–368, 404–409; 21 (1889): 121–132, 225–234, 255–265. On tuberculosis, see two cases that Victorino Pereira treated in 1889, *Gazeta Médica* 20 (1889): 512–516; and "Osteo-artrite tuberculosa do joelho com supuração e dose fístulas, resecção completa, união perfeita dos ossos," *Gazeta Médica* 20 (1889): 443–451. See also "Congresso para o estudo de tuberculose," 20 (1888): 133–141, 186–190, 227–236; (1889): 414–425, 467–476, 524–527, 567–572; 21 (1889): 27–33.
80 A. Paterson, "Excisáo parcial da maxila inferior," *Gazeta Médica* 3 (1869): 280. Alexander Paterson was a student in Edinburgh at the time that Lister had a chair at the University of Glasgow and Lister's father-in-law, James Syme, was at the University of Edinburgh. Lister wrote his first article on his pioneering antiseptic method in surgery in the *Lancet* in 1867.
81 Dr. Vicente Sabóia from Rio de Janeiro also met Lister on a trip to Scotland in 1871 and it is after this date that Rio de Janeiro is usually credited with the introduction of antisepsis. See Luís da Cunha Feijó, Visconde de Santa Isabel, "Memória histórica da Faculdade de Medicina do Rio de Janeiro" for 1879, in Brazil, Ministério do Império, *Relatórios ministeriais,* Época do Império, 1880, reel 17.
82 See, for example, John Paterson, "Sobre a fístula do ânus," *Gazeta Médica* 8 (1876): 262–263; Affonso José Paraiso de Moura, "Estreitamento fibroso do recto: Cirurgia e cura," *Gazeta Médica* 9 (1877): 352–357. In the 1880s references to antiseptic measures were common. By then the need for antiseptic or aseptic measures was not in question. What there was still disagreement about, reflecting the European debates over the matter, was the best means to obtain aseptic conditions. Thus Dr. Moura used alcohol and phenic acid. Others argued for the advantages of carbolic acid as an antiseptic agent. See *Primeiro Congresso Brazileiro de Medicina e Cirurgia do Rio de Janeiro* (Rio de Janeiro: Imprensa Nacional, 1889): 86–90; and José Francisco da Silva Lima, "Anesthesia local," *Gazeta Médica* 1 (1866): 25–27, 49–51. In his biography on Victorino Pereira, Ordival Cassiano Gomes mistakenly attributes the introduction of antiseptic methods in Salvador to Victorino; see p. 209. While the latter undoubtedly did much to promote its regular use from his faculty chair in surgery and in practical demonstrations at the Santa Casa hospital, he was not responsible for its initial introduction. On the shift from antisepsis to asepsis, see T. H. Pennington, "Listerism,

Its Decline, and Its Persistence: The Introduction of Aseptic Surgical Techniques in Three British Teaching Hospitals, 1890–99," *Medical History* 39 (1995): 35–60.

83   See Santos Filho, *História geral*, 2: 34.

84   Antônio Pacífico Pereira, "Caso de febre perniciosa, comatosa, curado pela aplicação hipodérmica de sulfato de quinina," *Gazeta Médica* 3 (1868): 73–76. Another Tropicalista supporter, Jerônymo Sodré Pereira, was the first doctor in Brazil to set up a physiology laboratory with facilities for practical teaching. See Santos Filho, *História geral*, 2: 149. The Tropicalistas were also opposed to heavy bleeding therapy.

85   Moacyr quotes from the regulations: "The candidates [to the position of] *opositor* [assistant professor] must be Brazilian citizens, have full access of their civil and political rights, and be in possession of the degree of medical doctors given by either of the schools of the Empire." *Instrução,* 151. The usual way of entering the medical school faculty was as an *opositor* (also called *sustituto*) and from among these the full professors were appointed. In 1845 Horner noted that "none other than Brazilians can be appointed members to the faculty." Gustavus R. B. Horner, *Medical Topography of Brazil and Uruguay* (Philadelphia: Lindsay and Blakiston, 1845), 77.

86   Borges, *Family,* 88. In the 1870s this was true of many medical schools in Europe and the United States. See Stanley Joel Reiser, *Medicine and the Reign of Technology* (Cambridge: Cambridge University Press, 1978), 81. See also the criticisms made by Raimundo Nina Rodrigues, "Memória histórica do Professor Raimundo Nina Rodrigues sobre o anno letivo de 1896," *Gazeta Médica* 73 (1976): 14–15. Pacífico Pereira was the first professor to introduce widespread use of the microscope in his teaching. See Coni, *Escola Tropicalista,* 39 n. 25; and Manoel Pinto de Souza Dantas, "Memória histórica dos acontecimentos mais notáveis na Faculdade de Medicina da Bahia no anno 1880," in Brazil, Ministério de Império, *Relatórios ministeriais,* Época do Império, reel 18 (1881). The situation at the Bahian school was similar to that of the Rio medical school. See Stepan, *Beginnings,* 53–56.

87   Coni, *Escola Tropicalista,* 34–35; "A medicina no Brasil," *Quarto Congresso Médico Latino Americano,* 66.

88   "O jubileo do Dr. Silva Lima," 251; Coni, *Escola Tropicalista,* 38. Wucherer was responsible for introducing one of the earliest microscopes into Salvador. This was probably a compound lens microscope, the use of which became widely available in Europe in the 1840s and was responsible for spectacular advances in parasitology and biology. See Charles-Edward Amory Winslow, *The Conquest of Epidemic Disease: A Chapter in the History of Ideas* (Madison: University of Wisconsin Press, 1980), 293; Brian Bracegirdle, "The Microscopical Tradition," in *Companion Encyclopedia of the History of Medicine,* ed. Bynum and Porter, 102–119; Reiser, *Medicine and the Reign of Technology,* esp. chap. 4, "The Microscope and the Revelation of a Cellular Universe," 69–90.

89 For some articles written by the doctor-trainees at the Santa Casa hospital, see D. A. de Mello, "Aneurisma de arteria poplitea; compressão digital; cura," *Gazeta Médica* 8 (1876): 535–540; J. M. de Aguiar, "Comunicação a redação da *Gazeta Médica* sobre a história natural da araroba," *Gazeta Médica* 10 (1878): 353–360; E. M. Ferreira, "Tumor branco do cotovelo direito, duas fístulas, raspagem," *Gazeta Médica* 20 (1889): 512–516.

90 Gomes, *M. V. Pereira*, 136.

91 Pacheco Mendes wrote on beriberi and parasitology in the *Gazeta Médica;* in 1887 he was on the editorial board of the medical journal. Ezequiel Britto was an intern at the Santa Casa, and in 1887 he too joined the editorial board of the *Gazeta Médica,* becoming one of the most copious contributors to the journal. He was also a member of the Bahian Medical Association and gave a paper there in 1889. Braz H. do Amaral worked often with Silva Lima, Victorino Pereira, and Moura at the Santa Casa hospital; some of the subjects he wrote on were ainhum and hygiene in schools. Soon after coming to Salvador, Nina Rodrigues worked at the Santa Casa, published his first work in the *Gazeta Médica,* and worked with the Tropicalistas to ensure that the Third Brazilian Medical Congress was held in Salvador instead of Rio de Janeiro, its usual site. Some of the younger generation Tropicalistas became linked to the older ones through marriage: Victorino Pereira married Silva Lima's daughter in 1881; Nina Rodrigues and Alfredo Britto both married daughters of José Luís D'Almeida Couto.

92 Quoted by Coni, *Escola Tropicalista*, 76.

93 It should be made clear that the changes were small ones; indeed, despite their gains in some areas, the Tropicalistas continued to complain about the adverse conditions in which they worked. Remédios Monteiro reported in 1879 that despite strenuous efforts to keep the hospital clean, there was an unpleasant smell as one entered the hospital. For a criticism of the way the hospital still refused to give scientifically trained doctors their due place in the 1890s, see Raimundo Nina Rodrigues, *Memória histórica da Faculdade de Medicina e Farmácia da Bahia* (1897), 24.

94 See the title pages of the issues of the *Gazeta Médica da Bahia* for 1866–89.

95 See the list of editors in appendix 1.

96 Santos Filho lists fifty-five medical journals in Brazil in the nineteenth century. Thirteen of these were published in Salvador. These high numbers attest to the failure of the medical press, not to its success. The average duration for medical journals in Salvador, other than the *Gazeta Médica,* was less than a year. Those in Rio de Janeiro were hardly more successful. Two notable exceptions in Rio during the Empire, one medical and the other cultural, were the *Anais da Academia de Medicina do Rio de Janeiro* and the *Revista do Instituto Histórico e Geográphico do Rio de Janeiro.* However, both these journals, like the organizations they were a part of, were sponsored by the imperial state in its effort to encourage the science and education so dear to the heart of Emperor Pedro II. The *Anais da Academia*

de Medicina do Rio de Janeiro underwent several name changes in the course of the century. In 1841 it was the *Revista médica brasileira;* in 1845 it became the *Anais de medicina brasiliense;* in 1849, *Anais Brasilienses de Medicina;* in 1885, the first mentioned name. The name changes indicate failures in the journal, which was then started up again. See Santos Filho, *História da medicina,* 2: 261–270; Luiz Otávio Ferreira, "O nascimento de uma instituição científica: Os periódicos médicos brasileiros na primeira metade do século XIX" (Ph.D. dissertation, Universidade de São Paulo, 1996).

97 In 1869 the annual subscription to the journal in Salvador was 8$000 mil-réis; in 1872 this went up to 10$000 mil-réis. It remained the same price in 1889. As a point of comparison, in 1879 the *Anais Brasilienses* was 6$000, in 1882 the *União Médica* was 12$000 mil-réis, in 1887 *Brasil Médico* was 14$000 mil-réis, and in 1873 the student journal *Revista Médica do Rio de Janeiro* was 3$000 mil-réis. Ao Livro Azul, Largo das Princesas, 15, was one bookstore that advertised in the *Gazeta Médica;* among the drugstores were those of A. Dias Silva, Lima Irmãos, and Caldas.

98 *Gazeta Médica* 1 (1866): 3.

99 See Stepan, *Beginnings,* 51. That this was also a complaint in Rio de Janeiro can be seen from the following statement: "if the medical school (in Rio de Janeiro) can count its students in the hundreds, this is not because there are hundreds of young men who want to seriously study [medicine] but simply because they want to earn a degree that will qualify them for the high positions in society and a comfortable life." Conselheiro Vicente Cândido do Figueira de Sabóia, "Relatório da Escola de Medicina do Rio de Janeiro," Brazil, Ministério do Império, *Relatórios ministeriais,* Época do Império, reel 18 (1881), 25.

100 Freyre, *Order and Progress,* 121.

101 Senex [José Francisco da Silva Lima], "A Bahia de há 66 anos (Reminiscências de um contemporâneo)." *Revista do Instituto Geográfico e Histórico da Bahia* 15, 34 (1908): 112.

102 Silva Lima, "O Dr. Paterson," 482–483.

103 For a good example of the image of altruism the Tropicalistas sought to project, see Dr. Paterson's obituary, *Gazeta Médica* 14 (1882): 241–247. See also the obituary for P. da Costa Chastinet, long-time editor of the *Gazeta Médica:* "his friends, and especially the poor who constituted so large a part of his clientele and for whom he was always accessible, [will deeply feel his loss]." *Gazeta Médica* 19 (1887): 7.

104 For example, see Silva Lima, "A pharmácia professão e a pharmácia indústria: commércio de remédios secretos e privilegiados," *Gazeta Médica* 8 (1876): 241; also letter to the journal, *Gazeta Médica* 9 (1877): 90. On homeopathic healing in Brazil, see Donald Warren, "A medicina espiritualizada: A homeopatia no Brasil do século XIX," *Religião e Sociedade* 13 (1986): 88–107; and speech surveying the history of the homeopathic institute in Brazil—Instituto Hahnemanniano—

given on the occasion of the centenary of the birth of Samuel Hahnemann by Dr. Joaquim José da Silva Pinto in *Annaes de Medicina Homeopáthica* 1, 10 (April 1883): 84–96.

105 Senex, "A Bahia," 114.

106 For information on the development of pharmacy in Brazil, see Santos Filho, *História da medicina,* vol. 1, pt. 1, chap. 3; José Ribeiro do Valle, "A farmacologia no Brasil," in *História das Ciências no Brasil,* ed. Ferri Mário Guimarães and Shozo Motoyama (São Paulo: EPU, 1973), 175–190.

107 The government encouraged the pharmacists because it collected taxes on European patent medicines. See Silva Lima's discussion of an article from a Boston journal and its relevance to Brazil, "A pharmácia professão," 241; see also José Francisco da Silva Lima, "Abusos e irregularidades no exercicio da Farmacia e da Medicina," *Gazeta Médica* 10 (1878): 497–501, 544–551. In Brazil pharmacists were allowed to keep the ingredients of their personally concocted remedies secret provided they obtained permission to do so from the Board of Public Hygiene and then the provincial government. The *Gazeta Médica* was highly critical of this; "Remedios Secretos," *Gazeta Médica* 11 (1879): 582. However, overall the journal avoided confrontations with the pharmacists. Silva Lima's family owned a well-known drugstore in Salvador, so he very likely understood the pharmacists' interests.

108 The *Sociedade Médico-Pharmacêutica de Beneficência Mútua* was founded in 1867 by Goes Siqueira, Silva Lima, and Maia Bittencourt—all early Tropicalistas or supporters. Almeida Couto, Costa Chastinet, Ramiro Monteiro, Silva Araújo, Victorino Pereira, Rozendo Guimarães—all core or supporter Tropicalistas—were active on its board. The stated aim of the society was to succor the widows and children of medical and pharmaceutical men. Help was also provided to the men if they became disabled through age or illness. It was not particularly successful because few physicians and pharmacists joined it. This was probably linked to the fact that since the patronage and *compadrio* systems were so strong in Brazil they functioned as a form of social help. In 1885 there were 101 members, and an editorial in the *Gazeta Médica* complained of indifference toward the organization. See "Doctors' and Pharmacists' Mutual Aid Society," 193–196. The pharmacists did make use of the *Gazeta Médica.*

109 The Tropicalistas' interest in Brazilian pharmacopoeia deserves further study. They were aware of several important contributions Brazil's luxuriant flora had made to European medicine and that they could learn a good deal from folk medicine. Thus, while they wanted to introduce modern medical therapies from Europe and North America into Brazil, they were certain that Brazil had contributions to make. See, for example, Wucherer's use of the pulp of the *gameleira* of the fig species, which he learned about from Brazilian folk medicine; *Gazeta Médica* 1 (1866): 52, and noted by Thomas Spencer Cobbold, *Parasites: A Treatise on the Entozoa of Man and Animals Including Some Account of the Ectozoa* (Lon-

don: J. and A. Churchill, 1879). They also identified those items of European pharmacopoeia that were originally Brazilian and reported on experiments in Brazilian medical practice with local plants. See José Francisco da Silva Lima, "Apontamentos sobre a araroba," *Gazeta Médica* 10 (1878): 353–360; José Luís D'Almeida Couto, "Alguns casos de cura de pústula maligna obtida pelo emprego de folhas de nogueira," *Gazeta Médica* 8 (1876): 23–28, 64–68; and Joaquim dos Remédios Monteiro, "Apontamentos para a história natural e farmacêutica do cordão de frade (Leonotis nepetoefolia)," *Gazeta Médica* 10 (1878): 501–503.

110 See Pacífico Pereira's criticism of Lacerda for communicating his findings to the lay press; "Investigacões sobre a beriberi," *Gazeta Médica* 15 (1883): 159–170. For another scathing criticism of Brazilian physicians' use of the lay press instead of the specialized medical journals, see an editorial article, "A imprensa médica no Brasil: A propósito de uma carta do Sr. Professor Domingos Freire a um diário da corte," *Gazeta Médica* 15 (1883): 429–437.

111 Barão de Itapoan et al., "Caso de defloração post-nuptial negada pelo marido; contestação extra-judiciária do exame médico-legal; protesto e réplica dos peritos," *Gazeta Médica* 11 (1879): 8–48, 107–149, 164–191, 399–417. See also Borges, *Family,* 106, 205–207.

112 The authors said they were adamantly against the misuse of medical expertise that "falsifies the principles of science and adulterates the teachings of great men." Barão de Itapoan et al., "Caso de defloração," 48.

113 There are many examples of this in Salvador: for example, C. A. Caldas Morais was a doctor and poet (Santos Filho, *História da medicina,* 1: 286); Climério C. de Oliveira was an obstetrician and author of a drama titled "A maternidade"; F. Sabino Alves de Rocha Vieira was a doctor, politician, and revolutionary agitator who wrote frequently on such subjects as "Can Brazil Dispense with a Revolution?"

114 For example, in 1871 Pires Caldas described a surgical method he had used with a patient with a gall bladder stone. His method differed from those of several French authorities in this type of operation. See "Cálculo vesical extraído pela talha preretal," *Gazeta Médica* 5 (1871): 78–82. Silva Araújo was very interested in treatment by electric shock for parasites; see "Tratamento da elephancia pela electricidade," *Gazeta Médica* 11 (1879): 441–465; "Ainda o tratamento da elephancia pela electricidade," *Gazeta Médica* 12 (1880): 163–179.

115 Joaquim dos Remédios Monteiro, "Pasteur e as suas doutrinas," *Gazeta Médica* 14 (1882): 111, 251; Remedios Monteiro, "Luíz Pasteur," *Gazeta Médica* 15 (1883): 250–259, 341–347, 401–406, 454–458, 493–497; Rudolf Virchow, "Sobre o valor da experimentação em pathologia," *Gazeta Médica* 13 (1881): 332–35, 381–84, 431–435, 474–477, 527–533; Robert Koch, "Conferência sobre a cholera morbus," *Gazeta Médica* 16 (1884): 110–124, 166–173, 218–229, 278–284; Robert Koch, "A missão alemã encarregada do estudo do cólera na India," *Gazeta Médica* 16 (1884): 74–82.

116 Over the whole period (1866–90) there are entries in the *Gazeta Médica* from
     journals in France, Britain, Germany, the Austrian Empire, Portugal, Italy, and
     the United States. For review of French medicine in the first half of the nine-
     teenth century, see the classic article by Erwin H. Ackernecht, "Hygiene in
     France, 1815–1848," *Bulletin of the History of Medicine* 22 (1948): 117–155; Ann F.
     La Berge, "The Early Nineteenth-Century French Public Health Movement:
     The Disciplinary Development and Institutionalization of *Hygiene Publique*,"
     Bulletin of the History of Medicine 58 (1984): 363–379; for a brief overview of
     German medicine, Günter B. Risse, "German Medicine and the State: Histori-
     cal Perspectives" (unpublished manuscript). For French influence on Brazilian
     medicine, see Sérgio Buarque de Holanda, *História geral da civilizacão brasileira:
     o Brasil monárquico,* Tomo II, 30 vol. (São Paulo: Difusão Europeia do Livro,
     1969), 470–472. On the evolution of medical education in nineteenth-century
     Europe and the United States, see Bonner, *Becoming a Physician.*
117 R. Blanchard, "As universidades e laboratórios na Alemanha," *Gazeta Médica* 13
     (1881): 66–79, 118–125, 158–164, 200–219, 366–373, 420–429, 463–474, 517–527;
     14 (1882): 6–14. Manoel Victorino Pereira, "Ensino médico na Áustria," *Gazeta
     Médica* 14 (1882): 151–163; Pacífico Pereira, "As reformas do ensino médico no
     Brasil," *Gazeta Médica* 15 (1884): 308–309; Pacífico Pereira, "Aos médicos depu-
     tados," 241–249. In 1885 Victorino Pereira took over the "Variedade" section of
     the *Gazeta* and reported on German medical writings.
118 See, for example, Otto H. Wucherer, "Sobre as causas da crescida freqüência
     da phthisica," *Gazeta Médica* 2 (1868): 265–268, 290–293; 3 (1869): 28–29; and
     Pacífico Pereira's glowing account of Virchow and other German doctors in his
     speech to the Third Brazilian Medical Congress, *Gazeta Médica* 22 (1890): 196–
     197; also in his article "Hygiene das escolas," *Gazeta Médica* 10 (1878): 198–199,
     245.
119 Pacífico Pereira, "Aos médicos deputados," 1–6, 49–56, 96–105, 145–151, 193–199,
     241, 337–346; Bonner, *Becoming a Physician,* 109–114. The fact that the imperial
     government provided a building for a polyclinic to be set up in Rio de Janeiro
     in 1881, and not in Salvador, was another source of contention for the Bahian
     doctors. Ironically, the lead speaker at the inauguration of the Rio polyclinic,
     attended by the emperor, was Silva Araújo, a core Tropicalista who had moved
     to Rio. In his speech, he pointed out how Pacífico Pereira had been the first to
     call for such an innovation in the *Gazeta Médica,* an innovation that had fallen
     on deaf ears. The speech was reported in Dr. Silva Araújo, "Discurso Inaugural
     Proferido no dia 28 de Junho de 1882," *União Médica* 2 (1882): 265–266.
120 This was pointed out to me in a personal communication by Carlos Oliveira,
     February 13, 1996. On Victorino Pereira's Germanophile influence, see Gomes,
     M. V. Pereira, 53–54. On the unlikeliness of Teutonism in Salvador, see Freyre,
     Order and Progress, 128. On the Recife school, Maricela Medina, "Tobias Ba-
     rreto (1839–1889): The Intellectual Odyssey of a Nineteenth Century Brazilian"

(Ph.D. dissertation, University of Michigan, 1986). For the importance of the German community and its influence in Salvador, see Edelweiss, "A secular presença da Alemanha," 223–242; and for Germans in northern Brazil, Freyre, *Nós e a Europa germânica.*

121 Victorino Pereira, "Ensino médico na Áustria," 159–160.

122 "Serviço de clínica cirúrgica a cargo do Dr. M. M. Pires Caldas," *Gazeta Médica* 1 (1866): 153, 177, 185, 198. In 1882 Silva Lima wrote about a man who called him and another doctor to see his wife. When the doctors started to write out a prescription, the man informed them that he had only needed a diagnosis; for treatment he would consult a homeopath; "Medicina Anedótica: A Procura de un diagnóstico," *Gazeta Médica* 14 (1882): 139. Dundas gives a description of doctors tending to a patient in which family and friends also had a say in the medical decisions made about a patient; *Sketches of Brazil,* 388. See also Horner, *Medical Topography,* esp. chap. 5, 70.

123 For examples of women spurning the authority of physicians, see chap. 4.

124 Gaston, "Brazil in Its Relation to Medicine," 290.

125 Ibid., 292; L. Papillaud, "Lettre médicale sur le Brésil," *Gazette Médicale de Paris* 3, 4 (1849): 887.

126 This evidence calls into question the rather passive depiction of the poor as helpless victims given in the work of Roberto Machado and Jurandir Freire Costa. They posit an alliance between doctor and state that comes to control large sections of the population. See Roberto Machado, Angel Loureiro, Rógerio Luz, and Kátia Muricy, *Danação da norma: Medicina social e constituição da psiquiatria no Brasil* (Rio de Janeiro: Graal, 1978); J. F. Costa, *Ordem médica e norma familiar,* 2d ed. (Rio de Janeiro: Graal, 1979).

127 Dr. Demetrio, "Gazeta Médica," *Gazeta Médica* 6 (1872), 1.

128 Doctors from the Northeast who contributed to the journal include I. F. Lemos, Ignácio Alcibiades Velloso, M. da F. Alençar, and, the most prolific in the early years of the journal, B. Mamoré, a doctor from Pará. In this book I focus on hookworm, filariasis, and beriberi—in which the doctors made more significant contributions. For ainhum, see José Francisco da Silva Lima, "A propósito do ainhum: Observações colhidas na Ilha dos Pinheiros," *Gazeta Médica* 12 (1880): 245–262; and, under various headings, *Gazeta Médica* 12 (1881): 341–360; 15 (1883): 466–477. For dracunculiasis, Silva Lima, "Notas sobre a filaria medinense (bicho da costa): Endemicidade d'este parasita na província da Bahia, e seu ingresso no corpo humano pela água em bebida," *Gazeta Médica* 9 (1877): 301–316; and several other articles also by Silva Lima on the subject in *Gazeta Médica* 22 (1890), 297–305, 337–345, 385–396, 433–444, 481–491, 633–640.

129 José Francisco da Silva Lima, "Bibliographia," *Gazeta Médica* 19 (1888): 425–434.

130 Gomes, *M. V. Pereira,* 174.

131 Papillaud, "Lettre médicale sur le Brésil," 897.

132 There is a long and important debate in Brazilian historiography about why the

monarchy fell and the role of the new groups in its fall that is part of the question of the relationship between state and society in nineteenth-century Brazil. Was the imperial state the creature of the traditional plantocracy? Or was the plantocracy kept in check by a "bureaucratic" state where "mandarins" loyally served the imperial government? Were the new urban groups progressive groups who challenged a conservative imperial government? Emília Viotti da Costa argues, subtly, in favor of this view, but more recent revisionist scholarship disagrees. For a good summary and bibliography, see Richard Graham, "State and Society in Brazil, 1822–1930," *Latin American Research Review* 22 (1987): 223–236; Carvalho, *Construção da ordem;* Eul-Soo Pang and Ron L. Seckinger, "The Mandarins of Imperial Brazil," *Comparative Studies in Society and History* 14 (1972): 215–244; E. Costa, "Brazil: The Age of Reform, 1870–1889," in *Cambridge History of Latin America* ed. Leslie Bethell (Cambridge: Cambridge University Press, 1985); 5: 725–777, E. Costa, *Brazilian Empire,* esp. chaps. 7 and 8. Some recent works following the revisionist trend are Robert M. Levine, *Vale of Tears: Revisiting the Canudos Massacre in Northeastern Brazil, 1893–1897* (Berkeley: University of California Press, 1992); George Reid Andrews, *Blacks and Whites in São Paulo, Brazil, 1888–1988* (Madison: University of Wisconsin Press, 1991). I see the Tropicalistas as representing new demands for medical practice in Salvador. But, like others of the new urban groups, they did not have an independent power base and so they tred carefully making alliances where they could. Among their ranks can be found sons of some the wealthiest old families and they were honored when the emperor paid them attention—as was Paterson when he was asked to host Pedro II, who visited Scotland at the same time as the British doctor. Useful literature on the intellectual and political changes of the 1870s includes João Cruz Costa, *A History of Ideas in Brazil,* trans. Suzette Macedo (Berkeley: University of California Press, 1964), 82–202; Antônio Cândido de Melo e Souza, *Formação de literatura brasileira* (São Paulo, 1976); Roberto Ventura, *Estilo tropical: História cultural e polêmicas literárias no Brasil, 1870–1914* (São Paulo: Companhia das Letras, 1991); Emília Viotti da Costa, "Empire, 1870–1889," and Boris Fausto, "Society and Politics," in *Brazil: Empire and Republic, 1822–1930,* ed. Leslie Bethell (Cambridge: Cambridge University Press, 1989), 161–213, 257–307; Charles A. Hale, "Political and Social Ideas in Latin America, 1870–1930," in *Cambridge History of Latin America,* ed. Leslie Bethell (Cambridge: Cambridge University Press, 1985), 4: 382–414.

133   "A nova organisação do serviço sanitário," 385–386.

134   This attitude was identical to Virchow's position of the role of medicine.

135   See Pacífico Pereira's discussion of a book on the administration of health, "Organisação da hygiene administrativa," *Gazeta Médica* 12 (1881): 503–510; and his article "Aos médicos deputados," 51–53. In the early Republic, Tropicalista efforts continued to be resisted. For example, in 1892 three Tropicalistas—Silva Lima, Pacífico Pereira, and Nina Rodrigues—were appointed to head a newly created

Medical and Sanitation Council to link state health to a more centrally organized system. However, their high expectations were dashed when the council
was granted only an advisory role. See Luiz Antônio de Castro Santos, "Power,
Ideology, and Public Health in Brazil, 1889–1930" (Ph.D. dissertation, Harvard
University, 1987).

136 See the highly critical speeches both these men made in the medical school:
Manoel Victorino Pereira, "No acto da inauguração do gabinete de anatomia e
physiologia pathológica e do horto botânico da Faculdade de Medicina," *Gazeta
Médica* 13 (1881), 258–63; Braz H. do Amaral, "Discurso proferido no acto da
collação do grão de doutor em medicina," *Gazeta Médica* 18 (1887): 315–327.

137 The Tropicalistas were Demétrio C. Tourinho, Virgílio Damázio, José L. D'Almeida Couto, Victorino Pereira, Ramiro Affonso Monteiro de Carvalho. The
supporters were José Goes de Siqueira, Jerônymo Sodré Pereira, Luís Álvares
dos Santos. See Lycurgo Santos Filho, *História da medicina no Brasil: do século
XVI ao século XIX,* vol. 2 (São Paulo: Brasiliense, 1947), 403.

138 Almeida Couto was president of São Paulo in 1884–85, of Salvador in 1885, and
in 1889 when the Empire fell. Sodré Pereira was president of Sergipe in 1889.

139 Santos Filho, *História da medicina,* vol. 2, 391–392. Goes Siqueira was an early
supporter of the Tropicalistas but he soon had deep differences with them; see
chap. 2. He was a member of the Conservative Party.

140 It was Sodré Pereira who called for the immediate and total abolition of slavery
in 1879 after the issue had remained dormant since the Rio Branco law of 1871.
See Skidmore, *Black into White,* 16. The political slant of the articles in the *Gazeta
Médica* was liberal but sometimes the Tropicalistas' economic liberalism came
up against their demands for greater government regulation in health. A good
example of this is their argument against the imposition of restrictions on unlicensed pharmacists because it went against free trade. See Silva Lima et al.,
"Abusos e irregularidades no exercício da pharmacia e da medicina," *Gazeta Médica* 10 (1878): 497–501, 544–551; Santos Filho, *História da medicina,* vol. 2, pt. 4,
chap. 3. On political parties in Salvador, see Tavares, *História da Bahia,* 158–167.

141 "Noticiário," *Gazeta Médica* 9 (1887): 25; *Revista Médica do Rio de Janeiro* (1876):
104, 223. Some of the founding members of the Rio de Janeiro Medical Society
were Júlio de Moura, Baptista Lacerda, M. Costa, Felício dos Santos, Nuno de
Andrade, Carneiro da Rocha. For the 1886 Society, see Luiz Otávio Ferreira,
Marcos Chor Maio, and Nara Azevedo, "A Sociedade de Medicina e Cirurgia do
Rio de Janeiro: A gênese de uma rede institucional alternativa," *História, Ciência,
Saúde, Manguinhos* 4, 3 (1997): 475–491.

142 "Editorial," *União Médica* 1 (1881): 4; the first quote is from an editorial of *Revista
Médica do Rio de Janeiro* 1 (1876): 6.

143 "A classe médica," *Gazeta Médica* 21 (1889): 1–3. In 1890, referring to the journal *Gazeta Médica da Bahia* and how it had survived for twenty-four years, Silva
Lima stated that its survival was certainly not because of "the majority of our col-

leagues who were indifferent to [our efforts] and even disdainful [of them, for] they only hold as valuable and acceptable science that is imported from abroad, and they do not hesitate to proclaim our incapacity to cultivate [medical science] in our own country." Silva Lima, "Terceiro Congresso Brasileiro de Medicina e Cirurgia: Discurso Inaugural do Presidente, Dr. Silva Lima," *Gazeta Médica* 22 (1890): 157.

144   "A Gazeta Médica, o seu pasado e o seu futuro," *Gazeta Médica* 27 (1895): 50.

145   Ackerknecht, *Short History of Medicine,* 133.

146   Dr. Demetrio, "Gazeta Médica," *Gazeta Médica* 6 (1872): 1.

147   For example, there were Dr. Sigaud; Dr. T. J. H. Langaard, who wrote *Dicionário de medicina* (1865); Aristides Garnier, a French doctor who lived in Rio de Janeiro and directed the *Anais Brasilienses de Medicina;* the Englishman Jonattas Abbot, who taught and worked in Salvador and founded a small natural history museum in the medical school. For biographical details of the latter, see Dr. Remedios Monteiro, "Apontamentos para a biografia do conselheiro Dr. Jonathas Abbot," *União Médica* 2 (1882): 343–344.

Chapter Two   The Politics of Disease

1   These themes have been much covered. See Charles E. Rosenberg, "The Bitter Fruit: Heredity, Disease, and Social Thought," in *No Other Gods: On Science and American Social Thought,* ed. Charles E. Rosenberg (Baltimore: Johns Hopkins University Press, 1976), 25–53 and n. 14 below. On the humoral theory, see Vivian Nutton, "Humoralism," in *Companion Encyclopedia of the History of Medicine,* ed. W. F. Bynum and Roy Porter (London: Routledge, 1994), 281–291.

2   See, for example, Allan M. Brandt, *No Magic Bullet: A Social History of Venereal Disease in the United States since 1880* (New York: Oxford University Press, 1987), 4, 40–41. The theme of new scientific ideas unsettling old constituencies and authorities is explored by Jack Morrell and Arnold Thackray, *Gentlemen of Science: Early Years of the British Association for the Advancement of Science* (Oxford: Clarendon, 1981).

3   Jaime L. Benchimol and Luiz Antônio Teixeira, *Cobras, lagartos e outros bichos: Uma história comparada dos Institutos Oswaldo Cruz e Butantan* (Rio de Janeiro: Universidade Federal do Rio de Janeiro, 1993), 7–9.

4   The best example of the influence of French "hygienism" in Brazil continuing in the second half of the century can be found in the important, lengthy report by the Barão de Lavradio, "Estudo das epidemias que han grassado nesta côrte de 1871 até 1880," *Anais Brasilienses de Medicina* 34 (1882–83): 359–622.

5   Robert Ventura, *Escritores, escravos e mestiços em um país tropical: Literatura, historiografia e ensaísmo no Brasil* (Nürnberg: Wilhelm Fink Verlag München, 1987); Sílvio Romero, *História da literatura brasileira,* 3d ed., vol. 1 (Rio de Janeiro: José Olympio, 1943); E. Bradford Burns, *The Poverty of Progress: Latin America in the Nineteenth Century* (Berkeley: University of California Press, 1980), 62–63.

6 José Francisco da Silva Lima, "Contribuição para a história de uma moléstia que reina atualmente na Bahia, sob a forma epidemia e caracterisada por paralisia, edema e fraqueza geral," *Gazeta Médica* 1 (1866): 110–113, 125–128, 138–139; 158–160, 183–185, 196–198, 219–220, 232–235, 243–245, 268–270; 2 (1867): 2–6, 28–30, 49–55, 65–68, 99–104; 3 (1868): 55–56, 85–87, 109–111. In 1872 the articles were published in book form titled *Ensaio sobre o beriberi no Brazil* (Bahia: J. B. Martin, 1872). We know today that beriberi is a disease of malnutrition caused by the deficiency of Vitamin B$_1$, thiamine. See Robert R. Williams, *Toward the Conquest of Beriberi* (Cambridge: Harvard University Press, 1961); H. Harold Scott, *A History of Tropical Medicine*, 2 vols. (Baltimore: Williams and Wilkins, 1939), 858–897; Erwin H. Ackerknecht, *History and Geography of the Most Important Diseases* (London: Hafner, 1965), 144, 150–151; Melinda S. Meade, "Beriberi," in *The Cambridge World History of Human Disease*, ed. Kenneth F. Kiple (Cambridge: Cambridge University Press, 1993), 606–612; Anne Hardy, "Beriberi, Vitamin B$_1$, and World Food Policy, 1925–1970," *Medical History* 39 (1995): 61–67. On beriberi among slaves in the New World, see Todd L. Savitt, *Medicine and Slavery: The Diseases and Health Care of Blacks in Antebellum Virginia* (Urbana: University of Illinois Press, 1978), 88; Kenneth F. Kiple and Virginia Himmelsteib King, *Another Dimension to the Black Diaspora: Diet, Disease, and Racism* (Cambridge: Cambridge University Press, 1981), 117–133; Kenneth F. Kiple, *The Caribbean Slave* (Cambridge: Cambridge University Press, 1984), 96–103; for beriberi among slaves in Brazil, see Mary C. Karasch, *Slave Life in Rio de Janeiro, 1808–1850* (Princeton: Princeton University Press, 1987), 165–166, 175–177, 180–182.

7 His subsequent reading was mainly on the work of British doctors in India such as Dr. C. Morehead, *Clinical Researches on Disease in India*, 2 vols. (London, 1856); he also read Dr. Aitken and, in French publications, writings by Monneret de la Berge and Fonssagrives. Le Roy de Méricourt had a long association with several Bahian doctors and was one of the first European doctors interested in the work of the Tropicalistas. He visited Brazil several times, corresponded with the Tropicalistas, and translated their work into French for publication in the French medical journal, *Arch. Méd. Nav.*

8 Silva Lima had seen fifty-one patients when he wrote about the beriberi epidemic in Bahia. In 1870 the total number of beriberi patients in the Santa Casa de Misericórdia charity hospital was seven; in 1871, nine patients; and in 1872, twelve patients. *Gazeta Médica* 15 (1883): 222–224. As a point of comparison, the number of victims in the 1849 yellow fever epidemic in Bahia was estimated at three thousand and in the 1855 cholera epidemic at nine thousand. On the definition of epidemic, see Maryinez Lyons, who has noted that epidemic in the nineteenth century meant not so much high numbers of disorders transmitted from sick to healthy, but a disorder that was simultaneously affecting people because of atmospheric conditions. *The Colonial Disease: A Social History of Sleeping Sickness in*

Northern Zaire, 1900–1940 (Cambridge: Cambridge University Press, 1992), 249
n. 6.

9 All of the following writings stress the complex intertwining of political interests
   with the attempt to combat "epidemic" disease: Jeffrey D. Needell, "The *Revolta
   Contra Vaccina* of 1904: The Revolt against Modernization in 'Belle Époque' Rio
   de Janeiro," *Hispanic American Historical Review* 67 (1987): 233–270; Stephen
   Williams, "A River of Tears: Corporate Interests and Public Consequences during Rio de Janeiro's First Yellow Fever Outbreak, 1849–1850" (paper presented
   at the 1995 meeting of the Latin American Studies Association Congress, Washington, D.C., September 28–30); Charles E. Rosenberg, *The Cholera Years: The
   United States in 1832, 1849, and 1866* (Chicago: University of Chicago Press, 1987),
   20–29; Judith Walzer Leavitt, "Politics and Public Health: Smallpox in Milwaukee, 1894–95," in *Sickness and Health: Readings in the History of Medicine and
   Public Health,* ed. Judith Walzer Leavitt and Ronald L. Numbers (Madison: University of Wisconsin Press, 1985), 372–384; Martin S. Pernick, "Politics, Parties,
   and Pestilence: Epidemic Yellow Fever in Philadelphia and the Rise of the First
   Party System," in *Sickness and Health,* ed. Leavitt and Numbers, 356–371.

10 On the concept of miasma, see Caroline Hannaway, "Environment and Miasmata," in *Companion Encyclopedia of the History of Medicine,* ed. Bynum and Porter,
   292–308; Vivian Nutton, "The Seeds of Disease: An Explanation of Contagion and Infection from the Greeks to the Renaissance," *Medical History* 27
   (1983): 1–34; Major Greenwood, "Miasma and Contagion," in *Science, Medicine,
   and History: Essays on the Evolution of Scientific Thought and Medical Practice,* ed.
   E. Ashworth Underwood (London: Oxford University Press, 1953), 500–507;
   Dennis G. Carlson, *African Fever: A Study of British Science, Technology, and Politics in West Africa, 1787–1864* (New York: Science History Publications, 1984);
   Charles-Edward Amory Winslow, *The Conquest of Epidemic Disease: A Chapter
   in the History of Ideas* (Madison: University of Wisconsin Press, 1980), 73–74,
   193–290; Oswei Temkin, "An Historical Analysis of the Concept of Infection,"
   in *The Double Face of Janus* (Baltimore: Johns Hopkins University Press, 1977),
   456–471; Richard B. Sheridan, *Doctors and Slaves: A Medical and Demographic
   History of Slavery in the British West Indies, 1680–1834* (Cambridge: Cambridge
   University Press, 1985), 17–41; Robert Dundas, *Sketches of Brazil; Including New
   Views on Tropical and European Fever* (London: John Churchill, 1852); Nancy
   Tomes, "The Private Side of Health: Sanitary Science, Domestic Hygiene, and
   the Germ Theory, 1870–1900," *Bulletin of the History of Medicine* 64 (1990): 503–
   539; Erwin H. Ackerknecht, "Anticontagionism between 1821 and 1867," *Bulletin of the History of Medicine* 22 (1948): 562–593; Robert P. Hudson, *Disease and
   Its Control: The Shaping of Modern Thought* (Westport: Greenwood, 1983), 141–
   144; Royston Lambert, *Sir John Simon (1816–1904) and English Social Administration* (London: MacGibbon and Kee, 1963); Richard A. Lewis, *Edwin Chadwick
   and the Public Health Movement, 1832–1854* (London: Longmans, Green, 1952);

Ann F. La Berge, "The Early Nineteenth-Century French Public Health Movement: The Disciplinary Development and Institutionalization of *Hygiene Publique*," *Bulletin of the History of Medicine* 58 (1984): 363–379; M. W. Flinn, ed., *Report on the Sanitary Condition of the Labouring Population of Great Britain by Edwin Chadwick, 1842* (Edinburgh: University of Edinburgh Press, 1965).

11   Silva Lima, "Contribuição," *Gazeta Médica* 2 (1867): 101, 109. For a summary of the various theories on the etiology of beriberi held by Brazilian doctors, see Antônio Augusto de Azevedo Sodré, "Considerações históricas sobre o beriberi," *Brasil Médico* 75, 1–2 (Jan–July 1961): 51–56.

12   José Francisco da Silva Lima, "Notícias acerca do Kakke, ou beriberi das Indias orientais," *Gazeta Médica* 19 (1888): 289–299, 337–343, 385–391. This observation was quite plausible since only upper-class Brazilians would have been able to afford the more polished, and thus less nutritious, white rice at this time. It is likely that the timing of the epidemic was related to the war against Paraguay (1865–70), which created a large demand for staple foods inland and raised the price of manioc flour and dried beef, the staple diet of poor Brazilians in the Northeast, and already low in vitamin B_1. Carlos Roberto Oliveira, "Medicine e estado: Origem e desenvolvimento da medicina social no Brasil, Bahia, 1866–1896" (master's thesis, Universidade do Estado do Rio de Janeiro, 1982), 244–247. For price fluctuations of manioc flour in relation to epidemics, but especially the cholera of 1855, see Kátia M. de Queirós Mattoso and M. Johildo de Athayde, "Epidemias e flutuações de preços na Bahia no século XIX," *L'Histoire Quantitative du Brésil de 1800 a 1930* (Colloques Internatinaux du Centre National de la Recherche Scientifique, 1971), 183–202. For a discussion of the nutritional values in the nineteenth-century Brazilian diet, see Kenneth F. Kiple, "The Nutritional Link between Slave Infant and Child Mortality in Brazil," *Hispanic American Historical Review* 69 (1989): 677–690.

13   Silva Lima, "Notícias," 388. For an interesting treatment of the theoretical compatibility between the germ theory and miasma, see Tomes, "Private Side of Health," 514–515, 528–530.

14   On resisting the new bacteriology, see Lambert, *Sir John Simon;* see also Winslow's discussion of Pettenkofer, *Conquest of Epidemic Disease,* 311–336; George Rosen, *From Medical Police to Social Medicine: Essays on the History of Health Care* (New York: Science History Publications, 1974); Steven J. Novak, "Professionalism and Bureaucracy: English Doctors and the Victorian Public Health Administration," *Journal of Social History* vol. 6, no. 4 (1973): 440–462; Howard D. Kramer, "The Germ Theory and the Early Public Health Program in the United States," *Bulletin of the History of Medicine* 22 (1948): 233–247; Russell C. Maulitz, "Physician versus Bacteriologist: The Ideology of Science in Clinical Medicine," in *The Therapeutic Revolution: Essays in the Social History of American Medicine,* ed. Morris J. Vogel and Charles E. Rosenberg (Philadelphia: University of Pennsylvania Press, 1979), 91–108. On a healthy skepticism regarding the huge claims

made for bacteriology, see Erwin H. Ackerknecht, *Rudolf Virchow: Doctor, States-man, Anthropologist* (Madison: University of Wisconsin Press, 1953), 105–118. For the transition in Brazil, see Jaime L. Benchimol, "Domingos José Freire e os primórdios da bacteriologia no Brasil," *História, Ciências, Saúde, Manguinhos* 2, 1 (1995): 67–98; Eduardo César Marques, "Da higiene à construção da cidade: O estado e o saneamento no Rio de Janeiro," *História, Ciências, Saúde, Manguinhos* 2, 2 (1995): 51–67.

15 See *Siglo Médico* 14 (April 28, 1867): 257–260, and A. Le Roy de Méricourt, "O beriberi não é uma moléstia exclusivamente própia da Índia; observa-se nas An-tilhas a no Brasil," *Gazeta Médica* 2 (1867): 49–55; (1868): 157, 162–163, cited by Kenneth F. Kiple, "The Nutritional Link between Slave Infant and Child Mor-tality in Brazil," *Hispanic American Historical Review* 69 (1989): 679.

16 O. Carnêiro Giffoni, *Diccionário bio-bibliográfico brasileiro de escritores médicos (1500–1899)* (São Paulo: Livraria Nobel, 1972), 237; Lycurgo Santos Filho, *Histó-ria da medicina no Brasil: Do século XVI ao século XIX* (São Paulo: Brasiliense, 1947), 1: 284; see also the obituary for Goes Siqueira in *Anais Brasilienses* 28 (1877): 204–210.

17 See, for example, his discussion of the work of the British sanitarian Dr. South-wood Smith in "Falla do Presidente da Província da Bahia, Francisco Xavier Pães Barreto," in Brazil, *Relatórios da Província da Bahia*, annex on health, reel 10 (March 1859), 2–3. Even his 1835 graduating dissertation showed his inclination toward public health; it was titled "Sobre a influência que exerce a civilização sobre a saúde pública."

18 "Falla do Presidente da Província da Bahia, João Antônio de Araújo Freitas Henriques," in Brazil, *Relatórios da Província da Bahia*, annex of the Inspetoria da Saúde Pública da Bahia, January 31, 1871, reel 11 (1872): 3–14.

19 Some of his writings included "Estudos sobre hygiene pública" (1872); "Relações da medicina com a metafísica" (*O Ateneu*, 1849); "Necrológio do D. Malaquias Álvares dos Santos" (Bahia, 1858); "Memória histórica dos acontecimentos mais notáveis na Faculdade de Medicina da Bahia no anno 1858"; "Algumas considera-ções sobre o Hospital dos Lázaros da Cidade da Bahia" (*Arquivo Médico Brasileiro* 4, 12 [1848]: 285–287).

20 There are several laudatory references to the good work accomplished by Goes Siqueira in this field. See, for example, A. Pacífico Pereira, "Organisação da hy-giene administrativa," *Gazeta Médica* 12 (1881): 506. This may also have been the Tropicalistas' "careful handling" of a powerful man.

21 R. V. "La medicina en el Brasil," *Siglo Médico* 14 (1867): 257–260.

22 Günter B. Risse, "History of Western Medicine from Hippocrates to Germ Theory," in *Cambridge World History of Human Disease*, ed. Kiple, 18. The intro-duction of laboratory medicine to Brazil came after the turn of the century be-cause it was dependent on big investment and thus needed government or phil-anthropic investment such as that provided by the Rockefeller Foundation. But

the Tropicalistas began to move medical thinking into the new era of medicine in Brazil.

23   Reprinted in Jose Goes Siqueira, "Relatório acerca do estado santário d'esta província durante o ano de 1866," *Gazeta Médica* 1 (1867): 189–192.

24   Ibid., 191.

25   For comments on Littré's influence on Brazilians, see João Cruz Costa, *A History of Ideas in Brazil,* trans. Suzette Macedo (Berkeley: University of California Press, 1964), 98–104.

26   Quoted by Goes Siqueira from "De quelques causes des maladies particulieres a notre temps," *Gazeta Médica* 1 (1867): 192.

27   However, in the 1880s conditions in the city probably worsened because of the severe drought in the Northeast that drove many people into Salvador. On the drought, see Gerald Michael Greenfield, "The Great Drought and Elite Discourse in Imperial Brazil," *Hispanic American Historical Review* 72 (1992): 375–400.

28   Added to this was the difference in their political affiliations. Siqueira belonged to the Conservative Party while most of the other Tropicalistas belonged to the Liberal Party or had politically liberal tendencies. See chap. 1.

29   Elias José Pedrosa, "Memória histórica dos acontecimentos mais notáveis na Faculdade de Medicina da Bahia no anno 1871," *Gazeta Médica* 6 (1872): 66–67.

30   "Falla do Presidente da Província da Bahia, Conselheiro Luíz Antônio da Silva Nunes," in Brazil, *Relatórios da Província da Bahia,* annex 2, Inspetoria da Saúde Pública, reel 14 (February 5, 1877), 14; *Gazeta Médica* 11 (1879): 579–580. Besides Silva Lima and Paterson, the commissions included the Tropicalistas José Luis De' Almeida Couto, Ramiro Affonso Monteiro de Carvalho, and Demétrio Ciríaco Tourinho, and were later joined by Pacífico Pereira.

31   See Domingos Pedro dos Santos, "Bibliographia do beriberi no Brazil," *Gazeta Médica* 15 (1883): 497–514, 543. Professors competing for chairs also worked on beriberi. Dissertations on beriberi at the school, presented either for graduating or for faculty competitions, included those of the Bahians Augusto Pinto (1869) and Almeida Couto (1871), two Pará doctors, Lemos (1868) and Jaime Brício (1868), and the Pernambucan Cosmé de Sá (1871).

32   Antônio Januário de Faria, "Algumas considerações sobre a moléstia denominada beriberi, a propósito do artigo do Sr. Le Roy de Méricourt," *Gazeta Médica* 3 (1869): 169–170.

33   Antônio Pacífico Pereira, "Estudo sobre a etiologia e natureza do beriberi," *Gazeta Médica* 12 (1881): 308–317, 453–462, 485–498, 533–543; 13 (1882): 1–12, 49–66, 97–106, 145–153, 193–200, 308–317, 409–419, 496–502. For biographical details on Pacífico Pereira, see Lycurgo Santos Filho, *História geral da medicina brasileira* (São Paulo: Hucitec, 1991), 2: 152; "Professor Pacífico Pereira," *Brasil Médico* 35 (1922): 378.

34   Pacífico Pereira also examined other aspects, such as changes in the urine and

kidneys of beriberi victims. He used Nachet, Vérick, and Hartnack lenses with a magnification of 600–1500 diameters and aniline dyes according to Koch's and Ogston's methods ("Estudo," *Gazeta Médica* 13 [1882]: 148, 194). At this time Robert Koch was still in the process of working to perfect staining methods in bacteriology although in general histology they were already in use.

35 Ibid., 13 (1882): 9–10, 48, 97–106.

36 Ibid., 12 (1881): 533–534.

37 Pacífico Pereira was familiar with the German sources because he had spent a year in Germany and because he drew on information from articles he read in *Virchow's Archiv.* Some of the authors he discussed (other than Pettenkofer) were M. Litten from the University of Berlin; Sanders-Ezn, who worked at the laboratory of Professor Carl F. W. Ludwig, one of the creators of modern physiology; M. Schultze and Wertheim; A. Schmidt, a physiologist who experimented on pigs in India; Ernst Felix I. Hoppe-Seyler, a physiological chemist and student of Virchow's well known for his work on hemoglobin and the red blood cell; and Ernst von Leyden, professor of medicine at Berlin.

38 Pacífico Pereira, "Estudo," *Gazeta Médica* 12 (1881): 535–536; 13 (1882): 102, 106. For his experimentation on animals, see 13 (1882): 97–106. On key nineteenth-century discoveries on the blood, see André Cournand, "Air and Blood," in *Circulation of the Blood: Men and Ideas,* ed. Alfred P. Fishman and Dickinson W. Richards (New York: Oxford University Press, 1964), 48–63.

39 Pacífico Pereira, "Estudo," *Gazeta Médica* 12 (1881): 533.

40 Ibid., 13 (1882): 58–65.

41 Ibid., 152; for an English translation of the article, see "Study of the Etiology and Nature of Beriberi," *St. Louis Medical and Surgical Journal* 42 (1882): 35–38, 263–266, 365–368, 590–593; 43 (1882): 33–35, 140–142. His interest in both bacteriology and hemoglobin shows him to be aware of the avant-garde medicine of his day. Bacteriology in the 1880s was only just beginning its spectacular advances and clinical bacteriology was in the process of being established as a specialty largely by Koch.

42 It is interesting to note that when notice of Pacífico Pereira's findings was given in the foreign press, his findings on microorganisms were most commented on. See "Pereira on the Blood in Beriberi," *British Medical Record* 10 (November 1882): 464–465.

43 Pacífico Pereira, "Investigações sobre o beriberi," *Gazeta Médica* 15 (1883): 159–170.

44 He was not alone in his balancing act. As Ackerknecht has noted, there were many physicians, or "contingent contagionists," who, in theory, allowed that epidemics may be caused by contagion (through "fomites" and later through bacteria) but in their practical considerations followed the miasmatists in advocating cleaning up the environment in order to destroy miasmatic emanations that caused disease. Ackerknecht, "Anticontagionism," 562–593.

45 Antônio Pacheco Mendes, "Contribuição ao estudo do beriberi," *Gazeta Médica* 16 (1884–85): 129–135, 157–160, 208–213, 260–264, 299–304, 347–351, 400–405; 17 (1885): 6–10, 157–162; 18 (1887): 299–306.

46 As Eric Cassell has argued, the tension between these two views of disease is present even today; see "Ideas in Conflict: The Rise and Fall (and Rise and Fall) of New Views of Disease," *Daedalua* 115 (1986): 21–22. On the differentiation between the "old" tropical medicine and the "new" in Brazil, see Ilana Lowy, "Yellow Fever in Rio de Janeiro and the Pasteur Institute Mission (1901–1905): The Transfer of Science to the Periphery," *Medical History* 34 (1990): 161–163.

47 Another important study in Bahia was by Raimundo Nina Rodrigues, "O beriberi e as polinevrites: Diagnóstico diferencial," *Gazeta Médica* 21 (1889): 550–556; 22 (1890): 9–14, 66–72, 108–113, 164–168, 211–218, 250–254. In 1873 the eminent court physician José Pereira Rego Filho praised Silva Lima's work on beriberi, which the latter forwarded to the Imperial Academy of Medicine seeking membership in the prestigious society, a membership he received. See "Relatório apresentado à Academia de Medicina do Rio de Janeiro, em sessão de 6 de maio de 1872, pelo Dr. José Pereira Rego Filho, sobre o trabalho do Sr. Dr. José F. da Silva Lima intitulado, 'Ensaios sobre o beriberi no Brasil,'" *Anais Brasilienses* 24 (1873): 407–429. But, in general, Rio physicians considered beriberi to be a disease of the northern regions of the country and thus of little concern to the capital. R. Nina Rodrigues, "o Beriberi," 552; A. Sodré, "Considerações históricas" 54.

48 For details on Lacerda's work and a bibliography of his main writings, see Ricardo Ventura Santos, "Edgar Roquette-Pinto; Os tipos antropológicos e a questão da degeneração racial no Brasil no início do século" (Paper presented at the Twentieth Annual Meeting of ANPOCS, Caxambu, Minas Gerais, October 1996). See also Nancy Leys Stepan, *Beginnings of Brazilian Science: Oswaldo Cruz, Medical Research, and Policy, 1890–1920* (New York: Science History Publications, 1981), 31–32; Simon Schwarzman, *Formação da comunidade científica no Brasil* (São Paulo: Companhia Editora Nacional, 1979), 60–62; Fernando de Azevedo, ed., *As Ciências no Brasil,* vol. 2 (Rio de Janeiro: Editora UFRJ, 1994), 215–221.

49 His interest in beriberi was probably not altogether unrelated to his professional closeness to the Tropicalista Silva Araújo.

50 *União Médica* 3 (1883): 449–459.

51 Pacífico Pereira, "Investigações," 159.

52 Ibid., 159–170.

53 Ibid., 161.

54 Ibid., 161–169.

55 Pacífico Pereira, "As investigacóes sobre o beriberi pelo Dr. S. Baptista de Lacerda," *Gazeta Médica* 15 (1884): 450; J. Baptista de Lacerda, "O microorganismo de beriberi," *União Médica* 3 (1883): 449–459; 4 (1884): 113–119.

56   *União Médica* 3 (1883): 456–462.

57   Ibid., 465, 466.

58   On Lacerda's preference for laboratory work over clinical, see Renato Clark Bacellar, *Brazil's Contribution to Tropical Medicine and Malaria: Personalities and Institutions* (Rio de Janeiro: Olímpica, 1963), 291–292; on the rise of laboratory medicine in Brazil, see Jaime L. Benchimol, *Manguinhos do sonho à vida: A ciência na belle époque* (Rio de Janeiro: FIOCRUZ, 1990), 12–18; Benchimol and Teixeira, *Cobras, lagartos*, 13–18; Benchimol, "Domingos José Freire," 53–86.

59   Stepan, *Beginnings*, 31–32.

60   R. Nina Rodrigues, "O Beriberi," 550–556.

61   Otto Wucherer, "Patologia interna sobre a moléstia vulgarmente denominada opilação ou cansaço," *Gazeta Médica* 1 (1866): 27–29, 39–41, 52–54, 63–64. For an English translation of parts of this article, see B. H. Kean et al., eds., *Tropical Medicine and Parasitology: Classic Investigations* (Ithaca: Cornell University Press, 1978), 1: 294–297. The disorder was known in various parts of the world as cachexia africana, tropical chlorosis, mal d'estomac, mal de coeur; Ackerknecht, *History and Geography* 130. In 1869 Wucherer summarized and commented on a book by R. Leuckart giving a detailed description of the structure of the parasite; "Sobre o anckylostoma duodenale ou strongylus duodenalis Dubini," *Gazeta Médica* 3 (1869): 170–172, 183–184, 198–220.

62   There is a discrepancy in the historical and medical literature as to who the main victims of the disorder were. In Brazil the disease was always associated with slaves and field workers whereas in North America and the Caribbean what is believed to have been hookworm was viewed as successfully resisted by blacks and contracted more easily by whites. The Tropicalistas held that most of the victims of the disease were from the poorest elements of the society. Jansen de Melo, "Pathogenia da hipoemia tropical," *Gazeta Médica* 15 (1883): 264, 272. Adolfo Lutz stated he saw no difference in the incidence between different ethnic groups; "Anckylostoma duodenale e anckylostomiase," *Gazeta Médica* 19 (1888): 162–163. However, research by the Rockefeller Foundation in the twentieth century demonstrated that blacks have relative immunity to hookworm. For the history of hookworm eradication in the American South, see John Ettling, *The Germ of Laziness: Rockefeller Philanthropy and Public Health in the South* (Cambridge, Mass.: Harvard University Press, 1981).

63   Wucherer's discovery initiated a whole cycle of investigations in Bahia beyond the core Tropicalista group. Thus, for example, by the 1870s, as Tropicalista disciples began moving into positions on the faculty of the medical school, there were theses on the subject. See, for example, Júlio R. de Moura, "Do hipoemia intertropical considerada como moléstia verminosa," *Gazeta Médica* 5 (1871): 6–9; J. de Moura, "O Dr. Davaine e sua doctrina parasitária da hypoemia intertropical," *Gazeta Médica* 14 (1882): 102–111; and Manoel Victorino Pereira, "Anchylostoma duodenal: Chlorose de Egypto—hypoemia intertropical," *Gazeta*

Médica 9 (1877): 19–31, 68–82. In 1871 Demétrio C. Tourinho won his chair in internal pathology with a work on hypoemia tropical.

64   Kean et al., eds., *Tropical Medicine*, 2: 297; Wucherer, "Patologia," *Gazeta Médica* 1 (1866): 64.

65   The disease is a very old one and was first reported in Brazil by Piso in 1648. H. Scott, *Tropical Medicine*, gives 1611 as the date of Piso's report, 2: 840. After malaria and tuberculosis, hookworm is believed to have been the most widespread disorder in hot climates until the advent of effective therapies. Thousands of worms attach themselves to a host's small intestine, where they suck blood for nutrition, producing severe anemia in the host, and sometimes causing the victim to have an urge to consume earth (geophagy). On the disorder generally, see H. Scott, *Tropical Medicine*, 2: 841; Ackerknecht, *History and Geography*, 131–132. For writings contemporary with the Tropicalistas, see Thomas Spencer Cobbold, *Parasites: A Treatise on the Ectozoa of Man and Animals Including Some Account of the Ectozoa* (London: J. and A. Churchill, 1879), 211–212; and Kean et al., eds., *Tropical Medicine*, 1: 287–324.

66   Ackerknecht, *History and Geography*, 131–132; Wucherer's work on hookworm was first published in Germany by Griesinger, who communicated the results of Wucherer's work in *Archiv für Physiologie Heilkunde* (1866): 387. The St. Gotthard epidemic was very severe indeed. According to Adolfo Lutz, in Brazil the average number of worms found in patients was between three hundred and four hundred. In the St. Gotthard workers the numbers of worms were between two thousand and three thousand. Lutz, "Anckylostoma duodenale e anckylostomiase," *Gazeta Médica* 20 (1888): 454.

67   See chap. 1.

68   Victorino Pereira, "Anchylostoma duodenale," 19–31, 68–82.

69   Ibid., 27, 78, 81.

70   For the abolition of Brazilian slavery, see Emília Viotti da Costa, *Da senzala à colônia* (São Paulo: Ciências Humanas, 1982); Rebecca J. Scott et al., *The Abolition of Slavery and the Aftermath of Emancipation in Brazil* (Durham: Duke University Press, 1988); Robert B. Toplin, *The Abolition of Slavery in Brazil* (New York: Atheneum, 1975).

71   Elizabeth Fee deals with the practical implications of the different styles in understanding and studying diseases in "Sin versus Science: Venereal Disease in Twentieth Century Baltimore," in *AIDS: The Burdens of History*, ed. Elizabeth Fee and Daniel M. Fox (Berkeley: University of California Press, 1988), 121–146.

72   "Discurso sobre as moléstias que mais afligem a classe pobre do Rio de Janeiro," published in *Revista Médica Fluminense*.

73   The discussion of Jobim's ideas is taken from Reginaldo Fernandes de Oliveira, *O conselheiro Jobim e o espírito da medicina do seu tempo* (Senado Federal: Centro Gráfico, 1982); James D. Goodyear, "Agents of Empire: Portuguese Doctors in Colonial Brazil and the Idea of Tropical Disease" (Ph.D. dissertation, Johns

Hopkins University, 1982), 323–325; Santos Filho, *História geral*, 2: 271–272; and Jobim's obituary in *Anais Brasilienses de Medicina* 30 (1879): 81–83.

74 Jobim quoted in Goodyear, "Agents of Empire," 330.

75 Ibid., 332.

76 Jansen de Melo, "Pathogenia da hipoemia tropical," 262–272.

77 *Jahrbücher* 96; Jobim's view of the disorder was noted by Hirsch in the 1859–62 German edition of the book but not in the 1883 English edition.

78 R. Oliveira, *O conselheiro Jobim*, 67.

79 Otto Wucherer, "Anchylostoma duodenães," *Gazeta Médica* 2 (1867): 151.

80 *Gazeta Médica* 14 (1882): 103–109. Júlio Rodrigues de Moura helped disseminate Tropicalista ideas on beriberi. He published his earliest work on beriberi not in Rio de Janeiro, where he lived, but in Bahia.

81 Lutz, "Anckylostoma duodenale e anckylostomiase," 118.

82 See, for example, his articles in *Archiv für Pathologische Anatomie und Physiologie und für Klinische Medecin* (1861): 345–363; (1872): 379–400; *Schmidt's Jahrbücher der in - und Ausländischen Gesammten Medecin* (1857): 119–125; (1858): 237–245.

83 Otto Wucherer, "A moléstia como parte do plano de creação," *Gazeta Médica* 1 (1866): 5–8. I deal more fully with Darwin's ideas in Bahia in chap. 5.

84 Wucherer sent his former teacher Griesinger specimens of the *Ancylostoma*. He also sent specimens to Spencer Cobbold, the British parasitologist, to Dr. Weber, and to Dr. Leuckhart. He sent specimens from his herpetology collection to the British Museum and the London Zoological Garden; see Kean et al., eds., *Tropical Medicine*, 1: 294. Cobbold published a description of the samples sent to him by Wucherer; see *Parasites*, 215. Wucherer also corresponded with Le Roy de Méricourt; Mr. Reed, a young English naturalist; Benjamin E. Cotting, a colleague of Agassiz; and John O'Neill, who practiced in West Africa and wrote on craw-craw.

85 Michael Worboys, "The Emergence and Early Development of Parasitology," in *Parasitology: A Global Perspective*, ed. Kenneth S. Warren and John Z. Bowers (New York: Springer-Verlag, 1983), 5. One need only peruse the 1883 edition of August Hirsch's *Handbook of Geographical and Historical Pathology* under the headings of the leading tropical ailments of the time to find constant references to the work and opinions of the Tropicalistas, especially Wucherer.

86 Wucherer noted that he had read about Griesinger's work in *Schmidt's Jahrbücher;* see Cobbold, *Parasites*, 214. Wucherer also published in the *Archiv für Physiologie Heilkunde,* a journal in which Griesinger also published.

87 A good example of such thinking can be seen in the writings of José Pereira Rego, Barão de Lavradio, who, as head of Rio de Janeiro's Board of Public Hygiene, wrote that if the authorities expected "improvement to continue they must not relax their efforts to . . . root out certain vices that have become rooted in society . . . of tobacco and spiritous liquors, and especially the vice of prostitution." Quoted by T. P. Corbally, "Rio de Janeiro," *Sanitarian* 10, 116 (November

1882): 642. On Lavradio, see Lourival Ribeiro, *O Barão de Lavradio e a higiene no Rio de Janeiro imperial* (Belo Horizonte: Itatiaia, 1992).

88 Otto Wucherer, "Sobre as causas da crescida frequência da tísica no Brasile especialmente na Bahia," *Gazeta Médica* 2 (1868): 267–268.

89 Otto H. Wucherer, "Preliminary Report on a Species of Worm, Found in the Urine of Patients with Tropical Hematuria in Brazil," in Kean et al., eds., *Tropical Medicine*, 1: 378.

90 Filariasis is a very old disorder caused by a family of parasites; the variety that Wucherer studied was known to the ancient Hindus, to the Arabs, and to the Europeans, where it produced a disorder commonly called elephantiasis arabum. Filariasis is caused by long threadworms that block human lymph channels, causing a general constitutional weakening and, often, immense swelling of the legs, arms, scrotum, and breasts. Because of their similar deforming symptoms, doctors often confused Arabian elephantiasis with Greek elephantiasis, which was, in fact, leprosy. The French doctor Jean Nicolas Demarquay had also discovered the embryonic filaria in 1863 in a patient who had spent time in Cuba. But when he showed the helminths to the expert Dr. Casimir Joseph Davaine, the latter doubted their significance. Thus the discovery was forgotten until Wucherer prompted interest in the parasite once again.

91 Quoted in Kean et al., eds., *Tropical Medicine*, 1: 379. According to Cobbold, *Parasites*, 200, it had long been posited that there was a relation between elephantiasis and hemochyluria. However, Silva Lima stated that in Bahia it was rare to find both symptoms together; "Memória sobre a hematuria chylosa, ou gordurosa dos países quentes, pelo Dr. J. Crevaux, médico da marinha franceza, com annotações e commentários," *Gazeta Médica* 8 (1876): 50.

92 For a good account of the early research into filariasis in Bahia, see José Francisco da Silva Lima, "Nova phase na questão da natureza verminosa da chyluria: Descoberta do representante adulto da filaria de Wucherer," *Gazeta Médica* 9 (1877): 387–396, 481–492; Pedro S. de Magalhães, "Descripção de uma espécie de filarias encontradas no coração humano," *Gazeta Médica* 19 (1887): 49–65, 109–130, 152–165, 200–211.

93 Wucherer introduced his work on the filaria in "Nota preliminar sobre vermes de uma espécie ainda não descripta, encontrados na urina de doentes de hematuria intertropical no Brazil," *Gazeta Médica* 3 (1868): 97–99; and "Sobre a hematuria no Brazil," *Gazeta Médica* 4 (1869): 39–40, 49–50, 61–62, 73–74, 85–86.

94 Otto Wucherer, "Anchylostomos duodenães encontradas em cadaveres de hypoemicos na ilha Mayotti, uma das Comoras," *Gazeta Médica* 2 (1868): 229.

95 E. Mauriac, "Coup-d'oeil sur la littérature médicale bresilienne," *Journal de Medecin de Bourdeau* 11 (1882): 326–329. A Brazilian translation of the article is in *União Médica* 3 (1883): 182–188.

96 This was the Metropolitan Counties Branch of the British Medical Association; see Magalhães, "Descripção de uma espécie de filarias," 55. For English transla-

tion of the key articles in the early unraveling of the filaria puzzle, see Kean et al., eds., *Tropical Medicine*, 1: 374–405. See also Le Roy Méricourt, "De l'hematurie intertropicale observee au Brezil," *Archives de Médecine Navale* (1870): 141; *Deutsches Archiv für Klinische Medicin* (Sept. 27, 1872): 379–400; Paul Bourel-Ronciere, "Resume of a Commentary upon the Writings of Silva Lima, Silva Araújo, and Others," *Archives de Médecine Naval* (1878); for further references up to 1878, see Cobbold, *Parasites*, 202–205. It should be noted that although the Tropicalistas were most interested in introducing the German model of medical teaching and practice, they were most recognized by the French and British medical communities where interest in tropical and naval medicine preceded German interest in those fields. Only German parasitologists like Griesenger, Leuckhart, and Virchow (whose breadth of interests was astounding) were alert to the Brazilians.

97 A number of physicians from different parts of the world reported sighting the parasites: in 1863, the French doctor Demarquay (see n. 91 above); in 1868, Dr. Salisbury in the United States; in 1870, Dr. Crevaux on board ship returning to France from the West Indies; in 1874, the Italian Dr. Sonsino in Egypt; in 1875, the British Dr. John O'Neill in a craw-craw patient in West Africa. See José Luís D'Almeida Couto, "Sobre a pathogenia da chyluria a propósito da monografia do Sr. Dr. Martins da Costa," *Gazeta Médica* 9 (1877): 58–59; Cobbold, *Parasites*, 190; Hirsch, *Handbook* (1883), 2: 321–323.

98 H. Scott, *Tropical Medicine*, 1: 159; Ronald Ross, *Memories of Sir Patrick Manson* (London: Harrison and Sons, n.d.), 9–10; Silva Lima, "Nova phase," 389; Cobbold, *Parasites*, 184–185; Timothy Richards Lewis, "The Nematoid Haematozoa of Man," *Quarterly Journal of Microscopical Science* 19 (1879): 245–269. Lewis called the parasite he found in human blood *Filaria sanguinis hominis*.

99 Cobbold, *Parasites*, 190, 192; Ross, *Memories*, 15.

100 Manson's biographers report that Manson found out about the filaria from reading Timothy Lewis's work on the *Filaria sanguinis hominis* at the British Museum. Indeed, they do not credit Wucherer with the discovery at all. See Philip H. Manson-Bahr and A. Alcock, *The Life and Work of Sir Patrick Manson* (London: Cassell, 1927), 39–41. It is tempting to speculate that Cobbold told Manson about the Brazilians' work. At the time, Cobbold, based in London, was the leading parasitologist in Britain and a nexus for all the work appearing on the filaria, as on other parasites. It is no coincidence that Lewis, Manson, and the Brazilian Tropicalistas all sent specimens to, and corresponded with, Cobbold. The latter knew Wucherer's work well because he had reported on it at scientific meetings and translated parts of it from the German. See *Parasites*, 181–211. For more on Cobbold, see Douglas M. Haynes, "From the Periphery to the Center: Patrick Manson and the Development of Tropical Medicine as a Medical Specialty in Britain, 1870–1900" (Ph.D. dissertation, University of California at Berkeley, 1992), 16–19.

101 Manson also discovered the "periodicity" of the parasites and thus explained why they were so difficult to find in the bloodstream. It had been a puzzle to Brazilian and other doctors in the tropics why the parasite could sometimes be found in the bloodstream and sometimes not. Manson discovered that the parasite only appears in the bloodstream at night. Today it is held that there are two forms of the filaria: one with nocturnal periodicity transmitted by night-biting mosquitoes and another with diurnal periodicity transmitted by day-biting mosquitoes. P. E. C. Manson-Bahr and F. I. C. Apted, *Manson's Tropical Diseases,* 18th ed. (London: Bailliere Tindall, 1982), 149.

102 John L. Paterson's assessment of filariasis research in 1878 is typical: "There are many zealous researchers of filariasis, as many here [in Brazil] as in other countries. We can, therefore, wait confidently for more definite answers." "Helmintologia; fatos relativos à filariose," *Gazeta Médica* 10 (1878): 536.

103 Silva Lima also kept in touch with European physician-researchers and he sent specimens of the *Ancylostoma duodenale* to the Hunterian Museum in Britain and to European doctors interested in tropical diseases. See Silva Lima, "Memória sobre a hematuria chilosa ou gordurosa dos países quentes pelo Sr. Dr. J. Chevaux, médico da marinha franceza com anotaçóes e comentários," *Gazeta Médica* 8 (1876): 7–22, 49–63, 97–111. The same issue also reproduced graphics of microorganisms associated with filariasis and bilharzia. See also Cobbold, *Parasites,* 213–215. Silva Lima received a paper from Duane Simmons on beriberi (kak-ke) in Japan. A. Pacífico Pereira, "Estudo sobre a etiologia e natureza do beriberi," *Gazeta Médica* 12 (1881): 494, n. 1.

104 A. J. P. Silva Araújo, "Casa de chyluria, elefancia de escroto, escroto linfático, craw-craw e erisepela em um mesmo indivíduo; Descobrimento da wucheria filaria na linfa no excroto; tratamento pela electricidade com excelentes resultados," *Gazeta Médica* 9 (1877): 492–504, 538; "*Filaria Sanguinis* Hominis in Relation to Elephantiasis, Chyluria, and Allied Diseases," *Lancet* 1 (March 30, 1878): 465.

105 Silva Araújo, "A muriçoca e as filarias wucheri," *Gazeta Médica* 10 (1878): 382, 385–389.

106 Silva Araújo, "Casa de chyluria," *Gazeta Médica* 9 (1877): 492–504; "Do tratamento da elefancia pela electricidade," *Gazeta Médica* 13 (1882): 350–355; "*Filaria Sanguinis* Hominis in Relation to Elephantiasis, Chyluria, and Allied Diseases," *Lancet* 1 (March 30, 1878): 465.

107 Magalhães, "Descripção de uma espécie de filarias," 49–51; *British Medical Record* 15 (June 1887): 273.

108 Magalhães, "Ainda algumas palavras sobre filariose de Wucherer," *Gazeta Médica* 11 (1879): 537–546; John L. Paterson, "Sobre o envólucro da filaria sanguinis hominis," *Gazeta Médica* 11 (1879): 97–107, 265–271, 345. See also the disagreement between Pires Caldas and Paterson over whether a surgical procedure for scrotal elephantiasis could succeed or not. Pires Caldas, "Elefancio do escroto:

Operação," *Gazeta Médica* 1 (1867): 245–246; J. L. Paterson, "Caso de elefancia tratado sem proveito pela ligadura da artéria femoral," *Gazeta Médica* 1 (1867): 220.

109 John L. Paterson, "Fatos relativos a filariose," *Gazeta Médica* 10 (1878): 529–536. They also looked at the relevance of age and gender. See also Silva Lima, "Sobre alquns casos de linfangile filariosa," 30 (1899): 457.

110 Quoted in *British Medical Record* (May 1885): 205.

111 Julio de Moura, "Dr. Otto Wucherer," *União Médica* 1 (1881): 228.

112 *Gazeta Médica* 12 (1880): 49.

113 Silva Lima, "Memória sobre a hematuria," 63.

114 Silva Lima, "Nova phase," 481.

115 Ibid., 395. Cobbold, *Parasites*, 186–187.

116 Silva Lima, "Nova phase," 481; Cobbold, *Parasites*, 191.

117 Cobbold, *Parasites*, 186–187; *Journal of the Quekett Microscopical Club* 6 (1879–81): 58–64; see also the obituary for Cobbold, *Gazeta Médica* 18 (1886): 170–171. All except Felício dos Santos, a doctor in Rio de Janeiro, were members of the Tropicalistas. As a result of Silva Lima's intervention, the parasites are today known as *Wucheria bancrofti.*

118 For example, in a paper presented on his behalf to the Medical Society of London in 1878, Cobbold acknowledged Brazilian contributions and then stated dryly, "Manson arrived independently at the same conclusion. Wucherer would, were he alive, be the last to claim priority to Lewis, Bancroft, and Manson in this matter [of the relationship between the filaria and elephantiasis]." *Lancet* 1 (March 30, 1878): 465. A review some years later of a Brazilian monograph on filariasis noted, "The major part of the pamphlet is occupied by an historical résumé of the whole subject of filarial disease in man, dating from Wucherer's discovery in 1868 of the immature form in the haematochylous urine. . . . We are glad to note that full credit is given to Manson for his laborious investigations, conducted, as they were, under conditions of great difficulty, and crowned by the really brilliant identification of the mosquito as the intermediary host." *British Medical Record* 15 (June 1887): 273.

119 For European journals reprinting and discussing the Brazilians' work, see the bibliography in Cobbold, *Parasites*, 202–205.

120 Manson-Bahr and Alcock, *Life and Work of Sir Patrick Manson*, 39–41. Manson's article "Tropical Medicine and Hygiene," *British Medical Journal* 2 (July–December 1917): 103–109, does mention Wucherer and Demarquay.

121 Ross, *Memoirs*, 10.

122 These included Wucherer, Silva Lima, Silva Araújo, Tourinho, Carvalho, Almeida Couto, Álvares dos Santos. This was probably in part to do with the fact that French doctors had taken note of the Tropicalistas and listed them among of a handful of doctors who were making scientific contributions in Brazil. See Mauriac, "Coup-d'oeil sur la littérature médicale bresilienne," 326–329; see also

comments by Pedro L. N. Chernoviz, a French doctor who was resident in Brazil, who praised the Tropicalistas in the *Guia Médico.*

123 They were Silva Araújo and Pedro S. de Magalhães. The former came from a wealthy Bahian family. He learned microscopy from Wucherer and his main interest was filariasis. He moved to Rio de Janeiro in 1879, becoming a member of the Imperial Academy of Medicine, then its secretary, speaker, and, finally, president. The latter came from a humble background. He graduated in Bahia in 1873 and became interested in cardiology, parasitology, and surgery. He spent a year in Berlin at the clinic of Ernst von Leyden and moved to Rio de Janeiro in 1883, where he joined the medical school faculty as professor in clinical surgery. He continued to work in tropical parasitology, especially the filaria, and a number of his writings on the latter subject became well known internationally. Both men worked at the General Polyclinic.

124 "Noticias varias," *Gazeta Médica* 18 (1887): 378.

125 These were held in Rio de Janeiro in 1888 and 1889.

126 Silva Lima, "Memória sobre a hematuria," 111.

127 Worboys, "Emergence and Early Development of Parasitology," 4.

128 Lowy, "Yellow Fever," 145. Once people gained an understanding of insect vectors and complex life cycles of the microorganisms involved in tropical disorders, researchers moved into schools of tropical medicine that increasingly studied protozoology, helminthology, and entomology, hoping to locate specific agents that could be isolated and eradicated. According to Worboys, when this happened, researchers of tropical medicine in Europe parted company with researchers in bacteriological centers. This separation does not seem to have occurred in Brazil at this time. The Oswaldo Cruz Institute, for example, carried out research on vaccination and immunological studies typical of bacterial disease, as well as on vector control and life of protozoa. See Worboys, "Emergence and Early Development of Parasitology," 6–11; John Farley, "Parasites and the Germ Theory of Disease," *Millbank Quarterly* 67 (1989): 50–68.

129 Lowy, "Yellow Fever," 162. The anomaly was the Pasteur Institute, which was financed entirely by private donations. Louis Pasteur was the consummate entrepreneur as well as brilliant scientist and, as such, an exception to the rule.

Chapter 3 Race, Climate, and Medicine: Framing Tropical Disorders

1 *Primeiro Congresso Brazileiro de Medicina e Cirurgia do Rio de Janeiro* (Rio de Janeiro: Imprensa Nacional, 1889), 4; Júlio de Moura, "A possibilidade de reunirse um congresso médico no Brasil," *Gazeta Médica* 2 (1868): 193.

2 *Primeiro Congresso Brazileiro,* 3.

3 Ibid., 6.

4 Ibid., 7, 8.

5 The papers given at the congress are in *Gazeta Médica* 20 (1888): 171–186, 216–227, 379–387; 21 (1889): 99–111.

6   On this question, see P. S. de Magalhães, "Reforma do ensino médico: O ensino da medicina tropical," *Brasil Médico* 37 (1923): 340–341. What was also at stake here were jobs and job definitions, which some viewed as threatening and others as new opportunities.

7   The medical questions about the nature of tropical medicine were mirrored by debates over whether a tropical society, personality, and race existed. See, for example, Roberto Ventura, *Escritores, escravos e mestiços em um país tropical: Literatura, historiografia e ensaísmo no Brasil* (Nürnberg: Wilhelm Fink Verlag München, 1987), 1–49; Thomas E. Skidmore, *Black into White: Race and Nationality in Brazilian Thought* (New York: Oxford University Press, 1974), 98–123.

8   David J. Bradley, "Tropical Medicine," in *The Oxford Companion to Medicine,* ed. John Walton, Paul B. Beeson, and Ronald Bodley Scott (Oxford: Oxford University Press, 1986), 2: 1393.

9   Ibid.

10 Michael Worboys, "The Emergence of Tropical Medicine: A Study of the Establishment of a Scientific Specialty," in *Perspectives on the Emergence of Scientific Disciplines,* ed. G. Lemaine et al. (The Hague: Mouton, 1976); Worboys, "Tropical Diseases," in *Companion Encyclopedia of the History of Medicine,* ed. W. F. Bynum and Roy Porter (London: Routledge, 1994), 1: 512.

11 Bradley, "Tropical Medicine," 2: 1397; Brian Maegraith, "Tropical Medicine: What It Is Not, What It Is," *Bulletin of the New York Academy of Medicine* 48 (1972): 1214; Worboys, "Tropical Diseases." The scare and reaction to the ebola virus is, in some ways, returning us yet again to the older notion of exotic disorders of the tropics from which the West must shield itself.

12 Michael Worboys, "Tropical Medicine and Colonial Imperialism, 1895–1914," in "Science and British Colonial Imperialism, 1895–1940" (Ph.D. dissertation, University of London, 1979); Martin F. Shapiro, "Medicine in the Service of Colonialism: Medical Care in Portuguese Africa, 1885–1974" (Ph.D. dissertation, University of California at Los Angeles, 1983); Mark Harrison, "Tropical Medicine in Nineteenth-Century India," *British Journal for the History of Science* 25 (1992): 299–318; Harrison, *Public Health in British India: Anglo-Indian Preventive Medicine, 1859–1914* (Cambridge: Cambridge University Press, 1994); David Arnold, *Colonizing the Body: State Medicine and Epidemic Disease in Nineteenth-Century India* (Berkeley: University of California Press, 1993).

13 For an interesting discussion on the evolution of the idea of tropical disorders as universal or distinctive, see Worboys, "Tropical Diseases," 1: 512–536; Bradley, "Tropical Medicine," 2: 1393–1399.

14 For a good introduction to the idea of degeneration in the nineteenth century, see J. Edward Chamberlin and Sander L. Gilman, eds., *Degeneration: The Dark Side of Progress* (New York: Columbia University Press, 1985), esp. the essay by Eric T. Carlson, "Medicine and Degeneration: Theory and Praxis," 121–143. For a discussion of the idea of degeneration in Brazil, see Dain Edward Borges,

"'Puffy, Ugly, Slothful, and Inert': Degeneration in Brazilian Social Thought, 1880–1940," *Journal of Latin American Studies* 25 (1993): 239–241.

15   Philip D. Curtin, *The Image of Africa: British Ideas and Actions, 1780–1850* (Madison: University of Wisconsin Press, 1964), and *Death by Migration: Europe's Encounter with the Tropical World in the Nineteenth Century* (Cambridge: Cambridge University Press, 1989). For a discussion on yellow fever in blacks and whites, see Kenneth F. Kiple and Virginia Himmelsteib King, *Another Dimension to the Black Diaspora: Diet, Disease, and Racism* (Cambridge: Cambridge University Press, 1981), 29–49; David N. Livingstone, "Human Acclimatization: Perspectives on a Contested Field of Inquiry in Science, Medicine, and Geography," *Human Science* 25 (1987): 359–394; Karen Ordahl Kupperman, "Fear of Hot Climates in the Anglo-American Colonial Experience," *William and Mary Quarterly* 41, 2 (April 1984): 213–240; Warwick Anderson, "Immunities of Empire: Race, Disease, and the New Tropical Medicine, 1900–1920," *Bulletin of the History of Medicine* 70 (1996): 94–118; Mark Harrison, "'The Tender Frame of Man': Disease, Climate, and Racial Difference in India and the West Indies, 1760–1860," *Bulletin of the History of Medicine* 70 (1996): 68–93. For some earlier writings on climate by Brazilians, see Afrânio Peixoto, *Minha terra, mi gente* (Rio de Janeiro: F. Alves, 1929) and Sílvio Romero, *História da literatura brasileira,* 3d ed. (Rio de Janeiro: José Olympio, 1949) I: 56–82.

16   Romero, *História* 359, 361; Nancy Leys Stepan, "Biological Degeneration: Races and Proper Places," in *Degeneration,* ed. Chamberlin and Gilman, 97–102; Robert J. C. Young, *Colonial Desire: Hybridity in Theory, Culture, and Race* (London: Routledge, 1995), 142–143.

17   See James D. Goodyear, "Agents of Empire: Portuguese Doctors in Colonial Brazil and the Idea of Tropical Disease" (Ph.D. dissertation, Johns Hopkins University, 1982), esp. chap. 2, "Brazil: 'Terrestrial Paradise?'" 34–73.

18   This view is borne out by the British physician Dr. Robert Dundas, who in a series of lectures in Liverpool in 1849 on tropical fevers praised the beneficial qualities of Bahia's climate, a judgment he had formed after twenty-three years of medical service to the British community in Bahia and before the epidemics struck. Donald B. Cooper, "Brazil's Long Fight against Epidemic Disease, 1849–1917, with Special Emphasis on Yellow Fever," *Bulletin of the New York Academy of Medicine* 51, 5 (1975): 672–696; Dundas, *Sketches of Brazil: Including New Views on Tropical and European Fever* (London: John Churchill, 1852), 201–208.

19   European concerns about degeneration in the tropics are well illustrated by a series of questions French doctors asked the Bahian Society of Medicine to respond to: Was the Bahian climate unhealthy? Do foreigners living there have a shorter life span than people living in the great European cities? Are Europeans more subject to contracting disease than the natives of the region? Is the European's fertility changed by climate, food, or work conditions? There were a total of twenty-two questions. *Gazeta Médica* 20 (1888): 45–48. An interesting paper

given at the First Brazilian Medical Congress at Rio de Janeiro, and published in the *Gazeta Médica,* was on the frequency of European patients with vesicular stones in Brazil, which a French study explained as linked to tropical climate. The Brazilian speaker stated that the French study, based on erroneous statistics, was incorrect. The article is a good example of Brazilian doctors rejecting the determinism of climate and the idea that whites fared badly in the tropics. Oscar Bulhões, "Frequencia dos cálculos visicais no Brasil, resultados operatórios," *Gazeta Médica* 20 (1889): 458–466. Goodyear notes that in the colonial period there were people who worried about how climate in Brazil could "undermine the social morality of the colony," inducing idleness and moral lapse. "Agents of Empire," 273–275. See also Nancy Leys Stepan, *"The Hour of Eugenics": Race, Gender, and Nation in Latin America* (Ithaca: Cornell University Press, 1991), 44–46; and Stepan, "Biological Degeneration," 97–120; Harrison, "Tropical Medicine," 306.

20   Skidmore, *Black into White,* 29–30; see also Moema Parente Augel, *Visitantes estrangeiros na Bahia oitocentista* (São Paulo: Cultrix, 1980), 214. For contemporary views, see Louis Agassiz and Elizabeth Agassiz, *A Journey in Brazil* (New York: Praeger, 1969), 529–532; and medical students' dissertations, for example, Guarino Aloysio Ferreira Freire, "Qual o papel que desempenha a civilisação no movimento das molestias mentaes?" (Faculdade de Medicina da Bahia, 1888).

21   For literature examining race in Brazil, see Artur Ramos, *O negro na civilização brasileira* (Rio de Janeiro: Casa do Estudante no Brasil, 1956); José Honório Rodrigues, *Brazil and Africa* (Berkeley: University of California Press, 1965); Romero, *História da literatura brasileira* (Rio de Janeiro: Gernier, 1888), esp. vol. 2; Florestan Fernandes, *The Negro in Brazilian Society* (New York: Columbia University Press, 1969); Jeffrey D. Needell, "History, Race, and the State in the Thought of Oliveira Vianna," *Hispanic American Historical Review* 75 (1995): 1–30; Dain Edward Borges, "The Recognition of Afro-Brazilian Symbols and Ideas, 1890–1940," *Luso-Brazilian Review* 32, 2 (1995): 59–78; Célia Maria Marinho de Azevedo, *Onda negra, medo branco: O negro imaginário das elites, século XIX* (Rio de Janeiro: Paz e Terra, 1987); and Lília K. Schwarcz, *Retrato em branco e negro: Jornais, escravos e cidadãos em São Paulo no final do século XIX* (São Paulo: Companhia das Letras, 1987); Skidmore, *Black into White;* Ventura, *Escritores, escravos e mestiços;* Ricardo Ventura Santos, "Edgar Roquette-Pinto: Os tipos antropológicos e a questão da degeneração racial no Brasil no início do século" (paper presented at the Twentieth Annual Meeting of Associação Nacional de Pós-Graduaçãoe Pesquisa em Ciências Sociais, Caxambu, Minas Gerais, October 1996); Marshall C. Eakin, "Race and Identity: Sílvio Romero, Science, and Social Thought in Late Nineteenth-Century Brazil," *Luso-Brazilian Review* 22, 2 (1985): 151–174; Marcos Chor Maio and Ricardo Ventura Santos, *Raça, ciência e sociedade* (Rio de Janeiro: FIOCRUZ, 1996). For a recent summary on theoretical approaches to race in Brazil, see Howard Winant, *Racial Conditions:*

Politics, Theory, Comparisons (Minneapolis: University of Minnesota Press, 1994),
130–148. For literature on racial science elsewhere, see Nancy Leys Stepan, *The
Idea of Race in Science: Great Britain, 1800–1960* (London: MacMillan, 1982);
George M. Frederickson, *The Image of the Black in the White Mind* (New York:
Harper and Row, 1971); William Ragan Stanton, *The Leopard's Spots: Scientific
Attitudes towards Race in America, 1815–1859* (Chicago: University of Chicago
Press, 1960); George W. Stocking, "The Persistence of Polygenist Thought in
Post-Darwinian Anthropology," in *Race, Culture, and Evolution: Essays in the His-
tory of Anthropology,* ed. Stocking (New York: Free Press, 1968, 42–68); Stephen
Jay Gould, *The Mismeasure of Man* (New York: Norton, 1981).

22 Stepan, "Biological Degeneration," 98; Skidmore, *Black into White,* 48–49.

23 Skidmore, *Black into White,* 49.

24 Young, *Colonial Desire,* 11.

25 Todd L. Savitt, *Medicine and Slavery: The Diseases and Health Care of Blacks in
Antebellum Virginia* (Urbana: University of Illinois Press, 1978), 8; Savitt, "Black
Health on the Plantation: Master, Slaves, and Physicians," in *Sickness and Health:
Readings in the History of Medicine and Public Health,* ed. Judith Walzer Leavitt
and Ronald L. Numbers (Madison: University of Wisconsin Press, 1985), 315,
318. As Curtin notes, "in this way the misunderstanding of the medical men came
ultimately to be enshrined at the core of scientific 'racism.'" *Image of Africa,* 84.

26 Stepan, "Biological Degeneration," 98.

27 For background on the intertwining of medicine and racial science in Latin
America, see Stepan, *"Hour of Eugenics,"* 41–46.

28 See, for example, John S. Haller Jr., "The Physician versus the Negro: Medical
and Anthropological Concepts of Race in Late Nineteenth Century," *Bulletin of
the History of Medicine* 44 (1970): 154–167; John S. Haller Jr. and Robin Haller,
The Physician and Sexuality in Victorian America (Urbana: University of Illinois
Press, 1974), 47–87. Some prominent doctors in colonial Brazil blamed slavery
for exacerbating ill health; Goodyear, "Agents of Empire," 275–277.

29 Curtin, *Image of Africa,* 67, notes that some European observers believed that
blacks were better suited to the tropics because they were able to throw off poisons (phlogiston) produced in the heat through greater perspiration. Such Europeans believed that blacks "paid a price for this physical adjustment. [T]his price
was a weaker power of mind plus an extreme tendency to indolence. Therefore,
no high civilization had ever occurred, nor was one possible, in any part of the
tropical world." See also Stepan, "Biological Degeneration," 99; Todd L. Savitt,
"Slave Health and Southern Distinctiveness," in *Disease and Distinctiveness in the
American South,* ed. Todd L. Savitt and James Harvey Young (Knoxville: University of Tennessee Press, 1988), 132; Douglas M. Haynes, "From the Periphery to the Center, Patrick Manson and the Development of Tropical Medicine
as a Medical Specialty in Britain, 1870–1900" (Ph.D. dissertation, University of
California at Berkeley, 1992), 76–77, notes that some observers believed that the

tropical sun had a degenerative affect on the brain; Dane Kennedy, "The Perils of the Midday Sun: Climatic Anxieties in the Colonial Tropics," in *Imperialism and the Natural World,* ed. John M. MacKenzie (Manchester: Manchester University Press, 1990), 118–140; Livingstone, "Human Acclimatization," 359–394; W. Anderson, "Immunities of Empire," 94–118; Harrison, "'Tender Frame of Man,'" 68–93.

30 Henry Thomas Buckle (1821–1862), quoted in Skidmore, *Black into White,* 28–29. Gilberto Freyre quotes the Austrian traveler Mauricio Lamberg, who wrote in 1896 that the backwardness of Brazil should be attributed "not to 'lack of intelligence and good intentions,' but rather 'to the nature of the inhabitants of the tropics, who lack the capacity of learned men in colder climates to devote their entire existence to the examination of a single scientific problem, even when such a course means the sacrifice of many of the comforts of life' "; *Order and Progress: Brazil from Monarchy to Republic,* trans. Rod W. Horton (Berkeley: University of California Press, 1986), 124. Another opinion came from the German traveler Johann Jacob Tschudi, who noted that "with blacks there was introduced into Brazil a bad element in the mixture of races. . . . In all countries where there has been [African] slavery, racial mixing with blacks has brought backwardness." See Augel, *Visitantes,* 199.

31 Skidmore, *Black into White,* 30.

32 E. Bradford Burns, *A History of Brazil,* 2d ed. (New York: Columbia University Press, 1980), 255.

33 The figures are from Herbert S. Klein, *African Slavery in Latin America and the Caribbean* (New York: Oxford University Press, 1986), 126–128. There were 1.5 million slaves if the noneconomically active ones are included.

34 That is, São Paulo, Rio de Janeiro, and Minas Gerais. Ibid., 130; Klein, "The Internal Slave Trade in Nineteenth Century Brazil: A Study of Slave Importations into Rio de Janeiro in 1852," *Hispanic American Historical Review* 51 (1971): 567–585.

35 Skidmore, *Black into White,* 14; Burns, *History of Brazil,* 257. Emília Viotti da Costa, *Da senzala à colônia* (São Paulo: Ciências Humanas, 1982), 329–340, gives the fullest account of these early voices raised against slavery. See especially her interesting analysis of the thinking of Federico Leopoldo César Burlamaque, who anticipates in many ways the thinking and contradictions of the abolitionists.

36 This was true as early as the 1830s. See, for example, Darwin's antislavery stance, *The Voyage of the Beagle* (New York: Dutton, 1959), 480.

37 Emília Viotti da Costa, *The Brazilian Empire: Myths and Histories* (Chicago: University of Chicago Press, 1985), 178–179.

38 Ordival Cassiano Gomes, *Manuel Vitorino Pereira: Médico e Cirurgião* (Rio de Janeiro: Agir, 1957), 161.

39 João Cruz Costa, *A History of Ideas in Brazil,* trans. Suzette Macedo (Berkeley:

University of California Press, 1964), 82–202; Ivan Lins, *História do positivismo no Brasil,* 2d ed. (São Paulo: Companhia Editora Nacional, 1967); Charles A. Hale, "Political and Social Ideas in Latin America, 1870–1930," in *The Cambridge History of Latin America,* ed. Leslie Bethell (Cambridge: Cambridge University Press, 1985), 4: 382–414.

40 Burns, *History of Brazil,* 208–9.

41 Nearly all of the theses and writings of doctors that I have looked at condemn slavery when they mention it. As one medical student put it: "In Brazil the trade in slaves has led to the happiness of few and the misfortune of many, and [it has] introduced into the heart of the population immorality, prostitution, and innumerable diseases—all of which has dammed our civilization still in its cradle." Francisco Tavares da Cunha Mello, "Algumas considerações psycho-physiológicas acerca do homem," (Ph.D. dissertation, Faculdade de Medicina da Bahia, 1851), 17 n. 1. Other students also condemned the institution from the point of view of how it acted as a degenerating force on the slaves themselves. See, for example, Eugênio Guimarães Rebello, "As raças humanas descendem de uma só origem" (Ph.D. dissertation, Faculdade de Medicina da Bahia, 1869), 13: "No radical difference exists among human groups. The European, Kaffir, Hottentot, [and] Polynesian are all as capable of the same perfectability as of the same physical degradation and moral perversion." For other dissertations referring to slavery in critical terms, see Ignácio Firmo Xavier, "Reflexões sobre o médico" (Ph.D. dissertation, Faculdade de Medicina da Bahia, 1850), 17–18; João Carlos Balthasar de Silveira, "Influência dos climas sobre a intelligência humana" (Ph.D. dissertation, Faculdade de Medicina da Bahia, 1874), 51. Jurandir Freire Costa, *Ordem médica e norma familiar,* 2d ed. (Rio de Janeiro: Graal, 1979), 121, however, holds the opposite to be true.

42 José Francisco da Silva Lima, "Notícia sobre o ainhum," *Gazeta Médica* 12 (1881): 341. See the explanation commonly given of another fatal slave disorder, *tétano traumático,* in Mary C. Karasch, *Slave Life in Rio de Janeiro, 1808–1850* (Princeton: Princeton University Press, 1987), 152–153.

43 For the abolition of slavery in Brazil, see chap. 2 n. 71. See also the bibliographical essay by Klein in *African Slavery,* 292–294. For debates on the caliber of the labor force, see Borges, "Puffy, Ugly"; C. Azevedo, *Onda negra, medo branco* 33–37, 97–104; Skidmore, *Black into White,* 21–27.

44 "Falla do Governador da Província da Bahia, Antônio Cândido da Cruz Machado," in Brazil, *Ministério do Império, Relatórios ministeriais,* Época do Império, reel 12 (March 1874), 131; "Falla do Governador da Província da Bahia, João Antônio de Araújo Freitas Henriques," *Relatórios ministeriais,* reel 11 (March 1872), 136.

45 Barão de Sergimirim, "Imperial Instituto Bahiano de Agricultura," annex to "Falla do Governador da Província da Bahia, Gonçalves Martins, Barão de S.

Lourenço," in Brazil, *Ministério do Império, Relatórios ministeriais,* Época do Imperio, reel 10 (March 1871), 3–4.

46 José Goes Siqueira, annex to "Relatório . . . pelo Presidente o Desembargador
    João Lins Vieira," in Brazil, *Ministério do Império, Relatórios ministeriais,* Época
    do Império, reel 4 (May 1859), 7–8.

47 Klein notes that "Brazil imported over 1 million slaves in the 19th century and
    had a resident slave population of only 1.7 million in the late 1850s, whereas the
    United States imported a few hundred thousand slaves and ended up with a resi-
    dent population of 4 million slaves on the eve of the Civil War." *African Slavery,*
    157; see also Carl Degler, *Neither Black nor White: Slavery and Race Relations in
    Brazil and the United States* (Madison: University of Wisconsin Press, 1986). For
    a discussion on the meaning of manumission and the stages in the passage to free-
    dom, see Kátia M. de Queirós Mattoso, *To Be a Slave in Brazil, 1550–1888,* trans.
    Arthur Goldhammer (New Brunswick: Rutgers University Press, 1986).

48 Klein, *African Slavery,* 220.

49 I am using Klein's definition for free coloreds: that is, "inclusive of both blacks
    and mulattos." Ibid., viii, 223. For population figures, see n. 62 below.

50 Ibid., 235–236. Examples include the musician Emerico Lobo de Mesquita and
    the writers Machado de Assis and Gonçalves Dias. Well-known Bahian doctors
    were Lino Coutinho, his grandson Jerônymo Sodré Pereira, Anselmo de Fon-
    seca, and Domingos Carlos da Silva; in Rio the most prestigious doctor in the last
    decades of the Empire was Torres Homem, a mulatto. Other mulattoes promi-
    nent in Brazil were the jurist Tobias Barreto; the archbishop Dom Silveiro Gomes
    Pimenta, the engineer André Pereira Rebouças; and the lawyer Luís Gonzaga
    de Pinto Gama. Such evidence, of course, has been used to fuel the myth of
    racial democracy in Brazil and led to arguments by Freyre about the possibility
    of social mobility for blacks in a society where, he held, the racial system was
    fluid. Building on this idea, Carl Degler called the intermediate racial category
    that, he believed, allowed for mobility the "mulatto escape hatch." Other social
    scientists rejected this approach to race in Brazil, providing evidence that even if
    the racial system operated differently from that of the United States, it was still
    a dichotomous one in which, as George Reid Andrews has noted, "movement
    within the black racial category is common . . . but . . . movement across the
    barrier separating the white and black racial groups is relatively rare." Andrews,
    Blacks and Whites in São Paulo, Brazil, 1888–1988 (Madison: University of Wis-
    consin Press, 1991), 253. However, as Andrews himself goes on to point out, the
    dichotomous racial classification system in the Empire years may be less accurate
    than the three-tier racial hierarchy proposed by Degler. The existence of slavery,
    the still early development of capitalism and industrialization, the limited elec-
    toral system, and the checks of patronage were all ways to control the popular
    (mainly black) classes and allow for limited numbers of (light) blacks to rise up

in the society. With the loosening of these controls under the Republic, new restrictions developed, among them the subtle myth of racial democracy that obscured the real barriers of a dichotomous racial system. For a discussion on the myth of racial democracy in the Empire, see E. Costa, *Brazilian Empire,* 234–246; for discussions of the myth after the Empire, Andrews, *Blacks and Whites,* esp. appendix B, 249–258; Winant, *Racial Conditions,* 150–151; Jan Fiola, "Race Relations in Brazil: A Reassessment of the 'Racial Democracy' Thesis" (Program in Latin American Studies, Occasional Paper Series No. 24, University of Massachusetts at Amherst, 1990); Pierre-Michel Fontaine, ed., *Race, Class, and Power in Brazil* (Los Angeles: Center for Afro-American Studies, University of California at Los Angeles, 1985); Charles H. Wood and José Alberto Magno de Carvalho, *The Demography of Inequality in Brazil* (Cambridge: Cambridge University Press, 1988). On race and science, see Lília K. Schwarcz, *O espetáculo das raças: Cientistas, instituições a questão racial no Brasil, 1870–1930* (São Paulo: Companhia das Letras, 1993). For an important series of articles that update and provide an overview of the evolution of racial thinking in Brazil, see Maio and Santos, *Raça, ciência e sociedade.* For more, see n. 21 above.

51 Quoted by Pierre Verger, *Notícias da Bahia—1850* (Salvador: Corrupio, 1981), 58. See also the comments by the American Reverend James C. Fletcher: "If a man has freedom, money, and merit, no matter how black may be his skin, no place in society is refused him," quoted in Freyre, *Order and Progress,* 170–171.

52 Skidmore, *Black into White,* 23. Brazilians also favored their approach because they believed that through racial assimilation Brazilians would become whiter, 70.

53 Ibid., 54. This is a theme Freyre focuses on in his analysis of Brazilian society. See, for example, *Order and Progress,* 198–216; and Frank Tannenbaum, *Slave and Citizen* (Boston: Beacon, 1992), 120–126.

54 Herbert S. Klein, "Colored Freedman in Brazilian Slave Society," *Journal of Social History* 3 (1969): 30–52. Klein also notes that slave owners manumitted Africans and mulattoes in almost equal proportion when self-purchase was involved, but when only the white owner's preference was involved, then mulattoes were invariably chosen. Klein, *African Slavery,* 228.

55 Degler, *Neither Black nor White,* 226–239, summarizes the debate.

56 "Whitening" is the historian's term for a process not self-consciously defined in the nineteenth century. For a discussion of the concept, see Skidmore, *Black into White,* 64–77; E. Costa, *Brazilian Empire,* 237; Degler, *Neither Black nor White,* 105–107, 191–195; Kátia M. de Queirós Mattoso, *Bahia: A Cidade do Salvador e seu mercado no século XIX* (São Paulo: Hucitec, 1977), 202; Needell, "History, Race, and the State," 11–16; Antônio Sérgio Alfredo Guimarães, "Cor, classes e status nos estudos de Pierson, Azevedo e Harris na Bahia: 1940–1960," in *Raça, ciência e sociedade,* ed. Maio and Santos, 143–158. Brazil was not the only country that adopted the system of whitening. It was very much a centerpiece of Latin

American race relations historically. See Winthrop R. Wright, *Café con Leche: Race, Class, and National Image in Venezuela* (Austin: University of Texas Press, 1995), 1–12; Peter Wade, *Race and Ethnicity in Latin America* (London: Pluto, 1993), 84–87.

57 This theme was a key preoccupation of North American biologists and racial "scientists" like Josiah Nott, Samuel Morton, Louis Agassiz, George Gliddon, and J. Aitken Meigs, who were writing at a time of crisis in the system of slavery in the United States, in a milieu of utter distaste for black-white unions, so that their primary aim was to foreclose the possibility of an interracial society. See Stepan, "Biological Degeneration," 98.

58 On European immigration, see Boris Fausto, "Society and Politics," in *Brazil: Empire and Republic, 1822–1930,* ed. Leslie Bethell (Cambridge: Cambridge University Press, 1989), 262; Jeffrey Needell, *A Tropical Belle Epoque: Elite Culture and Society in Turn-of-the-Century Rio de Janeiro* (Cambridge: Cambridge University Press, 1987), 32–33; Thomas H. Holloway, *Immigrants on the Land: Coffee and Society in São Paulo, 1886–1934* (Chapel Hill: University of North Carolina Press, 1980); Andrews, *Blacks and Whites,* 85–88. For the idea of improving the national population, see Greenfield, "Great Drought," 375–400, esp. 383–385, 398–399. See also Belisário Penna, *O saneamento do Brasil* (Rio de Janeiro: Typ. Revista dos Tribunaes, 1918); Luiz Antônio de Castro Santos, "Power, Ideology, and Public Health in Brazil, 1889–1930" (Ph.D. dissertation, Harvard University, 1987).

59 Skidmore, *Black into White,* 77. E. Costa, *Brazilian Empire,* 239; Skidmore has quoted J. B. Lacerda, the physician and scientist, who stated: "Contrary to the opinion of many writers, the crossing of black with the white does not generally produce offspring of an inferior intellectual quality," *Black into White,* 65. See also Stepan, *"Hour of Eugenics,"* 154–161.

60 Silveira, "Influência dos climas sobre a inteligência humana," 34, 35.

61 Brazilian fears of degeneration as a result of "tropicality" had their counterpart in Britain, where G. Steadman Jones has noted the belief that urban squalor and poverty created a vicious circle of biological degeneration; in France, where the humiliation of 1871 raised many self-searching questions about alcoholism, prostitution, suicide, insanity, and syphilis as signs of degeneration; and even in Germany, which was fearful that the processes of rapid industrialization and urbanization might weaken the stock. See Robert A. Nye, *Crime, Madness, and Politics in Modern France: The Medical Concept of National Decline* (Princeton: Princeton University Press, 1984), 132–170, 322–336.

62 In 1807 the total population was 51,112, of which 20 percent was mulatto, 52 percent black, and 28 percent white. In 1872 of a total of 108,138, more than 44 percent was mulatto, more than 18 percent black, and 35 percent white. Mattoso, *Bahia,* 147. See also Donald Pierson, *Negroes in Brazil: A Study of Race Contact in Bahia* (Carbondale: Southern Illinois University Press, 1967), 126–130; Thales de Azevedo, *Povoamento da Cidade do Salvador* (Bahia: Itapua, 1969), 235. In *Bahia,*

154, Mattoso argues that the binary opposition model of rich, white slave-owner versus poor, black slave or freedman, used for so long in the historiography of Bahia, in fact masks a deep negation of the real blurring of racial categories.

63　My information has been drawn from remarks made by nineteenth-century travelers; from secondary sources, such as those by Gilberto Freyre and Santos Filho, which do not always give the sources of their statements; and from obituaries. For an informative discussion of the occupational categories in Salvador, see Mattoso, *Bahia*, 159–167.

64　Freyre, *Order and Progress*, esp. the chapter "Education and Urban Culture," 103–165; Verger, *Notícias*, 57.

65　This is a key thesis in Gilberto Freyre's *Mansions and the Shanties: The Making of Modern Brazil*, trans. Harriet de Onis (Berkeley: University of California Press, 1986), 355–399, where he discusses the transfer of power and influence from the colonial and rural aristocracy to "the aristocracy of cap and gown," that is, the urban university graduate. He expands on this theme in *Order and Progress*, 103–165. See also Dain Edward Borges, *The Family in Bahia, Brazil, 1870–1945* (Stanford: Stanford University Press, 1992), 85–111, for an exploration of how the family doctor, supplanting the priest, became a central influence in a new, urban-based, middle- and upper-middle-class family.

66　Freyre, *Mansions*, 355–358.

67　In Brazil natural sons (i.e., not from adulterous liaisons) had full legal rights. Mattoso, *Bahia*, 205.

68　"Identidade da espécie humana," quoted by Freyre, *Mansions*, 398.

69　Freyre, *Order and Progress*, 185–187.

70　Octávio Torres, *Esboço histórico dos acontecimentos mais importantes da vida da Faculdade de Medicina da Bahia, 1808–1946* (Salvador: Vitória, 1952). See pictures and captions, no page number.

71　See, for example, the obituary of Dr. Manuel Joaquim Saraiva in *Revista do Instituto Geográfico e Histórico da Bahia* 16, 35 (1909): 188–191.

72　See chap. 2, n. 123 for his bibliographical details.

73　Charles E. Rosenberg, "The Bitter Fruit: Heredity, Disease, and Social Thought," in *No Other Gods: On Science and American Social Thought* (Baltimore: Johns Hopkins University Press, 1976), 33.

74　On neo-Lamarckianism, see Peter J. Bowler, *The Eclipse of Darwinism: Anti-Darwinian Evolution Theories in the Decades around 1900* (Baltimore: Johns Hopkins University Press, 1983), 58–117; George W. Stocking, "Lamarckism in American Social Science: 1890–1915," *Journal of the History of Ideas* 27, 2 (1962): 239–256; Edward J. Pfeifer, "The Genesis of American Neo-Lamarckism," *Isis* 56 (1965): 156–167.

75　Silva Lima, "Terceiro Congresso Brasileiro de Medicina e Cirurgia," *Gazeta Médica* 22 (1890): 151, 152.

76　Bowler, *Eclipse*, 66.

77 Júlio de Moura, "Apontamentos para servirem de base ao estudo das estações climatéricas brasileiras mas aconselhadas para o tractamento da tísica pulmonar," *União Médica* 1 (1881): 603–604, 606–607.

78 Moura, "Apontamentos," *União Médica* 2 (1882): 9–10.

79 For an interesting discussion of the universal-distinctive notion, see Worboys, "Tropical Diseases," 1: 512–536.

80 This was a very old idea in medical literature. See Curtin, *Image of Africa,* 66–67; Dennis G. Carlson, *African Fever: A Study of British Science, Technology, and Politics in West Africa, 1787–1864* (New York: Science History Publications, 1984).

81 Antônio Pacífico Pereira, "Estudo sobre a etiologia e natureza do beriberi," *Gazeta Médica* 12 (1881): 533–536.

82 Ibid., 535–536.

83 Antônio Pacífico Pereira, "Hygiene das escolas," *Gazeta Médica* 10 (1878): esp. 246. Freyre mistakenly attributes the article to Antônio's brother, Manoel Victorino; *Order and Progress,* 126 n. 1.

84 Pacífico Pereira, "Hygiene," 193–194.

85 Ibid., 199–200; my emphasis. See Schwarcz, *Espetáculo das raças.*

86 Braz H. do Amaral, "A gymnásia nas escolas," *Gazeta Médica* 21 (1889): 157–158.

87 Otto Wucherer, "Sobre as causas da crescida frequência da tísica no Brasil especialmente na Bahia," *Gazeta Médica* 2 (1868): 266. It should be noted that Wucherer was writing in the 1860s before tuberculosis came to be generally associated with the tropics.

88 Ibid., 268.

89 Ibid., 2.

90 Creoles here refer to the children of Africans born in Brazil.

91 Otto H. Wucherer, "Sobre a moléstia vulgarmente denominada 'opilação'," *Gazeta Médica* 1 (1866): 64; Manoel Victorino Pereira, "Anchylostoma duodenal," *Gazeta Médica* 9 (1877): 78, 82.

92 He considered ainhum a disease peculiar to the African race because it was a disorder contracted in Africa and brought over in the slave trade. After the slave trade ended in 1850, the disorder, according to Silva Lima, began to die out, so that by the 1880s he saw very few cases, "Um caso excepcional de ainhum," *Gazeta Médica* 15 (1884): 469. Going barefoot exacerbated the ailment because, in its last stages, the small toe would drop off, usually as a result of "accidental injury or gangrene." Silva Lima, "Estudo sobre o 'ainhum,' moléstia ainda não descrita, peculiar à raça etiópica e afetando os dedos mínimos dos pés," *Gazeta Médica* 1 (1867): 146–151, 172–176; Silva Lima, "Notícia sobre o ainhum," 341–360. On slaves going barefoot, see Augel, *Visitantes,* 205; Freyre, *Mansions,* 193.

93 R. da Cunha, "Caso de tétanos traumático," *Gazeta Médica* 6 (1872): 35–40; for a discussion of the various ailments probably included under *tétano traumático,* also known as *mal de sete dias,* see Karasch, *Slave Life,* 153–154.

94 Otto H. Wucherer, "A chamada geophagia on chlorose tropical, ou antes chlorose

(oriunda) de malária, considerada como moléstia de todos os climas," *Gazeta Médica* 2 (1867): 30–33, 40–42.

95 Ibid., 33.

96 Ibid., 42.

97 See Hirsch, *Handbook*, 1: 344–346.

98 Savitt, "Black Health on the Plantation," 315–319; Savitt, *Medicine and Slavery*, 7–8, 47; Hirsch, *Handbook*, 1: 344–345.

99 Curtin, *Image of Africa*, 66.

100 Quoted by Freyre, *Order and Progress*, 185.

101 For example, as Pacífico Pereira reminded his audience, "We should not forget that the progress of the country [is] heavily dependent on public hygiene. . . . [Otherwise] all [our] descendants will, in the end, be made up of those types, already common, with miserable constitutions who look wasted before their youth." In "Hygiene das escolas," GM, 10 (1878): 198.

102 José de Patrocínio, 1887, quoted by Skidmore, *Black into White*, 24.

103 For well-known mulatto Bahian doctors, see n. 50 above.

104 E. Costa, *Brazilian Empire*, 241–242.

105 Ibid., 241. Degler, *Neither Black nor White*, 93–138, deals extensively with the question "Who is black?" in the Brazilian context; and Skidmore shows how color was related to a person's social function, "Racial Ideas and Social Policy in Brazil, 1870-1940," in *The Idea of Race in Latin America, 1870-1940,* ed. Richard Graham (Austin: University of Texas Press, 1990), 9. For a useful discussion on perceptions of race and color, see Wright, *Café con Leche*, 1–10.

106 From his commencement speech to the Bahian School of Medicine, quoted in *Gazeta Médica* 18 (1886): 315–327.

107 Dr. Satyro de Oliveira Dias, "Discurso pela Sessão Magna Anniversária," *Revista do Instituto Geográphico e Histórico do Bahia* 18–20, 37–39 (1913): 132. For a discussion of this trend in the early Republic, see Nísia Trinidade Lima and Gilberto Hochman, "Condenado pela raça, absolvido pela medicina: O Brasil descoberto pelo movimento sanitarista da Primeira República," in *Raça, ciência e sociedade,* ed. Maio and Santos, 23–40.

108 Brazil was not alone in this heightened concern of the nation. See, for example, Benedict Anderson, *Imagined Communities: Reflections on the Origin and Spread of Nationalism* (London: Verso, 1990); E. J. Hobsbawm, *Nations and Nationalism since 1780: Programme, Myth, Reality* (Cambridge: Cambridge University Press, 1990). For more local reasons for the increased interest in foreign models as solutions to Brazilian problems, see Skidmore, "Racial Ideas," 10–11.

109 Raimundo Nina Rodrigues, "Memória histórica do Professor Raimundo Nina Rodrigues sobre o anno letivo de 1896," *Gazeta Médica* 73 (1976): 14; Freyre, *Order and Progress*, 121.

110 Lamartine de Andrade Lima, "Roteiro de Nina Rodrigues," *Centros de Estudos Afro-Orientais,* 2 (April 1980): 1–12, states that Nina Rodrigues was a Sephardic

Jew; other authors, such as E. Costa, *Brazilian Empire,* 242, and Skidmore, *Black into White,* 57, indicate that he was a mulatto. For a study of Nina Rodrigues's ideas, see Mariza Corrêa, "As ilusões da liberdade: A Escola Nina Rodrigues e a antropologia no Brasil" (Ph.D. dissertation, Universidade de São Paulo, 1982); Pedro Motta de Barros, "Alvorecer de uma nova ciência: A medicina tropicalista bahiana," *História, Ciências, Saúde, Manguinhos* 4, no. 3 (1997: 411–459; Marcos Chor Maio, "A medicina de Nina Rodrigues: Análise de uma trajetória científica," *Cadernos de Saúde Pública* 11, 2 (1995): 226–237; Ventura, *Escritores, escravos e mestiços,* 139–142. See also Nina Rodrigues's obituary in *Gazeta Médica* 38 (1906): 57–63.

111 L. Lima, "Roteiro," 2.

112 See the news items on the congress in *Gazeta Médica* 21 (1889): 45–46, 146.

113 Nina Rodrigues's publications include *O animismo fetichista dos negros bahianos* (São Paulo: Companhia Editora Nacional, 1935); *As raças humanas e a responsabilidade penal no Brasil* (Salvador: Progresso, 1957); "Um caso de surdez verbal com parafasia," *Gazeta Médica* 20 (1889): 551–555; "O beriberi e as polinevrites: Diagnóstico diferencial," *Gazeta Médica* 21 (1889): 550–556; 22 (1890): 9–14, 66–72, 108–113, 164–168, 211–218, 250–254.

114 Quoted by Antônio Caldas Coni, *A Escola Tropicalista Bahiana: Paterson, Wucherer, Silva Lima* (Salvador: Progresso, 1952), 76.

115 Raimundo Nina Rodrigues, "Contribuição para o estudo da lepra na província do Maranhão," *Gazeta Médica* 20 (1888): 105–113, 205–211, 301–314, 358–368, 404–409; 21 (1889): 121–132, 225–234, 255–265; "Os mestiços brasileiros," *Gazeta Médica* 21 (1890): 401–407, 497–503.

116 Erwin H. Ackerknecht, *History and Geography of the Most Important Diseases* (New York: Hafner, 1965), 110.

117 The Tropicalistas carried out several studies of leprosy at this time, for example, Antônio Pacífico Pereira, "Contágio da lepra: Investigações histológicas e bacteriológicas que demonstram sua natureza parasitária," *Gazeta Médica* 19 (1887): 527–541; 20 (1888): 1–10, 51–60, 99–104, 149–156, 245–253; J. L. Magalhães (who was not a Tropicalista although he published in their journal), "A mórphea no Brasil especialmente na província de São Paulo," *Gazeta Médica* 15 (1884): 358–365, 497–506, 557–569.

118 In this he sided with the Tropicalistas Pacífico Pereira, Silva Lima, and Júlio de Moura, against the anticontagionist stance of the Rio de Janeiro physician Lourenzo de Magalhães. Nina Rodrigues, "Contribuição," 304, 405; this disagreement reflected a debate in the French Academy of Medicine between the anticontagionist Le Roy de Méricourt and the contagionist Ernest Bernier in 1886. See Pacífico Pereira's reference to it in "Contágio," *Gazeta Médica* 19 (1888): 527–541.

119 Nina Rodrigues, "Contribuição," *Gazeta Médica* 20 (1888): 313–314. For Lombroso's concept of atavism, see Gould, *Mismeasure of Man,* 122–145. For the

introduction of Darwin's ideas into Brazil, see chap. 5 below and Therezina Alves Ferreira Collichio, *Miranda Azevedo e darwinismo no Brasil* (Belo Horizonte: Itatiaia, 1988); Afrânio Coutinho, *An Introduction to Literature in Brazil*, trans. Gregory Rabassa (New York: Columbia University Press, 1969), 163–169; Roque Spencer Maciel de Barros, *A illustração brasileira e a idéia de universidade* (São Paulo: Universidade de São Paulo, 1959).

120 Nina Rodrigues, "Contribuição," *Gazeta Médica* 20 (1888): 359; he quoted the Frenchman Bouchard in support of this.

121 Like many at the time, he used terms like "ethnic group" and "race" indiscriminately.

122 Two exceptions, he noted, were those of Professor Érico Coelho, with his work on puerperal fever in black women, and that of Nina Rodrigues's own colleague at the Rio de Janeiro school, Justo Jansen Ferreira, who had written "Labor and Its Consequences in the Black Species." See Nina Rodrigues, "Contribuição," *Gazeta Médica* 20 (1888): 360. Others who had touched on the topic were Paula Rodrigues, *Glaucoma* (Rio de Janeiro, 1887); Teixeira Brandão, "Influência das raças sobre a alienação mental," *Gazeta Médica* 19 (1888): 571; Moura Brazil, "Estudo do campo visual nas raças diversas do Brazil," *Gazeta Médica* 19 (1888): 572. See also "Da natureza do tétano e sua freqüência no Brazil nas diversas raças" (paper given at Third Medical Congress), *Gazeta Médica* 21 (1890): 442; and "Diagnóstico comparativo das dermatoses nos indivíduos das diferentes raças," *Gazeta Médica* 21 (1890): 445.

123 Nina Rodrigues, "Mestiços," 405.

124 Nina Rodrigues, "Contribuição," *Gazeta Médica* 20 (1888): 365.

125 Nina Rodrigues, "Mestiços," 497–503. His categories were branco (white), negro (black), mulatto, mameluco (white and Indian), caboclo (poor backlander, usually Indian), cafuso, pardo (the two latter: different shades of black). For a discussion of the theory of racial types, see Young, *Colonial Desire*, 13–15.

126 By the end of the nineteenth century Armand de Quatrefages remained almost alone among European biologists and anthropologists in his belief that racial crossing strengthened races; Stepan, "Biological Degeneration," 111.

127 Skidmore, *Black into White*, 59; Dain Edward Borges, "Medical Ideas, Class and Race in Brazil, 1830–1930" (paper presented to the Latin American Studies Association, Albuquerque, New Mexico, April 18–20, 1985), 13.

128 Raimundo Nina Rodrigues, *Os africanos no Brasil* (São Paulo: Companhia Editora Nacional, 1935) 20.

129 Ibid., 25 n. 4.

130 L. Lima, "Roteiro," 5; Skidmore, *Black into White*, 58.

131 Nina Rodrigues was, of course, also assaulting collegial etiquette. See his "Memória histórica," 7–30.

132 *Candomblé* by then was an Afro-Catholic syncretic ritual. For doctors from the

medical school involved in Afro-Brazilian ritual some decades later, see Ruth Landes, *City of Women* (Albuquerque: University of New Mexico Press, 1994).

133   Freyre held that many whites consulted the witch doctors and *orixás* (deities) of the African religions and that Nina Rodrigues spoke openly about this fact but in very scathing terms, for the consultations, according to Nina Rodrigues, were to deal with personal afflictions and not for scientific study; *Order and Progress,* 304. See also Dale T. Graden, "'So Much Superstition among These People!': Candomblé and the Dilemmas of Afro-Bahian Intellectuals, 1864–1871," 57–73; and Kim D. Butler, "Ginga Baiana: The Politics of Race, Class, Culture, and Power in Salvador, Bahia," in *Afro-Brazilian Culture and Politics: Bahia, 1790s to 1990s,* ed. Hendrik Kraay (Armonk: M. E. Sharpe, 1998), 158–175.

134   For a discussion of racial classification systems, see n. 50 above. See also Ricardo Ventura Santos, "Da morfologia às moléculas, de raça à população: Trajetórias conceituais em antropologia física no século XX," in *Raça, ciência e sociedade,* ed. Maio and Santos, 125–142; Roger Bastide, *The African Religions of Brazil: Toward a Sociology of Interpretation of Civilizations,* trans. Helen Sebba (Baltimore: Johns Hopkins University Press, 1978); Edison Carneiro, *Candomblés da Bahia* (Rio de Janeiro: Coquetel, n.d.).

135   As a result Europeans were forced to consider problems of health in the tropics, which led to the setting up of schools of tropical medicine in Liverpool and London in 1899, in Hamburg in 1901, and in Portugal and France in 1902. See Shapiro, "Medicine in the Service of Colonialism," 19; Worboys, "Tropical Diseases," 1: 520.

136   Prime Minister Joséph Chamberlain (1899), quoted by Worboys, "The Emergence of Tropical Medicine: A Study of the Establishment of a Scientific Specialty," in *Perspectives on the Emergence of Scientific Disciplines,* ed. G. Lemaine et al., p. 94. Of course it is true that, ultimately, the bacteriological theory of disease would also work toward neutralizing the idea of the inevitable unhealthiness of the tropics. But the connection was made slowly not only because of a lack of understanding of transmission but because many doctors had vested interests, intellectually and professionally, in the old explanations.

137   "Discurso do Dr. Theodoro Sampaio," *Revista do Instituto Geográfico e Histórico da Bahia* 21 (1914): 126–128.

Chapter Four Physicians and Women in Bahia

1   A. J. R. Russell-Wood, "Female and Family in the Economy and Society of Colonial Brazil," in *Latin American Women: Historical Perspectives,* ed. Asunción Lavrin (Westport: Greenwood, 1978), 68; Ann L. Stoler, "Making Empire Respectable: The Politics of Race and Sexual Morality in 20th-Century Colonial Cultures," *American Ethnologist* 16, 2 (1989): 634–659; Helen Callaway, *Gender, Culture, and Empire* (London: Macmillan, 1987).

2   There was, of course, a lucrative aspect of this expansive policy. See, for example, histories on how male midwives and doctors pushed into the sphere of female midwives. Adrian Wilson, *The Making of Man-Midwifery: Childbirth in England, 1660–1770* (London: University of California Press, 1995); Charles E. Rosenberg and Carroll Smith-Rosenberg, eds., *The Male Midwife and the Female Doctor* (New York: Arno, 1974).

3   For a portrayal of this sort of strong woman who often also dealt with "spiritual" health, see Ruth Landes, *The City of Women* (Albuquerque: University of New Mexico Press, 1994).

4   For the eclipse of the planter patriarchal family, see the classic work by Gilberto Freyre, *Order and Progress: Brazil from Monarchy to Republic,* trans. Rod W. Horton (Berkeley: University of California Press, 1986), and *New World in the Tropics* (New York: Vintage, 1963). For more, see n. 18 below. For a discussion of evolving ideas on educating women to be good mothers, see Rima D. Apple, "Constructing Mothers: Scientific Motherhood in the Nineteenth and Twentieth Centuries," *Society for the Social History of Medicine* 8, 2 (1995): 161–178.

5   For some examples of these writings, see Álvaro Bruno Cavalcanti de Britto, "Higiene da mulher no estado de gravidez" (Ph.D. dissertation, Faculdade de Medicina da Bahia, 1870); Antônio Pedro da Silva Castro, "Hygiene da mulher no estado de gravidez" (Ph.D. dissertation, Faculdade de Medicina da Bahia, 1870); João Pinheiro de Lemos, "Do celibato professado pelas mulheres" (Ph.D. dissertation, Faculdade de Medicina da Bahia, 1851); Joaquim Januário dos Santos Pereira, "Pathologia da hemorragia puerperal" (Ph.D. dissertation, Faculdade de Medicina da Bahia, 1869); Elpídio Joaquim Barauna, "Hygiene da mulher em estado de gravidez" (Ph.D. dissertation, Faculdade de Medicina da Bahia, 1868). For graduating dissertations in Rio de Janeiro on similar topics, see Jurandir Freire Costa, *Ordem médica e norma familiar,* 2d ed. (Rio de Janeiro: Graal, 1979).

6   How far the normative standards of this group of men were accepted by women and society generally is the central problem of this type of primary source. On this, see the remarks by Stuart B. Schwartz, "Somebodies and Nobodies in the Body Politic: Mentalities and Social Structures in Colonial Brazil," *Latin American Research Review* 31 (1996): 129–130.

7   For a discussion of this idea, see the seminal article by Carroll Smith-Rosenberg and Charles Rosenberg, "The Female Animal: Medical and Biological Views of Woman and Her Role in Nineteenth Century America," in *Women and Health in America,* ed. Judith Walzer Leavitt (Madison: University of Wisconsin Press, 1984), 12–27; and Carroll Smith-Rosenberg, "Puberty to Menopause: The Cycle of Femininity in Nineteenth-Century America," in *Disorderly Conduct: Visions of Gender in Victorian America,* ed. Smith-Rosenberg (New York: Knopf, 1985), 182–196. For an earlier period, see Hilda Smith, "Gynecology and Ideology in Seventeenth Century England," in *Liberating Women's History: Theoretical and*

Critical Essays, ed. Berenice E. Carroll (Urbana: University of Illinois Press, 1976), 97–114; Ludmilla J. Jordanova, *Sexual Visions: Images of Gender in Science and Medicine between the Eighteenth and Twentieth Centuries* (Madison: University of Wisconsin Press, 1989), esp. chap. 3, "Body Image and Sex Roles"; Ornella Moscucci, *The Science of Woman: Gynaecology and Gender in England, 1800–1929* (New York: Cambridge University Press, 1990), 75–101.

8   Lindolpho Cavalcanti de Abreu, "Tumores de útero" (Ph.D. dissertation, Faculdade de Medicina da Bahia, 1885), 5.

9   Frederico Augusto da Silva Lisboa, "Hygiene da mulher em estado da gravidez" (Ph.D. dissertation, Faculdade de Medicina da Bahia, 1870), 5. Silva Lima also pointed to the health hazards of young sexually overactive women or unchaste widows; see "Prenhez extra-uterina de 18 meses," *Gazeta Médica* 1 (1866): 260.

10 The passages on the healthy nature of women's sexual desire in these dissertations conflicts with the Victorian image of "passionless" women. See Nancy F. Cott, "Passionlessness: An Interpretation of Victorian Sexual Ideology, 1790–1850," in *Women and Health,* ed. Leavitt, 57–69.

11 Lisboa, "Hygiene da mulher," 3–4.

12 A. P. Castro, "Hygiene da mulher," 16. Some of the degenerative consequences of masturbation were idiocy and madness; of excessive sexual pleasures, asthma, coughs, and nervous disorders. See Ladislau José de Carvalho e Araújo, "Influência do celibato sobre a saúde do homen" (Ph.D. dissertation, Faculdade de Medicina da Bahia, 1870), 15. On onamism, see Paula Bennett and Vernon A. Rosario II, eds., *Solitary Pleasures: The Historical, Literary, and Artistic Discourses of Autoeroticism* (New York: Routledge, 1995).

13 A. P. Castro, "Hygiene da mulher," 16; Francisco Borges de Barros, "Influência do celibato sobre a saúde do homen" (Ph.D. dissertation, Faculdade de Medicina da Bahia, 1869), 6.

14 A. Britto, "Hygiene da mulher," 6; Carvalho e Araújo, "Influência do celibato," 10.

15 Carvalho e Araújo, "Influência do celibato," 17; Guarino Aloysio Ferreira Freire, "Qual o papel que desempenha a civilisação no movimento das molestias mentaes?" (Ph.D. dissertation, Faculdade de Medicina da Bahia, 1888), 13–14; F. Barros, "Inflência do celibato," 2–3. For a good discussion on the question of consanguinity and marriage strategies, see Linda Lewin, *Politics and Parentela in Paraíba: A Case Study of Family-Based Oligarchy in Brazil* (Princeton: Princeton University Press, 1987); Lewin, "Some Historical Implications of Kinship Organization for Family-Based Politics in the Brazilian Northeast," *Comparative Studies in Society and History* 21 (1979): 262–292.

16 For more on this contrast, see J. F. Costa, *Ordem médica e norma familiar;* Dain Edward Borges, *The Family in Bahia, Brazil, 1870–1945* (Stanford: Stanford University Press, 1992).

17 See Borges, *Family,* 90–99. For an exploration of the physician's influence

on women in the family, see Smith-Rosenberg, "Puberty to Menopause," and "The Hysterical Woman: Sex Roles and Role Conflict in Nineteenth-Century America," in *Disorderly Conduct,* 182–216.

18 There is a large literature on the patriarchal family in Brazilian historiography, including critiques of those who, like Freyre, see the traditional Brazilian family purely as a patriarchal one. See Gilberto Freyre, *The Masters and the Slaves,* trans. Samuel Putman (New York: Knopf, 1969); Freyre, *The Mansions and the Shanties: The Making of Modern Brazil,* trans. Harriet de Onis (Berkeley: University of California Press, 1986); *Order and Progress,* and *New World in the Tropics.* Other important contributions include Antônio Cândido, "The Brazilian Family," in *Brazil: Portrait of Half a Continent,* ed. T. Lynn Smith and Alexander Merchant (New York: Dryden, 1951), 291–312; Carmelita Junqueira Ayres Hutchinson, "Notas preliminares ao estudo da família no Brasil," in *Anais da II Reunião Brasileira de Antropologia, Bahia, Julho de 1955* (Bahia: Universidade da Bahia, 1957), 261–274; Charles Wagley, "Luso-Brazilian Kinship Patterns: The Persistence of a Cultural Tradition," in *Politics of Change in Latin America,* ed. Joseph Maier and Richard W. Weatherhead (New York: Praeger, 1964), 174–189; Emilio Willems, "Structure of the Brazilian Family," *Social Forces* 31 (1953): 339–345; Eni de Mesquita Samara, *A família brasileira* (São Paulo: Brasiliense 1985); Samara, *As mulheres, o poder, e a família: São Paulo, século XIX* (São Paulo: Marco Zero, 1989); Darrell Erville Levi, *The Prados of São Paulo, Brazil: An Elite Family and Social Change, 1840-1930* (Athens: University of Georgia Press, 1987); Muriel Nazzari, *Disappearance of the Dowry: Women, Families, and Social Change in São Paulo, Brazil, 1600-1900* (Stanford: Stanford University Press, 1991); Donald Ramos, "City and Country: The Family in Minas Gerais, 1804–1838," *Journal of Family History* (1978): 361–375; D. Ramos, "Marriage and Family in Colonial Vila Rica," *Hispanic American Historical Review* 55 (1975): 200–225; Elizabeth Anne Kuznesof, *Household Economy and Urban Development: São Paulo, 1765 to 1835* (Boulder: Westview, 1986); Kuznesof, "Sexual Politics, Race, and Bastard-Bearing in Nineteenth-Century Brazil: A Question of Culture or Power?" *Journal of Family History* 16 (1991): 241–260; Aida C. Metcalf, "Searching for the Slave Family in Colonial Brazil: Reconstruction from São Paulo," *Journal of Family History* 16 (1991): 283–298; Mariza Corrêa, "Repensando a família patriarcal brasileira," in *Colcha de retalhos: Estudos sobre a família no Brasil,* ed. Maria Suely Kofes de Ameida et al., São Paulo: Brasiliense, 1982), 13–38, and other essays in the same volume. On the family in Bahia, see Borges, *Family,* and Kátia M. de Queirós Mattoso, *Bahia: A cidade do Salvador e seu mercado no século XIX* (São Paulo: Hucitec, 1977), 205–224.

19 On the deficiencies of the colonial patriarchal family and the merits of the hygienic, nuclear family, see J. F. Costa, *Ordem médica e norma familiar,* 19–33, 215–218. For the politics of consanguineous marriages, see Lewin, *Politics and Parentela in Paraíba.*

20   Freyre, *Mansions,* 73–74; Borges, *Family,* 100–101; Mattoso, *Bahia,* 205.

21   See Russell-Wood, "Female and Family," 66–67, 79–80.

22   Lisboa, "Hygiene da mulher," 5.

23   Aprígio Ramos Proença, "Ensaio de estadística médica da Cidade de S. Salvador" (Ph.D. dissertation, Faculdade de Medicina da Bahia, 1852), 22.

24   Freire, "Qual o papel," 13.

25   Cândido, "Brazilian Family," 291–312.

26   Ibid., 300–304; Borges, *Family,* 79.

27   João José Reis, *Slave Rebellion in Brazil: The African Muslim Uprising in 1835 in Bahia,* trans. Arthur Brakel (Baltimore: Johns Hopkins University Press, 1993); Kátia M. de Queirós Mattoso, "Slave, Free, and Freed Family Structures in Nineteenth-Century Salvador, Bahia," *Luso-Brazilian Review* 25, 1 (1988): 69–84; Muriel Nazzari, "Concubinage in Colonial Brazil: The Inequalities of Race, Class, and Gender," *Journal of Family History* 21 (1996): 107–119.

28   Reis tells of one slave who had to borrow a room from friends in order to meet with the woman who was the mother of several of his children. *Slave Rebellion,* 179.

29   Mattoso, "Slave, Free, and Freed Family Structures," 69–70; for the colonial period, Nazzari, "Concubinage," 110; for another region of Brazil, Donald Ramos, "Single and Married Women in Vila Rica, Brazil, 1754–1838," *Journal of Family History* 16, 3 (1991): 261–282.

30   See, for example, D. Ramos, "Marriage and Family in Colonial Vila Rica"; and Sandra Lauderdale Graham, *House and Street: The Domestic World of Servants and Masters in Nineteenth-Century Rio de Janeiro* (Austin: University of Texas Press, 1992), 78–79.

31   Borges points also to a group of artisans, skilled workers, and small farmers of the Recôncavo, mainly colored and recent Iberian immigrants who formed families in many ways akin to those of the upper classes, particularly regarding male authority and the seclusion and supervision of women. See *Family,* 80.

32   Reis, *Slave Rebellion,* 178. See also Borges, *Family,* 177–178. Thales de Azevedo, "Democracia racial," in *Povoamento da Cidade do Salvador* (Bahia: Itapua: 1969), 220–221, says that neighborhood segregation by class started much earlier. For a brief history on the urbanization of Salvador, see Maria Raquel Matteo Mattedi et al., "Salvador: O processo de urbanização," in *Habitação e urbanismo em Salvador* (Bahia: Seplantec CPE, 1979), 341–364; see also Robert M. Levine, "The Singular Brazilian City of Salvador," *Luso-Brazilian Review* 30, 2 (1993): 59–70.

33   Borges, *Family,* 93.

34   For a description of the use of midwives in Brazil in the 1840s, see L. Papillaud, "Lettre sur l'état de la médecine au Brésil, en response a la refutation du docteur D.D.," *Gazette Médicale de Paris* 3, 4 (1849): 794–795; for doctors entering women's medicine, see Jane B. Donegan, *Women and Men Midwives: Medicine, Morality, and Misogyny in Early America* (Westport: Greenwood, 1978).

35 José Francisco da Silva Lima, "Eclâmpsia com albuminuria no sexto mês da gestação; aborto espontâneo; restablecimento completo: refloxões," *Gazeta Médica* 6 (1872): 75.

36 For developments in gynecology and obstetrics, see Charlotte G. Borst, *Catching Babies: The Professionalization of Childbirth, 1870–1920* (Cambridge, Mass.: Harvard University Press, 1995); Catherine M. Scholten, " 'On the Importance of the Obstetrik Art': Changing Customs of Childbirth in America, 1760–1825," Judith Walzer Leavitt and Whitney Walton, "Down at Death's Door," and Leavitt, "Birthing and Anesthesia," in *Women and Health,* ed. Leavitt, 142–154, 155–165, 175–184; Theodore Cianfrani, *A Short History of Obstetrics and Gynecology* (Springfield: Charles C. Thomas, 1960), 172–359; Walter Radcliffe, *Milestones in Midwifery* (Bristol: John Wright, 1967). See also several relevant chapters in Judith Walzer Leavitt and Ronald L. Numbers, eds., *Sickness and Health: Readings in the History of Medicine and Public Health* (Madison: University of Wisconsin Press, 1985); Judith Walzer Leavitt, *Brought to Bed: Childbearing in America, 1750–1950* (New York: Oxford University Press, 1986). For another region, see Moscucci, *Science of Woman,* esp. chap. 5, 134–165, "The 'Unsexing' of Women," on the introduction of ovariotomy.

37 This was due to a false opening between the bladder and the vagina that was often the result of a childbirth injury. Cianfrani, *Short History,* 321–330; Leavitt, *Brought to Bed,* 28–29.

38 Cianfrani, *Short History,* 341–357. These operations were performed without anesthesia or antisepsis and, after some early successes, had such high failure rates that advocates of abdominal gynecological surgery were dubbed "belly rippers" by their opponents, Alexander Paterson, "Dissertação sobre a ovariotomia e as moléstias para allívio ou cura das quaes esta operação é mais particularmente adopta," *Gazeta Médica* 3 (1868): 19. Only after the widespread use of anesthesia from midcentury on, and the slow recognition of Lister's antiseptic and aseptic methods from the 1870s on, did the above operations begin to have a higher rate of success.

39 For example, Vern Bullough and Martha Voght, "Women, Menstruation, and Nineteenth-Century Medicine," in *Women and Health,* ed. Leavitt, 29. This was a very old debate in European medical literature.

40 See, for example, Thomas Laqueur, "Orgasm, Generation, and the Politics of Reproductive Biology," in *The Making of the Modern Body: Sexuality and Society in the Nineteenth Century,* ed. Catherine Gallagher and Thomas Laqueur (Berkeley: University of California Press, 1987), 1–41; Laqueur, *Making Sex: Body and Gender from the Greeks to Freud* (Cambridge, Mass.: Harvard University Press, 1993); Mary Poovey, " 'Scenes of an Indelicate Character': The Medical 'Treatment' of Victorian Women," in *Making of the Modern Body,* ed. Gallagher and Laqueur, 137–68.

41   Leavitt, "Birthing and Anesthesia," 181.

42   José Francisco da Silva Lima, "Fístula vesico-vaginal; operação pelo processo americano: Resultado satisfactório," *Gazeta Médica* 3 (1869): 193.

43   José Francisco da Silva Lima, "Boletim bibliografico," *Gazeta Médica* 2 (1868): 256.

44   Alexander Paterson, "Dissertação sobre a ovariotomia," 19–21, 32–33.

45   Cianfrani, *Short History,* 285–287. He reports that until 1857 ovariotomy had only been performed 4 times in France, as opposed to 97 times in the United States and 123 times in England. See also Moscucci, *Science of Woman,* 143. For the influence of French medicine on Brazilian medical schools, see chap. 1.

46   José Francisco da Silva Lima, "Fístula vesico-vaginal": 193–198.

47   John L. Paterson, "Caso de pólipo fibróide de útero," *Gazeta Médica* 10 (1878): 201–06.

48   Manoel Maria Pires Caldas, "Quisto ovariano; ovariotomia; cura," *Gazeta Médica* 19 (1888): 391–405.

49   Rita Lobato Velho Lopes, "Parallelo entre os métodos preconisados na operação cesarina" (Ph.D. dissertation, Faculdade de Medicina da Bahia, 1887), 4.

50   Papillaud, "Lettre sur l'état de la médecine," 795, notes that midwives were usually mulattas and not African. For literature on midwives, see Jean Towler and Joan Bramall, *Midwives in History and Society* (London: Croom Helm, 1986); Jean Donnison, *Midwives and Medical Men: A History of the Struggle for the Control of Childbirth* (London: Historical Publications, 1988); and nn. 52 and 60 below.

51   Lycurgo Santos Filho, *História da medicina no Brasil: Do século XVI ao século XIX,* 2 vols. (São Paulo: Brasiliense, 1947), 200–201; Joana Maria Pedro, "Práticas abortivas e gestão do corpo feminino em Florianópolis entre 1900–1950" (paper presented at the Nineteenth LASA Congress, Washington, D.C., September 28–30, 1995), 2–4. For priestesses who were also healers, see Maria Andrea Loyola, *Médicos e curandeiros: Conflito social e saúde* (São Paulo: Difusão Européia do Livro, 1984).

52   For French midwives in Rio de Janeiro, see S. Graham, *House and Street,* 82, and Santos Filho, *História geral da medicina brasileira,* 2 vols. (São Paulo: Hucitec, 1991), vol. 2, 328–329. The Tropicalistas respected the work of these formally trained midwives. For more on midwifery, see Santos Filho, *História da medicina,* vol. 1, 199–209. For literature on midwives in contemporary Latin America, see Ronald A. Schwartz, "The Midwife in Contemporary Latin America," *Medical Anthropology* 5, 1 (1981): 51–71.

53   Santos Filho, *História da medicina,* 1: 227.

54   Santos Filho, *História geral* 2, 93, 331. On women's literacy, see n. 86 below.

55   Conselheiro Dr. Elias José Pedreira, "Memória histórica dos acontecimentos notáveis ocorridos no anno 1871 na Faculdade de Medicina da Bahia," in Brazil,

Ministério do Império, *Relatórios ministeriais,* Época do Império, 1832–1888, reel 11. This was an old complaint; Papillaud had also noted it. Santos Filho, *História geral* 2, 93. There are a few references to male midwives in Salvador. I have not discovered if they were formally trained or not. On the rise of male midwives in England, see Wilson, *Making of Man-Midwifery.*

56 Silva Lima, "Fístula vesico-vaginal," 193.

57 Silva Lima, "A farmacia Professão e a farmacia industria; comércío de remedios segrêdos," *Gazeta Médica* 8 (1876): 289. Midwives were also healers.

58 Silva Lima, "Fístula vesico-vaginal," 193.

59 José Francisco da Silva Lima, "Erysipela séptica: Seguida de abscessos múltiples e negrose do occiptal em uma crianza recém nacida," *Gazeta Médica* 13 (1882): 560–565.

60 Leavitt, *Brought to Bed,* 36–63; Donegan, *Women and Men Midwives;* Barbara Ehrenreich and Deidre English, *Witches, Midwives, and Nurses: A History of Women Healers* (Old Westbury: Feminist Press, 1973). Edward Shorter has contested the view of the noninterventionist midwife; see *A History of Women's Bodies* (New York: Basic, 1982).

61 Manoel Maria Pires Caldas, "Cálculo vesical; operação de litotrícia; fístula vesico vaginal; operação pelo método americano, cura completa de ambas enfermidades," *Gazeta Médica* 1 (1866): 100–104.

62 Ibid., 101.

63 For example, Pires Caldas held that the method of suturing he had used was more effective than the one advocated by a French physician, Dr. Couty, writing in the *Montpellier Medical Journal.*

64 For differing approaches to the "naturalness" of childbirth, see Frances E. Kobrin, "The American Midwife Controversy: A Crisis of Professionalization," in *Women and Health,* ed. Leavitt, 318–326; for a discussion on recent debates about the meanings of childbirth, see Paula A. Treichler, "Feminism, Medicine, and the Meaning of Childbirth," in *Body/Politics: Women and the Discourses of Science,* ed. Mary Jacobus, Evelyn Fox Keller, and Sally Shuttleworth (New York: Routledge, 1990), 113–138.

65 Deoclesiano Ramos, "Estado enfisematoso do feto complicando o trabalho do parto," *Gazeta Médica* 18 (1887): 344–351.

66 Antônio Pacífico Pereira, "Alguns casos d'eclampsia tratados pelo bromureto de potássio e hydrato de chloral," *Gazeta Médica* 11 (1879): 56.

67 Ibid., 57–58.

68 José Francisco da Silva Lima, "Prenhez extra-uterina de 18 meses; extração do feto pela in cição abdominal; morte no 19° dia depois da operação; autópsia; reflexóes," *Gazeta Médica* 1 (1867): 255–261.

69 Judith Walzer Leavitt, "'Science' Enters the Birthing Room," in *Sickness and Health,* ed. Leavitt and Numbers, 94.

70 Pacífico Pereira, "Alguns casos d'eclampsia," 53–59, 153–162.

71 See José Francisco da Silva Lima, "A farmácia Professáo e a farmácia industria; comercio de remedios secretos y privilegíados," *Gazeta Médica* 8 (1876): 289.

72 Cianfrani, *Short History,* 288–300; Leavitt, *Brought to Bed,* 36–63, 116–141. For some examples of cases of female patients in Bahia in which both anesthesia and antisepsis were used, see Antônio Pacífico Pereira, "Casos de cefalotiopsia repetida sem trações e de cranioclasia," *Gazeta Médica* 14 (1882): 1–6; Pacífico Pereira, "Alguns casos d'eclampsia," 53–55, 153–162; Pires Caldas, "Quisto ovariano," 391–405.

73 Despite this case, on the whole the Tropicalistas had reduced the practice of bleeding. See Pacífico Pereira, "Alguns casos d'eclampsia," 153–162; and Senex [José Francisco da Silva Lima], "A Bahia de há 66 anos," *Revista do Instituto Geográfico e Histórico da Bahia* 15, 34 (1908): 111–113. For a discussion of the effects of such therapies, see Edward Shorter, *Bedside Manners: The Troubled History of Doctors and Patients* (New York: Simon and Schuster, 1985), 44–48; Charles E. Rosenberg, "The Therapeutic Revolution: Medicine, Meaning, and Social Change in Nineteenth-Century America," in *The Therapeutic Revolution,* ed. Morris J. Vogel and Charles E. Rosenberg (Philadelphia: University of Pennsylvania Press, 1979), 3–26; John H. Warner, *The Therapeutic Perspective: Medical Practice, Knowledge, and Identity in America, 1820–1885* (Cambridge, Mass.: Harvard University Press, 1986); W. F. Bynum and V. Nutton, eds., *Essays in the History of Therapeutics* (Amsterdam: Rodopi, 1991); *Clio Médica* 22 (1991), a whole issue dedicated to aspects of the history of therapeutics.

74 See also Borges, *Family,* 91.

75 For the story of this process in the United States, see Leavitt, *Brought to Bed;* Leavitt and Walton, "'Down to Death's Door," 81–97; Scholten, "'On the Importance of the Obstetrik Art,'" 142–154; Donegan, *Women and Male Midwives,* 237–284; Judy Barrett Litoff, *American Midwives, 1860 to the Present* (Westport: Greenwood, 1978), 18–26; Jacques Gélis, *History of Childbirth: Fertility, Pregnancy, and Birth in Early Modern Europe* (Boston: Northeastern University Press, 1991).

76 See, for example, the contemporary situation for the district of Nova Iguaçu, in the state of Rio de Janeiro, in Loyola, *Médicos e curandeiros,* 117–121; Paula Montero, *Da doença à desordem: A magia na umbanda* (Rio de Janeiro: Graal, 1985). Both these works are by anthropologists studying the interrelationship between folk medicine and official medicine in contemporary Brazil. See also Pedro, "Práticas abortivas." The Bahian social scientist Thales de Azevedo informed me personally that birthing with midwives was still a common occurrence for his generation of Bahians. On current midwifery, see Nancy Scheper-Hughes, *Death without Weeping: The Violence of Everyday Life in Brazil* (Berkeley: University of California Press, 1992); R. Schwartz, "Midwife in Contemporary Latin America," 51–71. Borges cites a Bahian dissertation written in 1947 that accused unlicensed midwives of causing infant tetanus mortality to newborns that

they attended in home births probably through the application of "traditional plasters of spider web powder, dung and tobacco dust to the umbilicus." *Family*, 331, 25.

77 This factor accounts for the slow inroads Western medicine made generally in Brazil, not only in the case of women in Bahia.

78 Goodyear puts the total number of physicians in Brazil during the colonial era at about one hundred, most of whom attended the upper civil servants. See chap. 1. There were several medical regulating bodies under the Portuguese Crown: the Fisicatura in the sixteenth century; the Câmaras Municipais, which took over the duty in 1604; and the ProtoMédicato, set up in 1782. Although the duty of these bodies was to oversee the provision of health to the community and license healers, they were notoriously inefficient. For an analysis of folk medicine in Brazil, in particular the blends between African, Indian, and European folk traditions, see Alceu Maynard Araújo, *Medicina rústica* (São Paulo: Companhia Editora Nacional, 1979); Borges, *Family*, 94. Two other forms of healing were home medicine with popular medical manuals such as that of a French doctor who spent time in Brazil, Pedro Luís Napoleão Chernoviz, whose book went through many editions; the Danish doctor Theodor Laangard's medical dictionary was also popular in Brazil. Homeopathy was strong in Brazil because of its royal support. Much to "allopathic" doctors' disgust, homeopathy had its own center and journal. See the anniversary speech given at the Homeopathic Institute of Brazil in *Annaes de Medicina Homeopáthica* 1, 10 (April 1883): 84–96.

79 See Stanley J. Stein, *Vassouras, A Brazilian Coffee County, 1850–1900: The Roles of Planter and Slave in a Plantation Society* (Princeton: Princeton University Press, 1985), 188–195. But even in cities where more Western-trained doctors were to be found, there were also African and other folk healers. See, for example, Freyre, *Mansions*, 317–319. Moreover, such healers were used by both rich and poor alike.

80 The historical relationship between Western medicine and alternative forms of healing in Brazil is a subject that needs to be researched. Certainly the Tropicalistas were interested in folk healing and folk remedies because they, like all well-informed physicians, knew that some of the most effective therapies and techniques in scientific medicine had been derived from folk medicine. At the same time, they rejected most folk healing as based on superstition. For a sense of their appreciation of folk healing, see M. de F. Alencar, "Luxação direita do maxiliar inferior—difícil contensão na cavidade glenoide," *Gazeta Médica* 7 (1874): 162–163; for a more skeptical attitude, see Dr. José Goes Siqueira, "Hygiene Publica: Estado Sanitario da Cidade," *Gazeta Médica* 5 (1871): 76. See also Tammy Lynn Pertillar, "Afro-Brazilian Women and Medicine: A Nineteenth-Century Social Issue, 1808–1888" (master's thesis, Howard University, 1993). For studies of other countries, see Lilian R. Furst, *Women Healers and Physicians: Climbing a Long Hill* (Lexington: University of Kentucky Press, 1997).

81 Leavitt, *Brought to Bed,* 39.

82 This was a constant theme. See, for example, Antônio Pacífico Pereira, "Memória histórica dos acontecimentos mais notáveis do anno 1882," in Brazil, Ministério do Império, *Relatórios ministeriais,* Época do Império, reel 19 (1832–1888), 1–15. However, there were many graduating dissertations written on obstetrics. For a partial list, see Santos Filho, *História geral* 2, 332–336. Rio, according to Papillaud, "Lettre sur l'état de la médecine," 794, had better practical training. On "demonstrative midwifery," see Virginia G. Drachman, "The Loomis Trial: Social Mores and Obstetrics in Mid–Nineteenth Century," in *Women and Health,* ed. Leavitt, 166–174.

83 Dr. Mathias Moreira Sampaio, in writing his 1867 report for the Bahian medical school, saw fit to quote the words of a Rio de Janeiro doctor: "It is hard to believe that doctors emerge out of our school (and thus by definition are qualified obstetricians) who have not once practiced on or even felt a woman in labor." "Memória histórica dos acontecimentos mais notáveis na Faculdade de Medicina da Bahia no anno 1867," in Brazil, Ministério do Império, *Relatórios ministeriais,* Época do Império, reel 9 (1868), 14.

84 For the history of women's education in Brazil, see n. 116 below. For views of nineteenth-century Brazilian women, see Tânia Quintaneiro, *Retratos de mulher: O cotidiano feminino no Brasil sob olhar de viajeros do século XIX* (Petrópolis: Vozes, 1995); Maria Odila Leite da Silva Dias, *Quotidiano e poder em São Paulo no século XIX* (São Paulo: Brasiliense, 1984); S. Graham, *House and Street.*

85 Leavitt, *Brought to Bed,* 81, 109. Leavitt also mentions doctors' experimenting with the poorest patients to acquire expertise. But birthing, she argues, shifted into the hands of doctors through the demands made by upper-class urban women.

86 June E. Hahner, *Emancipating the Female Sex: The Struggle for Women's Rights in Brazil, 1850–1940* (Durham: Duke University Press, 1990), 13; Hahner, "Women and Work in Brazil, 1850–1920: A Preliminary Investigation," in *Essays Concerning the Socioeconomic History of Brazil and Portuguese India,* ed. Dauril Alden and Warren Dean (Gainesville: University of Florida Press, 1977), 90.

87 Hahner, 20–26, 42–65. The uses of literacy for women, for example, were viewed by most men in very narrow terms. Hahner notes Elizabeth Agassiz's comments about the head of the plantation where she was staying in the 1860s, who, coming upon her reading fiction, gave her a book he said would be far more suitable for a woman's reading. It was a "textbook of morals." See Hahner, *Emancipating,* 49–50.

88 Serafim Vieira de Almeida, "Responsabilidade médica" (Ph.D. dissertation, Faculdade de Medicina da Bahia, 1888), 27–28. This is an area for which it is difficult to find direct evidence in the historical record. I am drawing these conclusions mainly from later studies. See Loyola, *Médicos e curandeiros,* 56; Landes, *City of*

Women; Oswaldo Rodrigues Cabral, *A medicina teológica e as benzedeiras: Suas raízes na história e sua persistência no folclore* (São Paulo: Departamento de Cultura, 1958); Sônia Maluf, *Encontros nocturnos: Bruxas, bruxarias no Laigo da Conceição* (Rio de Janeiro: Rosa dos Tempos, 1993); Pedro, "Práticas abortivas;" Scheper-Hughes, *Death without Weeping,* 291–292. For the names of some abortifacients used by midwives, see also Scheper-Hughes, 334.

89 For a similar situation in Rio, see Hahner, *Emancipating,* 59.

90 See Drachman, "Loomis Trial," 168–169. In this article, Drachman shows how male doctors, who knew that a thorough medical examination should involve both touching the female genitals as well as looking at them, often sacrificed one of these activities in order not to affront female modesty and lose patients. See also Leavitt, *Brought to Bed,* 108–115; and Donegan, *Women and Men Midwives,* 18–19, 141–163.

91 Borges, *Family,* 199–205. On the question of women and honor in another region of Latin America, see Verena Martinez Alier, "Elopement and Seduction in Nineteenth Century Cuba," *Past and Present* 55 (May 1972), 91–129; Alier, *Marriage, Class, and Color in Nineteenth Century Cuba: A Study of Racial Attitudes and Sexual Values in a Slave Society* (New York: Cambridge University Press, 1974); Geoffrey E. Fox, "Honor, Shame, and Women's Liberation in Cuba: Views of Working Class Emigré Men," in *Female and Male in Latin America,* ed. Ann Pescatello (Pittsburgh: University of Pittsburgh Press, 1973), 273–292. For "dishonorable" women, see Donna J. Guy, *Sex and Danger in Buenos Aires: Prostitution, Family, and Nation in Argentina* (Lincoln: University of Nebraska Press, 1990); Engel Magali, *Meretrizes e doutores: Saber médico e prostituição no Rio de Janeiro, 1840–1890* (São Paulo: Brasiliense, 1989).

92 Borges, *Family,* 204–205; Susan K. Besse, *Restructuring Patriarchy: The Modernization of Gender Inequality in Brazil, 1914–1940* (Chapel Hill: University of North Carolina Press, 1996). For women and social change in other countries in South America, see Asunción Lavrin, *Women, Feminism, and Social Change in Argentina, Chile, and Uruguay, 1890–1940* (Lincoln: University of Nebraska Press, 1995).

93 Willems, "Structure of the Brazilian Family," 339–345.

94 Alier, "Elopement and Seduction," 108; for a similar theme in eighteenth-century Argentina, see Susan M. Socolow, "Acceptable Partners: Marriage Choice in Colonial Argentina, 1778–1810," in *Sexuality and Marriage in Colonial Latin America,* ed. Asunción Lavrin (Lincoln: University of Nebraska Press, 1989), 209–251.

95 Aquello Leite, "Prenhez extra-uterina; ulceração de parede abdominal," *Gazeta Médica* 9 (1877): 396–401.

96 Silva Lima, "Erysipela séptica," *Gazeta Médica* 13 (1882): 560–566.

97 José Francisco da Silva Lima, "Caso de gravidez com integridade de membrana hymen," *Gazeta Médica* 11 (1879): 397–399.

98   José Francisco da Silva Lima, "Abscesso intrapelvino: Ruptura pela vagina," *Gazeta Médica* 14 (1882): 49–50.

99   For the Tropicalista critique of the dissertations, see chap. 5.

100 Silva Lima, "Caso de gravidez," 397–399.

101 Ibid., 398.

102 Ibid., 397–399.

103 Borges, *Family*, 104. In his schema the lower classes are treated by the motley collection of folk and faith healers. While this framework has ingredients of truth, it is oversimplified in that it divides the practice of medicine into dichotomies: Western medicine for the rich and alternative healing for the poor. The opposition of Western and alternative healing does not capture the nuances at work in the Brazilian case; rather, the evidence shows that all classes used several different types of healing.

104 "Policlínica geral do Rio de Janeiro," *Gazeta Médica* 13 (1881): 335.

105 "Enfermaria de partos," *Gazeta Médica* 13 (1876): 389–390.

106 José Francisco da Silva Lima, "Caso de prenhez reputada extra-uterina; erro de diagnóstico motivado pela presença de um tumor fibroso intersticial do segmento inferior de útero," *Gazeta Médica* 8 (1876): 167–174.

107 Ibid., 171. *Casas de saúde* were private infirmaries where a patient usually paid. On *casas de saúde*, see also Steven Williams, "A River of Tears: Corporate Interests and Public Consequences during Rio de Janeiro's First Yellow Fever Outbreak, 1849–1850" (paper given at the 1995 meeting of the Latin American Studies Association, Washington, D.C., September 28–30); and Santos Filho, *História geral* 2: 473–480. In this case the African woman was there from October to late-January. She was single, had five children, and made her living as a cook, so it is unlikely that she would have been able to pay for her stay at the infirmary.

108 Silva Lima, "Caso de prehnez," 174.

109 The combined obstetrics and gynecology cases treated by Silva Lima, J. Paterson, Pires Caldas, Pacífico Pereira, and Victorino Pereira reported in the *Gazeta Médica* between 1866 and 1888 total sixty-five. Of these, thirty-four are lower-class patients, twelve upper-class, nineteen unknown.

110 For women as doctors in the United States, see Mary Roth Walsh, *"Doctors Wanted: No Women Need Apply": Sexual Barriers in the Medical Profession, 1835–1875* (New Haven: Yale University Press, 1977); Regina Markell Morantz, "The 'Connecting Link': The Case for the Woman Doctor in 19th-Century America," and Virginia G. Drachman, "The Dilemma of Women Doctors in Late 19th-Century America," in *Sickness and Health*, ed. Leavitt and Numbers, 161–172, 173–182. See also n. 120 below.

111 The Leôncio Carvalho decree 7247 of April 19, 1879, was a broad educational reform I deal with more fully in chap. 5. One part of it included opening both lower and higher education to women.

112 For her biography, see Alberto Silva, *A primeira médica do Brasil* (Rio de Janeiro:

Pongetti, 1954); see also Francisco Bruno Lobo, "A primeira médica formada no Brasil," *Revista de História* 42 (April–June 1971): 483–486. The first woman doctor in Brazil was Maria Augusta Generoso Estrela but she received her degree in the United States at New York Medical College in 1881.

113   Hahner, *Emancipating*, 62, tells of the debate over women's brains that took place in the pages of the *Gazeta Acadêmica da Bahia*. On the polluting nature of the streets, see S. Graham, *House and Street*, 10–30.

114   Hahner, "Women and Work in Brazil," 89–90; Russell-Wood, "Female and Family," 83–88. For more on the other Brazilian women doctors, see Hahner, *Emancipating*, 56–60; for legislation opening up women's education, 21–23.

115   Hahner, *Emancipating*, 100; S. Graham, *House and Street*; Dias, *Quotidiano e poder*; Miriam Moreira Leite, *A condição feminina no Rio de Janeiro, século XIX: Antologia de textos de viajeros estrangeiros* (São Paulo: Hucitec, 1993); Hahner, *Poverty and Politics: The Urban Poor in Brazil, 1890–1920* (Albuquerque: University of New Mexico Press, 1986); Dorothy do Rego Asevedo, "Estrutura ocupacional da população feminina da Cidade do Salvador segundo os dados do censo de 1872" (paper presented at the Universidade Federal da Bahia, 1975). On prostitution, see Luís Carlos Soares, "Da necessidade do bordel higienizado: Tentativas de controle da prostituição carioca no século XIX," in *História e sexualidade no Brasil*, ed. Ronaldo Vainfas (Rio de Janeiro: Graal, 1986), 143–168; and Engel, *Meretrizes e doutores.*

116   For the education of women during the Empire years, see Heleith I. B. Saffioti, *Women in Class Society,* trans. Michael Vale (New York: Monthly Review, 1978), 140–178; and Hahner, *Emancipating*, 42–76. For Latin America more broadly, see Francesca Miller, *Latin American Women and the Search for Social Justice* (Hanover: University Press of New England, 1991), 35–67.

117   For some of the efforts of individual women, see Hahner on such women as schoolteacher Luciana de Abreu, Violante Ximenes de Bivar e Vallasco, and Josefina Álvares de Azevedo. *Emancipating*, 50–55.

118   Joaquim Monteiro Caminhoá, "Memória histórica da Faculdade de Medicina do Rio de Janeiro relativa ao anno 1874," in Brazil, Ministério do Império, *Relatórios ministeriais*, Época do Império, reel 14 (1874), 25.

119   A. Silva, *Primeira médica*, 216.

120   On the limitations placed on women within the medical profession in nineteenth-century North America, see Regina Markell Morantz-Sanchez, *Sympathy and Science: Women Physicians in American Medicine* (New York: Oxford University Press, 1985); Cathy Luchetti, *Medicine Women: The Story of Early American Women Doctors* (New York: Crown, 1998). See also the essays in the section "Physicians," in *Women and Health,* ed. Leavitt, 391–452; and n. 110 above.

121   "A mulher médica," *Gazeta Médica* 3 (1868): 70.

122   Ibid., 72.

123   *Gazeta Médica* 6 (1872): 45. The Universities of Zurich in 1864 and of Paris in

1867 were the first European university schools of medicine to admit women. Bonner, *Becoming a Physician,* 313.

124 Conselheiro Dr. Antônio Januário de Faria, "Discurso do director da Faculdade de Medicina da Bahia no acto de collação de grão," *Gazeta Médica* 8 (1876): 567.

125 Antônio Pacífico Pereira, "Hygiene das escolas," *Gazeta Médica* 10 (1878): 436.

126 This position was in contrast, for example, to the *Gazeta Acadêmica da Bahia,* published by medical school professors (see n. 113 above). For the relation between Tropicalistas and medical school, see chap. 5.

127 José Alves de Mello, "Memória histórica dos acontecimentos mais notáveis do anno 1879," in Brazil, Ministério do Império, *Relatórios ministeriais,* Época do Império, reel 17 (1879), 8.

128 Antônio Pacífico Pereira, "Reforma das faculdades de medicina," *Gazeta Médica* 12 (1880): 200. In 1882 three women attended the medical school in Rio de Janeiro. The first woman to graduate from Rio de Janeiro's medical school was Ermelinda Lopes de Vasconcelos in 1881. In Bahia, Ephigênia Velga graduated in 1890 and Francisca Barretto Praguer in 1893.

129 Also helping to recast women's thinking was the emergence of a small but important women's press, and associations. See Hahner, *Emancipating,* 26–38. Susan K. Besse, *Restructuring Patriarchy,* deals with the opening up of new spaces for women but for a later period.

130 Of the nine doctors Lobato thanks in her graduating dissertation, four were Tropicalistas, including Pacífico Pereira, Barão de Itapoan, and Demétrio Cyríaco Tourinho. Besides a printed dedication, she appended a handwritten one to Pacífico Pereira and his family.

131 Maricela Medina, "Tobias Barreto (1839–1889): The Intellectual Odyssey of a Nineteenth Century Brazilian" (Ph.D. dissertation, University of Michigan, 1986), 292. One of the best illustrations of this sort of thinking comes from Joaquim Monteiro Caminhoá, who, writing in 1874 at the time of much debate about the importance of educational reform in Brazil, noted that Victor Hugo had forecast that America (the continent), and most especially Brazil, would be the future leader of the civilized world. In order to help make the promise come true, the doctor called for the immediate emancipation of women in Brazil and government legislation to allow women to become doctors: "Let Brazil . . . legislate now allowing students of both sexes to be included in its reform. It is better to be in the vanguard of civilization, than to be pushed by its waves. . . . Let me remind you that the . . . intellectual and social independence of women . . . [leads] to the independence of humanity, and is one of the . . . surest measures against prostitution and the decadence of behavior [costumes]." "Memória histórica," 25.

132 A. Silva, *Primeira médica,* 151.

133 Ibid., 138 n. 85.

134 Hahner, *Emancipating,* 59–60.

Chapter Five Moving into Mainstream

1   Coming from the lower ranks of society need not, in itself, have made doctors willing to follow the "modern" Tropicalistas. As I noted in chap. 1, the lower-class background of many students at the medical school probably made them favor the forces of conservatism and maintenance of the status quo. However, from the 1860s on, there were big changes in European medicine together with deep political questioning in Brazil, two factors that helped make for more critical young medical students and doctors who found the Tropicalistas an appealing alternative to the status quo.

2   For example, Pedro S. de Magalhães commented scathingly that *mulungu* (from which the medication erythrina was derived) was used by some Brazilian clinicians but not many. It seemed, he wrote, that Brazilian doctors were waiting for European confirmation before they fully accepted the medication. "Nota sobre o mulungu," *Gazeta Médica* 13 (1882): 357–365. The Tropicalistas consistently identified European medications derived from Brazilian pharmacopoeia; see chap. 1 n. 109.

3   For an interesting analysis of the changing strategies of different generations of scientists and industrialists to achieve the rewards of prestige and influence, see Arnold Thackray, "Natural Knowledge in Cultural Context: The Manchester Model," *American Historical Review* 79 (1974): 672–709; also, Jack Morrell and Arnold Thackray, *Gentlemen of Science: Early Years of the British Association for the Advancement of Science* (Oxford: Clarendon, 1981).

4   The greatest political debate of the period was abolition of slavery; as indicated in chap. 3, the Tropicalistas were favorable to abolition. However, the *Gazeta Médica* was not used as a platform to fight for abolition in the way it was for the right of provincial autonomy, especially the autonomy of the medical school.

5   The relationship between the Tropicalistas and new ideas like Darwinism is discussed below.

6   Antônio Caldas Coni, *A Escola Tropicalista Bahiana: Paterson, Wucherer, Silva Lima* (Salvador: Progresso, 1952), 34.

7   The directors to the school were appointed by the government. Primitivo Moacyr, *A instrução e o Império: Subsídios para a história da educação no Império, 1854–1889,* 3 vols. (São Paulo: Companhia Editora Nacional, 1938), 2: 152.

8   For a biographical note, see *União Médica* 2 (1882): 435–436.

9   He was one of the twelve members of the Council of Health that had played an important advisory role to the provincial government during the epidemics of 1849 and 1855. For information on the council, see chap. 1.

10   For information on the Sociedade de Beneficência, see chap. 1.

11   Some of the articles he contributed to the *Gazeta Médica* show him to be within an older framework of medical interests particularly linked to military medicine; see "Algumas considerações sobre as feridas por arma de fogo tratadas por meio

d'agua fria," *Gazeta Médica* 3 (1868): 29–32. He was also clearly interested in the environmental approach to medicine prominent in the nineteenth century; see "Breves considerações sobre a influência geológica dos terrenos no desenvolvimento das epidemias," *Gazeta Médica* 5 (1871): 45–46; and "Um exame de sanidade," *Gazeta Médica* 7 (1874): 185–187.

12 See Elias José Pedreira, "Memória histórica dos acontecimentos notáveis ocorridos no anno 1871 na Faculdade de Medicina da Bahia," in Brazil, Ministério do Império, *Relatórios ministeriais,* Época do Império, 1832–1888, reel 11.

13 His last name is sometimes rendered as Farias. Coni pits Faria versus the Tropicalistas but from my sources this is erroneous. See *Escola Tropicalista,* 35.

14 One man trained in Bahia who had been director of the medical school from 1836 to 1844 was Francisco de Paula Araújo e Almeida. The director from 1844 to 1854 was João Francisco de Almeida but it is uncertain where and when he graduated. Paula Araújo graduated in 1820, more than a decade before the medical faculties were properly constituted and when Portuguese influence and early nineteenth-century French medical paradigms were paramount.

15 Some of his articles in the *Gazeta Médica* were "Ascite dependente de lesão hepatica; operação de paracentese (pela segunda vez), seguida de peritenite; cura," *Gazeta Médica* 1 (1867): 270–271; "Algumas considerações sobre a moléstia denominada beriberi, a propósito do artigo do Sr. Le Roy de Méricourt," *Gazeta Médica* 3 (1869): 169–170. Further writings include "Memória histórica dos acontecimentos mais notáveis do anno 1858 na Faculdade de Medicina da Bahia"; "Lições de clínica médica, 1872."

16 José Affonso de Moura, "Memória histórica dos acontecimentos mais notáveis do anno 1873 na Faculdade de Medicina da Bahia," in Brazil, Ministério do Império, *Relatórios ministeriais,* Época do Império, 1874, reel 13 (1832–88).

17 His obituary appeared in the *Gazeta Médica* 15 (1883): 153–154. See also the speech given by Victorino Pereira on the occasion of Faria's death in which he refers to Faria as a man of his times, a cultivator of science, and claims "in the second phase of medical teaching [in Bahia] no one was better than [Faria] in honoring his teaching position [by] imparting a conviction and a love of science." *Gazeta Médica* 15 (1883): 156–157.

18 In debates over a rejected medical school report by Luís Álvares dos Santos, a pro-Darwinist, Rodrigues Silva sided with Rosendo Guimarães, who consistently attacked dos Santos. See Pedro Ribeiro de Araújo, "Memória histórica dos acontecimentos mais notáveis do anno 1875 na Faculdade de Medicina da Bahia," in Brazil, Ministério do Império, *Relatórios ministeriais,* Época do Império, reel 15 (1876), 5, 7, 8; and Egas Carlos Moniz Sodré de Aragão, "Memória histórica dos acontecimentos mais notáveis do anno 1876 na Faculdade de Medicina da Bahia," in Brazil, Ministério do Império, *Relatórios ministeriais,* Época do Império, reel 16 (1877), 3–11; and Elias de Figueiredo Nazareth, "Lyceu Provincial da Bahia," *Revista do Instituto Geográphico e Histórico da Bahia* 21, vol. 19, No. 40

(1914), 94–95. His obituary was published in the *Gazeta Médica* and mentioned him as an accomplished physician but it was not prominently placed in the journal; *Gazeta Médica* 18 (1886): 188. For the article in which Wucherer wrote about Darwin, see "A moléstia como uma parte do plano de creação," *Gazeta Médica* 1, 11–12 (1866): 128–130.

19 See Claudemiro Augusto de Morais Caldas, "Memória histórica dos acontecimentos mais notáveis do anno 1881 na Faculdade de Medicina da Bahia," in Brazil, Ministério do Império, *Relatórios ministeriais,* 1882, Época do Império, reel 18, appendix.

20 On beriberi, he wrote "Algumas das dificuldades no diagnóstico do beriberi e das nefrites," *Gazeta Médica* 22 (1891): 491–502.

21 See appendix 3 for the list of Tropicalistas who were faculty members. The total number of faculty varied between twenty-seven in 1869 and thirty-six in 1885.

22 The lists of faculty members are to be found in the introductory pages of the students' graduating dissertations.

23 After 1876 the congregation could no longer propose adjuncts for the posts of full professors. For an explanation of who made up the congregation and how decisions were handled, see n. 26 below.

24 According to Ordival Cassiano Gomes, "The role of the adjuncts in the development of scientific teaching in the Bahian school of medicine is a chapter still to be written, a chapter which will afford new light and interpretation on certain facts in the history of medicine in Bahia. . . . From these adjuncts came the great masters of Bahian medicine." *Manuel Vitorino Pereira: Médico e cirurgião* (Rio de Janeiro: Agir, 1957), 54.

25 The core members who were also faculty professors in the 1880s were Antônio Pacífico Pereira, Manoel Victorino Pereira, Demétrio Ciríaco Tourinho, Virgílio Clímaco Damázio, Ramiro Affonso Monteiro, and José Luís D'Almeida Couto.

26 The congregation was made up of both professors and adjuncts but the latter were not allowed to participate in the most important decision-making. See Moacyr, *Instrução,* 3: 153.

27 On Germanism, see João Cruz Costa, *A History of Ideas in Brazil,* trans. Suzette Macedo (Berkeley: University of California Press, 1964), 186–193; Lycurgo Santos Filho, *História geral da medicina brasileira,* 2 vols. (São Paulo: Hucitec, 1991), 2: 105–106.

28 See the illustration and caption on Luís Alvares's brother Malaquias in Octávio Torres, *Esboço histórico dos acontecimentos mais importantes da vida da Faculdade de Medicina da Bahia, 1808–1946* (Salvador: Vitória, 1952), 16–17.

29 His writings included "Museu Público de Buenos Aires," "Relatório sobre a Exposição de Cordova na República Argentina," "O passeio do mar," "Saudação poética ao Imperador e Imperatriz," "A emancipação."

30 Nazareth, "Lyceu Provincial," *Revista do Instituto Geográfico e Histórico da Bahia* 19, 40 (1914): 95.

31 "O Conselheiro Dr. Luís Álvares dos Santos," *Gazeta Médica* 17 (1886): 289–290.

32 Because this "Memória" was rejected, it was never published. I have therefore had to rely on the accounts of the "Memória" and the debates it provoked, which were noted in the following year's "Memória histórica" by Egas Carlos Moniz Sodré de Araújo. See also Santos Filho, *História geral,* 2: 97; Roque Spencer Maciel de Barros, *A illustração brasileira e a idéia de universidade* (São Paulo Universidade de São Paulo, 1959).

33 Cabral was allowed to graduate only after he had written a new dissertation called "Qual o melhor tratamento da febre amarella?" but he published his first dissertation in book form a year after graduating; see n. 46 below. Santos Filho, *História geral,* 2: 97, 106; Ribeiro de Araújo, "Memória histórica dos acontecimentos mais notáveis do anno 1875," 7. On the introduction of Darwinism into Brazil, see n. 44 below.

34 For the law, see Moacyr, *Instrução,* 3: 180; see also M. J. de Araújo, "Breve notícia sôbre a fundação e marcha do ensino médico na Bahia," *Gazeta Médica* 10 (1878): 510; Ribeiro de Araújo, "Memória histórica," 8.

35 Sodré de Araújo, "Memória histórica," 3.

36 Within European medicine, military and naval medicine was generally considered a low-status occupation until the interest in tropical medicine resulting from colonial expansion in the second half of the nineteenth century; see Dennis G. Carlson, *African Fever: A Study of British Science, Technology, and Politics in West Africa, 1787–1864* (New York: Science History Publications, 1984), 17. The *Gazeta Médica* reflected this image in several of its articles. For example, the journal recorded instances when men the Tropicalistas considered unqualified were given medical appointments in the army; "Á propósito da Promoção de um curandiero a cirurgiáo—mór da Guarda Nacional," *Gazeta Médica* 4 (1870): 145–150. It also recorded naval doctors colluding with authorities to cover up an outbreak of yellow fever; *Gazeta Médica* 4 (1869): 25–28. However, the Tropicalistas recognized the value of naval and military medicine because within European medicine it was naval medicine, more preoccupied with the disorders of hot countries than mainstream European medicine, that spoke directly to their own interests. Moreover, it must be remembered that Bahia was essentially a port-city that, according to the estimate of Kátia Mattoso, received approximately 800 to 1,000 ships per day; *Bahia,* 143. Some naval doctors were an important source of keeping the Tropicalistas updated. For a good history of medicine and the navy more generally, see John J. Keevil et al., *Medicine and the Navy, 1200–1900,* 4 vols. (Edinburgh: E. and S. Livingstone, 1957–63).

37 Regarding the idea of foreigners, Sodré de Araújo noted, "We have here professors . . . who have nothing to envy the most illustrious European." "Memória histórica," 3.

38 Ibid., 3, 6.

39 Ibid., 7.

40   Ibid., 9.

41   For a discussion of the radical nature of nineteenth-century German medicine,
     see Erwin H. Ackernecht, *Rudolf Virchow: Doctor, Statesman, Anthropologist*
     (Madison: University of Wisconsin Press, 1953), 159–166; Karl Figlio and Paul
     Weindling, "Was Social Medicine Revolutionary? Rudolf Virchow and the Rev-
     olutions of 1848," *Bulletin of the Society for the Social History of Medicine* 34 (June
     1984): 10–18.

42   Wucherer, "A moléstia," 128–131. He used this view of change to explain his belief
     that disorders, like organisms, underwent constant transformation.

43   Ibid., 130. Wucherer had befriended Dr. Cotting when the latter visited Bahia as
     a member of Dr. Agassiz's expedition to Brazil. When Darwin died the *Gazeta
     Médica* reproduced an obituary praising his achievements; see R. Blanchard,
     "Darwin: Biografia," 13 (1882): 567–575. It is interesting to note that Fritz Müller,
     whom Wucherer mentions, was a German Darwinist and political activist forced
     to leave Germany after the 1848 revolutions and lived in Brazil in Santa Cata-
     rina. For many years he was a naturalist with the National Museum. See Simon
     Schwartzman, *Formação da comunidade científica no Brasil* (São Paulo: Compan-
     hia Editora Nacional, 1979), 59. He wrote *Für Darwin* and corresponded with
     Darwin, who mentions Müller's work several times in *The Origin of Species*.

44   For the introduction of Darwin into Brazil, see Therezina Alves Ferreira Colli-
     chio, *Miranda Azevedo e darwinismo no Brasil* (Belo Horizonte: Itatiaia, 1988);
     Afrânio Coutinho, *An Introduction to Literature in Brazil,* trans. Gregory Ra-
     bassa (New York: Columbia University Press, 1969), 163–169. R. Barros, *Illus-
     tração,* 145, gives 1874 as the date Darwin was first discussed in Rio de Janeiro;
     Sílvio Romero gave 1869 as the year Darwin was first read in Pernambuco Bar-
     ros, 145. The introduction of Darwinian ideas into Brazil probably came from
     several sources: in the "Germanophile" Recife movement of the 1860s and 1870s,
     it is probable that Haeckel's popularization of Darwinian evolution was an im-
     portant source. In Bahia, Wucherer was one source. He was familiar with the lit-
     erature on evolution, including German literature. Finally, France was probably
     the most important source of Brazilian exposure to Darwin's ideas, particularly
     since, following the French pattern, Darwin's theories were usually referred to as
     transformisme. For the French reception of Darwin, see Linda Clark, *Social Dar-
     winism in France* (University, Ala.: University of Alabama Press, 1984); Robert E.
     Stebbins, "France" in *The Comparative Reception of Darwinism,* ed. Thomas F.
     Glick (Chicago: University of Chicago Press, 1988), 117–163.

45   R. Barros, *Illustração,* 145.

46   Domingos Guedes Cabral, "Funções do cérebro" (Bahia: Imprensa Econômica,
     1876). Cited in R. Barros, *Illustração,* 145; R. Barros, "As faculdades do Império e
     a renovação intelectual," *Estado de São Paulo* (February 9, 1958); Sílvio Romero,
     A filosofia no Brasil; ensaio crítica (Porto Alegre: Typ. do Deutsche Zeitung, 1878)
     118–136.

47 João Ferreira de Campos, "Funções de cérebro," (Ph.D. dissertation, Faculdade de Medicina da Bahia, 1876), cited in R. Barros, *Illustração*, 146 n. 122. In 1878 a group of students in the Bahian medical school started a journal titled *Evolução* that included literary and scientific topics; *Gazeta Médica* 11 (1878): 340.

48 R. Barros, *Ilustração*, 145.

49 Richard Graham, *Britain and the Onset of Modernization in Brazil, 1850–1914* (Cambridge: Cambridge University Press, 1968), 18; on religion in nineteenth-century Brazil, see Ralph dela Cava, *Miracle at Joaseiro* (New York: Columbia University Press, 1970), 20–26.

50 For the debate around the directions for change in Brazil, see R. Barros, *Illustração*, 32–33.

51 Barros argues that the rejection of the report and the dissertation is evidence of the strength of the Catholic reaction in Bahia. It should be noted that dos Santos's suggestions for improvement of the medical school brought the initiative for change into the heart of the medical school instead of waiting, safely, for the government to legislate more resources and a change in organization. Interestingly, the other "Memória histórica" that compounded the usual "safe" criticisms of the government with specific criticisms of local professors and that was also rejected came from another Tropicalista member, Nina Rodrigues. See chap. 3.

52 Of the critique of patronage by the liberal professionals, Emília Viotti da Costa states: "But in spite of their critique of the traditional society, these intellectuals continued to depend on the patronage of the elites—the same elites that constituted the intellectuals' main audience. So it is not surprising that when intellectuals criticized the system of patronage, what they seemed to be asking for was not that patronage be abolished, but that it be replaced by an enlightened patronage that would reward only merit and talent"; The *Brazilian Empire Myths and Histories* (Chicago: University of Chicago Press, 1985), 197. On the importance of patronage in nineteenth-century Brazil for success in almost any field, see E. Costa, *Brazilian Empire*, 180–190, 196–197; Richard Graham, *Patronage and Politics in Nineteenth-Century Brazil* (Stanford: Stanford University Press, 1990).

53 Silva, a mulatto, was also opposed to the abolition of slavery and even against the abolition of flogging. Gilberto Freyre, *Order and Progress: Brazil from Monarchy to Republic,* trans. Rod W. Horton (Berkeley: University of California Press, 1986), 186. The Tropicalistas also supported the idea of decentralized higher learning because that conformed more closely to the highly successful German model of medical teaching. See Thomas Neville Bonner, *Becoming a Physician: Medical Education in Britain, France, Germany, and the United States, 1750–1945* (New York: Oxford University Press, 1995), 182–279.

54 See the editorial "A Faculdade de Medicina da Bahia e o governo imperial," *Gazeta Médica* 15 (1883): 209–217, which tells of a discussion on finances in the Senate on August 21, 1882, during which Senator Correia raised the complaints

made in Pacífico Pereira's "Memória Histórica" about the favoritism toward the Rio de Janeiro school. The imperial minister defended the government saying it was common knowledge that the many improvements made in the Rio school were carried out by private donations secured by the director with the government's approval. If Bahia was unable to do the same, this was merely because she lacked the resources to do so, and had nothing to do with the government. The *Gazeta Médica* disputed the latter contention. Such complaints about regional favoritism were echoed in other fields such as agriculture. See Gerald Michael Greenfield, "The Great Drought and Elite Discourse in Imperial Brazil," *Hispanic American Historical Review* 72 (1992): 384.

55 See S. R., "A Faculdade de Medicina da Bahia e o Ministro do Império," *Gazeta Médica* 18 (1887): 529–532.

56 See, for example, the long article by Antônio Pacífico Pereira titled "Aos médicos deputados: Reformas necessárias à legislação e ao ensino médico," *Gazeta Médica* 9 (1877): 1–6, 49–56, 96–105, 145–151, 193–199, 241, 337–346.

57 For example, like the criticisms of the Tropicalistas, the "Memórias históricas" complained about overzealous central government interference, the lack of practical teaching facilities despite laws that promised the facilities, and the government's favoritism toward individuals who had not qualified for their degrees.

58 Louís Couty, "O ensino superior no Brasil," *Gazeta Médica* 15 (1884): 521–532. See also Nancy Leys Stepan, *Beginnings of Brazilian Science: Oswaldo Cruz, Medical Research, and Policy, 1890–1920* (New York: Science History Publications, 1981), 32, 56.

59 Couty, "Ensino superior," 529.

60 Ibid., 529.

61 *Primeiro Congresso Brazileiro de Medicina e Cirurgia do Rio de Janeiro* (Rio de Janeiro: Imprensa Nacional, 1889), 7.

62 Antônio Pacífico Pereira, "As reformas do ensino médico no Brasil," *Gazeta Médica* 15 (1884): 305–312, 401–407, 545–550.

63 Ibid., 547, 548–549.

64 Dr. Demetrio, "Gazeta Médica," *Gazeta Médica* 6, 121 (1872): 1.

65 See the introduction to Júlio Augusto Ferreira da Veiga's dissertation, "Considerações sobre o abortamento" (Faculdade de Medicina da Bahia, 1885).

66 Domingos Pedro dos Santos, "Bibliographia do beriberi no Brazil," *Gazeta Médica* 15 (1883): 498.

67 See, for example, Antônio Moreira Maia, "Considerações acerca do abortamento" (Ph.D. dissertation, Faculdade de Medicina da Bahia, 1883); Dionysio Ferreira da Silva, "Abortamento" (Ph.D. dissertation, Faculdade de Medicina da Bahia, 1885). Most of the dissertations discussed European disorders and cases.

68 See, for example, Francisco Tavares da Cunha Mello, "Algumas considerações psycho-physiológicas acerca do homem" (Ph.D. dissertation, Faculdade de Medicina da Bahia, 1851); Ignácio Firmo Xavier, "Reflexões sobre o médico"

(Ph.D. dissertation, Faculdade de Medicina da Bahia, 1850). For a student who was critical, see Hernani da Silva Pereira, "História da alimentação no Brasil" (Ph.D. dissertation, Faculdade de Medicina da Bahia, 1887).

69   Selections from Victorino Pereira's dissertation on hookworm were published in the *Gazeta Médica* 9 (1877): 19–20, 151–153; Domingos Pedro dos Santos's bibliography on beriberi in Brazil, *Gazeta Médica* 15 (1883): 497–514, 543. In 1878 the student J. M. de Aguiar's work on the therapeutic qualities of the Brazilian araroba was published, "Comunicação a redação da *Gazeta Médica* sobre a história natural da *araroba*," *Gazeta Médica* 10 (1878): 353–360. Pacheco Mendes's research on the etiology of beriberi was published in 1887; *Gazeta Médica* 18 (1887): 299–306. Nina Rodrigues's work on leprosy in Maranhão was published in 1888; *Gazeta Médica* 20 (1888): 105–113, 205–211, 301–314.

70   Quoted by Bonner, *Becoming a Physician,* 237.

71   Besides the two Pereira brothers mentioned in chap. 1, Pacheco Mendes spent time in Germany after graduating and later translated German medical writings into Portuguese. Pedro Severiano de Magalhães, who graduated from Bahia in 1873 and later moved to Rio de Janeiro, studied under Ernst von Leyden in Berlin. Pacífico Pereira also translated writings by Billroth. On German medicine, see Arleen Marcia Tuchman, *Science, Medicine, and the State in Germany: The Case of Baden, 1815–1871* (New York: Oxford University Press, 1993).

72   For students attending the meetings and assisting the doctors at the Santa Casa, see Manoel Maria Pires Caldas, "Aneurisma da carótida," *Gazeta Médica* 8 (1876): 439; and José Luís D'Almeida Couto, "Sobre a pathogenia da chiluria a propósito da manografia do Sr. Dr. Martins da Costa," *Gazeta Médica* 9 (1877): 59.

73   Schwartzman, *Formação da comunidade,* 76, 83–84.

74   For an account of the reform, see Flávio Coelho Edler, "As reformas do ensino médico e a profissionalização da medicina na corte do Rio de Janeiro, 1854–1884" (Master's thesis, Universidade de São Paulo, 1992); Santos Filho, *História geral* 2, 101.

75   R. Barros, *Illustração,* 274–279, esp. regarding the faculties, 277. On Protestant schools, see Freyre, *Order and Progress,* 317–318.

76   Fernando de Azevedo, *Brazilian Culture: An Introduction to the Study of Culture in Brazil,* trans. William Rex Crawford (New York: Macmillan, 1950), 403.

77   R. Barros, *Illustração,* 222, 317; Maria do Carmo Tavares de Miranda, *Educação no Brasil: Esboço de estudo histórico* (Recife: Imprensa Universitária, 1966), 56; E. Costa, *Brazilian Empire,* 33. The whole debate of ensino livre in Brazil drew on a similar debate then taking place in German, Austrian, and French medical schools. See Ackerknecht, *Virchow,* 123–136; Bonner, *Becoming a Physician,* 257.

78   See R. Barros, *Illustração,* 279. Other stipulations in the new law concerned women's right to enter the medical schools and the freedom to employ foreigners to teach in the faculties, "when it is found necessary," para. 25, art. 20, quoted

in *Ilustração* 278. There were other rules relating to specific institutions such as that the famous secondary school Colégio Pedro II no longer have compulsory religious education. See Azevedo, *Brazilian Culture*, 380 n. 15, 386 n. 19.

79 Nancy Leys Stepan, *Beginnings of Brazilian Science: Oswaldo Cruz, Medical Research, and Policy, 1890-1920* (New York: Science History Publications, 1981), 55; R. Barros, *Illustração*, 305–306; "Reforma das Faculdades," *Gazeta Médica* 11 (1879): 250, 261–64.

80 Antônio Pacífico Pereira, "Reforma das faculdades de medicina," *Gazeta Médica* 12 (1880): 149–162, 197–202; For my discussion in this section I am drawing on the most important articles and editorials written in the *Gazeta Médica* on the reform issue. Although the editorials and some articles have no author, it is likely they were written by A. Pacífico Pereira, the Tropicalista who was most expert on these matters. "Reforma das faculdades," *Gazeta Médica* 11 (1879): 201–219, 249–264; "A reforma de ensino médico no Brasil," *Gazeta Médica* 12 (1880): 101–108; "Projecto para a criação de uma universidade," *Gazeta Médica* 13 (1881): 241–258; (1882): 293–308, 329–350; "Parecer da comissão da Faculdade de Bahia sobre o proyecto . . . universidade . . . ," *Gazeta Médica* 13 (1882): 392–409; "A reforma do ensino médico," *Gazeta Médica* 14 (1882): 145–151; Pacífico Pereira, "As reformas do ension médico no Brasil," 305–312, 401–407, 545–550. Pacífico Pereira, "Apontamentos para a história da organisação do ensino médico na Bahia," *Gazeta Médica* 30 (1898): 154–163, 227–234, 260–264, 549–556; Pacífico Pereira, "Parecer da comissão da Faculdade de Medicina da Bahia sobre o projeto para a criação de uma Universidade da Corte," in "Memória histórica dos acontecimentos mais notáveis do anno 1882 na Faculdade de Medicina da Bahia," Brazil, Ministério do Império, *Relatórios ministeriais*, Época do Império, annex B (1883); reel 19 "Parecer" is discussed by R. Barros, *Illustração*, 333–334; see also *Gazeta Médica* 13 (1881) and (1882): 392–409.

81 See, for example, an editorial titled "Os diplomas de Philadelphia e os avisos do Ministério do Império," *Gazeta Médica* 9 (1877): 256–257.

82 "Reforma das Faculdades," *Gazeta Médica* 11 (1879): 260–261; Pacífico Pereira, "Apontamentos para a historia da organisação de ensino médico na Bahia," *Gazeta Médica* 30 (1898), 158–159, 227–229.

83 "Reforma das Faculdades," *Gazeta Médica* 11 (1879), 255–257.

84 "Reforma de ensino médico no Brasil," *Gazeta Médica* 12 (1880): 102; Pacífico Pereira, "Apontamentos," *Gazeta Médica* 30 (1898): 228.

85 Antonio Pacífico Pereira, "Reforma da Faculdade de Medicina," *Gazeta Médica* 12 (1880): 197.

86 It was drawn up by the viscount of Sabóia, director of the Rio de Janeiro medical school. Azevedo hailed it as "the greatest [reform] in its material and technical results, . . . [which] gave new statutes to the medical schools . . . and began a new epoch in the evolution of medical teaching in the country." F. Azevedo, *Brazilian Culture*, 386 n. 19.

87 Pacífico Pereira, "Apontamentos para a história da organisação do ensino médico," 260–263.

88 E. Bradford Burns mentions alliances between priests and the Republican Party, *A History of Brazil,* 2d ed. (New York: Columbia University Press, 1980), 281; Viotti da Costa has a more complex interpretation than the usual one given of the impasse between Church and Empire in 1874; *Brazilian Empire,* 209. On the Church question, see Percy A. Martin, "Causes and the Collapse of the Brazilian Empire," *Hispanic American Historical Review* 4 (1921): 4–48; George Boehrer, "The Church in the Second Reign, 1840–1889," in *Conflict and Continuity in Brazilian Society,* ed. Henry H. Keith and S. F. Edwards (Columbia: University of South Carolina Press, 1969), 115–143; Boehrer, "The Church and the Overthrow of the Brazilian Monarchy," *Hispanic American Historical Review* 48 (1968): 380–401. On the conflict between the military and the state in the nineteenth-century, see June E. Hahner, *Civilian-Military Relations in Brazil, 1889–1898* (Columbia: University of South Carolina Press, 1969); José Murilo de Carvalho, "As forças armadas na Primeira República: O poder desestabilizador," in *O Brasil republicano,* vol. 2 of *História geral da civilização brasileira,* ed. Boris Fausto (São Paulo, 1977), 183–234; W. S. Dudley, "Institutional Sources of Officer Discontent in the Brazilian Army, 1870–1889," *Hispanic American Historical Review* 55 (1975): 44–65; Hahner, "The Brazilian Armed Forces and the Overthrow of the Monarchy: Another Perspective," *Americas* 26, (1969): 171–182.

89 Luís Anselmo de Fonseca, "Discurso," *Gazeta Médica* 30 (1898): 255.

90 *Gazeta Médica* 15 (1883): 209–210.

91 "Congresso Pedagogico," *Gazeta Médica* 15 (1883): 291.

92 "Os ultimos decretos para as faculdades de medicina," *Gazeta Médica* 15 (1883): 302. Both articles are in the same issue of the *Gazeta Médica.* The journal notes that the former article had already been written when the journal received the official decrees.

93 "Discurso proferido pelo Dr. Manoel Victorino Pereira, no acto de tomar posse da 2a cadeira de clínica cirúrgica da Faculdade de Medicina da Bahia," *Gazeta Médica* 15 (1883): 60, 61, 62.

94 See S. R., "A Faculdade de Medicina da Bahia e o Ministro de Imperio," *Gazeta Médica* 18 (1887): 529–532; 19 (1887): 4–12. The candidate rejected by the minister was Antônio Pacheco Mendes, a younger Tropicalista, who was later confirmed in the chair of pathological physiology.

95 *Gazeta Médica* 18 (1887): 529.

96 Ibid., 529.

97 In 1877 the Bahian faculty congregation had turned down the validity of an American doctor's diploma that the government had accepted; "Os diplomas de Philadelphia," 289. That same year a student the Bahian faculty had suspended for one year was pardoned by the emperor. In 1885 a candidate who was listed as second in the outcome of a competition was appointed to the post by the central

government. All of these incidents, and others like them, ended up alienating much of the faculty from the government.

98 The eleven were Virgílio Damázio, Santos Pereira, Demétrio Tourinho, Augusto Maia Bittencourt, Almeida Couto, Rosendo Guimarães, Pacífico Pereira, Pacheco Mendes, José Antônio de Freitas, Manoel Victorino Pereira, and Manoel Joaquim Saraiva. The pattern of political sympathies among the Tropicalistas is similar to that of other regions with small republican Parties. That is, the progressive wing of the Liberal Party advocated republican positions on federalism and abolition. This helps explain why the transition to the Republic in 1889 in such regions was less painful than one would expect given the minuscule size of the formal republican movement.

99 See chap. 1.

100 Gomes, *M. V. Pereira,* 174.

101 *Revista do Instituto Geográphico e Histórico do Bahia* 16, 35 (1909): 211–215. These were Antônio Pacífico Pereira, Braz H. do Amaral, Deoclesiano Ramos, Satyro de Oliveira Dias, José Francisco da Silva Lima, José Luís D'Almeida Couto, Alfredo Tomé de Britto, Jerônymo Sodré Pereira, Raimundo Nina Rodrigues, and Francisco Pacheco de Mello.

102 Theodore Zeldin, *France, 1848–1945,* (Oxford: Clarenson, 1973) 42.

Conclusion

1 I am using Marcos Cueto's definition of what he terms "scientific excellence in the periphery." See "Science under Adversity: Latin American Medical Research and American Private Philanthropy, 1920–1960," *Minerva* 35 (1997): 233.

2 Luiz Otávio Ferreira, Marcos Chor Maio, and Nara Azevedo, "A Sociedade de Medicina e Cirurgia do Rio de Janeiro: A gênese de uma rede institucional alternative," *História, Ciência, Saúde, Manguinhos* 4, 3 (1997): 480–481.

3 Nancy Leys Stepan, *Beginnings of Brazilian Science: Oswaldo Cruz, Medical Research, and Policy, 1890–1920* (New York: Science History Publications, 1981), 159.

4 Michael Worboys, "The Emergence and Early Development of Parasitology," in *Parasitology: A Global Perspective,* ed. Kenneth S. Warren and John Z. Bowers (New York: Springer-Verlag, 1983), 4.

5 Ilana Lowy, "Yellow Fever in Rio de Janeiro and the Pasteur Institute Mission (1901–1905): The Transfer of Science to the Periphery," *Medical History* 34 (1990): 145.

6 Ibid., 162.

7 In the 1890s the Tropicalistas were already calling for eradication campaigns. See José Francisco da Silva Lima's demand for mosquito eradication after learning they were involved in the transmission of filariasis; "Sobre alguns casos de lymphangite filariosa," *Gazeta Médica* 30 (1899): 507–508.

8 From the 1890s through the 1920s, three events in particular served to inform

coastal Brazilians about the backlands and to give them a sense of urgency regarding reform: the millenarian Canudos revolt of the 1890s, popularized by Euclides da Cunha's best-selling masterpiece, *Rebellion in the Backlands* (1902); Artur Neiva and Belisário Penna's medical survey of the states of Goiás, Pernambuco, and Bahia in 1913, which led to Penna's *O saneamento do Brasil* (1918); and finally, a three-year march of rebels through the Brazilian backlands in 1924–27, led by Luís Carlos Prestes, later the leader of the Brazilian Communist Party. See Luíz Antônio de Castro Santos, "Power, Ideology, and Public Health in Brazil, 1889–1930" (Ph.D. dissertation, Harvard University, 1987); Nísia Trinidade Lima and Gilberto Hochman, "Descobrindo a nação, construindo o estado: O movimento pela reforma da saúde pública no Brasil da Primeira República" (Paper presented at the 1995 meeting of the Latin American Studies Association, Washington, D.C., September 28–30).

9   For why this happened, see L. Santos, "Power, Ideology."

10 For the new research institutions in the Republic and the influence of European science, see Simon Schwartzman, *Formação da comunidade científica no Brasil* (São Paulo: Companhia Editora Nacional, 1979), 83–136. This was true of the local traditions in other regions too. See, for example, Mark Harrison, *Public Health in British India: Anglo-Indian Preventive Medicine, 1859–1914* (Cambridge: Cambridge University Press, 1994).

11 Thomas E. Skidmore, *Black into White: Race and Nationality in Brazilian Thought* (New York: Oxford University Press, 1974); and "Racial Ideas and Social Policy in Brazil, 1870–1940," in *The Idea of Race in Latin America, 1870–1940,* ed. Richard Graham (Austin: University of Texas Press, 1990), 7–36; Emília Viotti da Costa, *The Brazilian Empire: Myths and Histories* (Chicago: University of Chicago Press, 1985); Jeffrey D. Needell, "History, Race, and the State in the Thought of Oliveira Vianna," *Hispanic American Historical Review* 75 (1995): 1–30.

12 Some of the successes of this period were a full understanding of filariasis, discovered by Patrick Manson in 1879; the malaria parasite by Laveran in 1880; *Vibrio cholera* by Koch in 1883; plague bacillus by Kitasato and Yersin in 1894; the malarial life cycle by Grassi and Ross in 1897; trypanosomiasis by Bruce in 1896–1902 and Chagas in 1908; and leishmaniasis by several researchers in 1900–11. See Worboys, "Emergence and Early Development of Parasitology," 7. On the history of therapeutics, see Morris J. Vogel and Charles E. Rosenberg, eds., *The Therapeutic Revolution: Essays in the Social History of American Medicine* (Philadelphia: University of Pennsylvania Press, 1979); W. F. Bynum and V. Nutton, ed., *Essays in the History of Therapeutics* (Amsterdam: Rodopi, 1991).

13 For example, in the case of hookworm, the International Health Board gave three dosages of oil of chenodium to cure the disorder and recommended wearing shoes and building latrines as means of prevention. On the rise of bacteriology in Brazil, see Schwartzman, *Formação da comunidade,* 119–136; Stepan, *Be-*

ginnings, 66–104; Jaime L. Benchimol and Luiz Antônio Teixeira, *Cobras, lagartos e outros bichos: Uma história comparada dos Instituos Oswaldo Cruz e Butantan* (Rio de Janeiro: Universidade Federal do Rio de Janeiro, 1993), 19–76.

14 Nancy Leys Stepan, *"The Hour of Eugenics": Race, Gender, and Nation in Latin America* (Ithaca: Cornell University Press, 1991), 35–54.

15 Skidmore, "Racial Ideas," 12.

16 A statement made in 1899 by Joseph Chamberlain, then the British colonial secretary. Quoted by Michael Worboys, "Science and British Colonial Imperialism, 1895–1940" (Ph.D. dissertation, University of London, 1979), 94.

17 Quoted by Stepan, "Tropical Medicine and Public Health in Latin America," in her summary of Jaime Benchimol's work on Domingos Freire, *Medical History* 42 (1998): 109.

18 For recent bibliography, see Introduction n. 6.

PRIMARY SOURCES

The most important primary sources used for this book are Brazilian medical journals for the second half of the nineteenth century, especially the *Gazeta Médica da Bahia*. The journal, which was published every two weeks (with a few breaks), describes the activities of the Tropicalistas, provides information on their medical interests and broader social and political interests, and is invaluable as a source of information on the activities of the Bahian medical community as a whole. Besides the *Gazeta Médica da Bahia*, I consulted Brazilian and European medical journals (listed below) at the library of the Memorial da Medicina da Bahia and the Faculdade de Medicina da Bahia, the library of the Facultad de Medicina de Buenos Aires, the National Library of Medicine in Bethesda, the New York Public Library, the New York Academy of Medicine Library, the Health Sciences Libraries of Columbia University and the Paul and Lydia Kalmanovitz Library at University of California at San Francisco, Stanford's Lane Library, the Berkeley libraries, and through Inter-Library Loan.

The medical journals were supplemented by several other types of sources. First were the graduating dissertations (1850–90) located at the Arquivo no Memorial da Medicina, Terreiro de Jesus, Salvador, which all medical students in Brazil were required to complete before being allowed to formally exercise the medical profession. I consulted more than one hundred dissertations. The earlier dissertations are disappointing because they tend to be directly imitative of French medical dissertations. However, in the 1870s and 1880s the Bahian dissertations became much more interesting, for some of the medical students refused to work on topics taken from the French agenda and concentrated on what they viewed as particularly Brazilian or Bahian medical problems. These were the most valuable dissertations for my purposes. But even the more "orthodox" dissertations written in the 1870s and 1880s contain frequent references to the Tropicalistas and their journal so that information could be gleaned as to the Tropicalistas' impact on the student community.

Other useful sources included official publications such as the annual medical health reports for Bahia contained in Brazil, *Relatórios da Província da Bahia* (1823–89). The annual reports for the medical schools in Bahia and Rio de Janeiro found in Brazil, Ministério do Império, *Relatórios ministeriais,* Época do Império (1832–88), provide vital information on the activities and grievances of doctors teaching in the medical schools, and about the debates within the schools on the status, objectives, and problems of medical teaching in Brazil.

The reports and papers presented at the first medical congresses ever held in Brazil were another particularly valuable source. These include the *Primeiro Congresso Brazileiro de Medicina e Cirurgia do Rio de Janeiro* (Rio de Janeiro: Imprensa Nacional, 1889); *Segundo Congresso Brazileiro de Medicina e Cirurgia* (Rio de Janeiro: Imprensa Nacional, 1890); and *Terceiro Congresso Brazileiro de Medicina e Cirurgia* (Salvador, 1891). A reading of the papers and discussion sessions at the congresses gives an idea of the growing acceptance of ideas pioneered by the Tropicalistas in Brazil.

Although this book is based primarily on published sources, I also consulted some manuscript sources. At the Arquivo Público do Estado da Bahia, Salvador, I consulted the documentation contained in the Secção Histórica, Presidência da Província, Série: Saúde Pública. This deals mainly with reports put out by the official Inspectoria de Hygiene da Bahia, and correspondence between the Inspectoria and doctors and pharmacists requesting payments for services rendered, describing work accomplished during vaccination drives or epidemic outbreaks, and other matters. The *Despatches from Consuls in Bahia, Brazil,* give a sense of the milieu in which the doctors worked, since the consuls often commented on the health of the city and gave anecdotal evidence on Bahian physicians. Similarly, travelers' accounts proved to be a useful supplementary source (listed in the general bibliography). Books written by foreign physicians who either visited or lived for a period of time in Brazil were also extremely informative, particularly the works of Sigaud, *Du climat et des maladies du Bresil* (1844); Robert Dundas, *Sketches of Brazil; Including New Views on Tropical and European Fever* (1852); and Gustavus R. B. Horner, *Medical Topography of Brazil and Uruguay* (1845). Finally, nineteenth-century writings on the subjects of interest to the Tropicalistas provided the broader context of their work. Two of the most important were Thomas Spencer Cobbold, *Parasites: A Treatise on the Ectozoa of Man and Animals Including Some Account of the Ectozoa* (1879), and August Hirsch, *Handbook of Geographical and Historical Pathology* (1883).

Nineteenth-Century Brazilian Journals Consulted:

Anais Brasilienses de Medicina (journal of the officially sponsored Academia Imperial de Medicina and originally titled *Anais de Medicina do Rio de Janeiro*)
Brasil Médico
Annaes de Medicina Homeopáthica
Gazeta Médica da Bahia
Progresso Médico
Revista Brasileira de Medicina

Revista do Instituto Geográfico e Histórico da Bahia
Revista do Instituto Histórico e Geográfico do Rio de Janeiro
Revista Médica do Rio de Janeiro
União Médica

Non-Brazilian Nineteenth-Century Journals Consulted:

Archives de Médecine Navale
Archiv für Pathologische Anatomie und Physiologie und für Klinische Medecin
Boston Medical and Surgical Journal
British Medical Record
Edinburgh Medical Record
Gaillard's Medical Journal of New York
Gazette Médicale de Paris
Journal of the Proceedings of the Linnean Society (Zoology)
Journal of the Quekett Microscopical Club
Lancet
London Medical Record
Medical Times and Gazette
Quarterly Journal of Microscopical Science
St. Louis Medical and Surgical Journal
Sanitarian, N.Y.
Schmidt's Jahrbücher der in - und Ausländischen Gesammten Medecin
El Siglo Médico: Boletin de Medicina y Gaceta Médica
Veterinarian

BIBLIOGRAPHY

Ackerknecht, Erwin H. "Anticontagionism between 1821 and 1867." *Bulletin of the History of Medicine* 22 (1948): 562–593.

———. "Hygiene in France, 1815–1848." *Bulletin of the History of Medicine* 22 (1948): 117–155.

———. *Rudolf Virchow: Doctor, Statesman, Anthropologist.* Madison: University of Wisconsin Press, 1953.

———. *History and Geography of the Most Important Diseases.* New York: Hafner, 1965.

———. *A Short History of Medicine.* Rev. ed. New York: Ronald, 1955.

Adamo, Sam C. "The Broken Promise: Race, Health, and Justice in Rio de Janeiro, 1890–1940." Ph.D. dissertation, University of New Mexico, 1983.

Agassiz, Louis, and Elizabeth Agassiz. *A Journey in Brazil.* New York: Praeger, 1969.

"AHR Forum: Subaltern Studies as Postcolonial Criticism." *American Historical Review* 99, no. 5 (1994): 1475–1490.

Alden, Dauril. "The Population of Brazil in the Late Eighteenth Century: A Preliminary Study." *Hispanic American Historical Review* 43 (1963): 173–203.

Alden, Dauril, ed. *Colonial Roots of Modern Brazil.* Berkeley: University of California Press, 1973.

Alier, Verena Martinez. "Elopement and Seduction in Nineteenth Century Cuba." *Past and Present* 55 (May 1972): 91–129.

———. *Marriage, Class, and Color in Nineteenth Century Cuba: A Study of Racial Attitudes and Sexual Values in a Slave Society.* New York: Cambridge University Press, 1974.

Amado, Jorge. *Tent of Miracles.* New York: Avon, 1971.

Anderson, Benedict. *Imagined Communities: Reflections on the Origin and Spread of Nationalism.* London: Verso, 1990.

Anderson, Robin L. "Public Health and Public Healthiness, São Paulo, Brazil, 1876–1893." *Journal of the History of Medicine* 41, 3 (July 1986): 293–307.

Anderson, Warwick. "Immunities of Empire: Race, Disease, and the New Tropical Medicine, 1900–1920." *Bulletin of the History of Medicine* 70 (1996): 94–118.

Andrade, Manuel Correia de. *A terra e o homem no nordeste.* 4th ed. São Paulo: Ciências Humanas, 1980.

Andrade, Maria José de Souza. *A mão de obra escrava em Salvador, 1811–1860.* São Paulo: Corrupio, 1988.

Andrews, George Reid. *Blacks and Whites in São Paulo, Brazil, 1888–1988.* Madison: University of Wisconsin Press, 1991.

Apple, Rima D. "Constructing Mothers: Scientific Motherhood in the Nineteenth and Twentieth Centuries." *Society for the Social History of Medicine* 8, 2 (1995): 161–178.

Araújo, Alceu Maynard. *Medicina rústica.* São Paulo: Companhia Editora Nacional, 1979.

Araújo, Carlos da Silva. *Fatos e personagens da história da medicina e da farmácia no Brasil.* Vols. 1 and 2. Rio de Janeiro: Revista Continente Editorial, 1979.

Arnold, David. "Cholera and Colonisation in British India." *Past and Present* 113 (1986): 118–151.

———. *Colonizing the Body: State Medicine and Epidemic Disease in Nineteenth-Century India.* Berkeley: University of California Press, 1993.

Arnold, David, ed. *Imperial Medicine and Indigenous Societies.* Manchester: Manchester University Press, 1987.

———. *Warm Climates and Western Medicine: The Emergence of Tropical Medicine, 1500–1900.* Amsterdam: Rodopi, 1996.

Asevedo, Dorothy do Rego. "Estrutura ocupacional da população feminina da Cidade do Salvador segundo os dados do censo de 1872." Paper presented at the Universidade Federal da Bahia, 1975.

Aufderheide, Patricia Ann. "Order or Violence: Social Deviance and Social Control in Brazil, 1780–1840." Ph.D. dissertation, University of Minnesota, 1976.

Augel, Moema Parente. *Visitantes estrangeiros na Bahia oitocentista.* São Paulo: Cultrix, 1980.

Azevedo, Célia Maria Marinho de. *Onda negra, medo branco: O negro imaginário das elites, século XIX.* Rio de Janeiro: Paz e Terra, 1987.

Azevedo, Fernando de. *Brazilian Culture: An Introduction to the Study of Culture in Brazil.* Trans. William Rex Crawford. New York: Macmillan, 1950.

Azevedo, Fernando de, ed. *As ciencias no Brasil.* 2 vols, 215–221. Rio de Janeiro: Editora UFRJ, 1994.

Azevedo, Thales de. "Family, Marriage, and Divorce in Brazil." In *Contemporary Cultures and Society of Latin America,* ed. Dwight B. Heath and Richard N. Adams, 288–310. New York: Random House, 1965.

———. *Povoamento da Cidade do Salvador.* Bahia: Itapua, 1969.

Bacelar, Jeferson Affonso. *Negros e espanhóis: Identidade e ideologia étnica em Salvador.* Salvador: Universidade Federal da Bahia, 1983.

Bacellar, Renato Clark. *Brazil's Contribution to Tropical Medicine and Malaria: Personalities and Institutions.* Rio de Janeiro: Olímpica, 1963.

Barker-Benfield, G. J. *The Horror of the Half-Known Life: Male Attitudes toward Women and Sexuality.* New York: Harper and Row, 1976.

Barman, Roderick J. *Brazil: The Forging of a Nation, 1798–1852.* Stanford: Stanford University Press, 1988.

Barman, Roderick J., and Jean Barman. "The Role of the Law Graduate in the Political Elite of Imperial Brazil." *Journal of Inter-American Studies and World Affairs* 18, 4 (November 1976): 423–450.

Barros, Pedro Motta de. "Alvorecer de uma nova ciência: A medicina tropicalista bahiana." *História, Ciências, Saúde, Manguinhos* 4, no. 3 (1997): 411–459.

Barros, Roque Spencer Maciel de. *A ilustração brasileira e a idéia de universidade.* São Paulo: Universidade de São Paulo, 1959.

Barroso, Carmen. *Mulher, sociedade e estado no Brasil.* São Paulo: Brasiliense/UNICEF, 1982.

Bastide, Roger. *The African Religions of Brazil: Toward a Sociology of Interpretation of Civilizations.* Trans. Helen Sebba. Baltimore: Johns Hopkins University Press, 1978.

Belo, José-Maria. *Inteligência do Brasil: Ensaios sobre Machado de Assis, Joaquim Nabuco, Euclides da Cunha e Rui Barbosa.* São Paulo: Companhia Editora Nacional, 1935.

Benchimol, Jaime L. *Manguinhos do sonho à vida: A ciência na belle époque.* Rio de Janeiro: FIOCRUZ, 1990.

———. "Domingos José Freire y los comienzos de la bacteriología en Brasil." In *Salud, cultura y sociedad,* ed. Marcos Cueto, 53–86. Lima: Instituto Estudios Peruanos, 1996.

———. "Do Pasteur dos micróbios ao Pasteur dos mosquitos: Febre amarela no Rio de Janeiro, 1880–1903." Ph.D. dissertation, Universidade Federal Fluminense, 1996.

Benchimol, Jaime L., and Luiz Antônio Teixeira. *Cobras, lagartos e outros bichos: Uma história comparada dos Institutos Oswaldo Cruz e Butantan.* Rio de Janeiro: Universidade Federal do Rio de Janeiro, 1993.

Bennett, Paula, and Vernon A. Rosario II, eds. *Solitary Pleasures: The Historical, Literary, and Artistic Discourses of Autoeroticism.* New York: Routledge, 1995.

Benton, Ted. "Social Darwinism and Socialist Darwinism in Germany, 1860–1900." *Revista di Filosofia* 73 (1982): 79–121.

Besse, Susan K. *Restructuring Patriarchy: The Modernization of Gender Inequality in Brazil, 1914–1940.* Chapel Hill: University of North Carolina Press, 1996.

Bethell, Leslie. *The Independence of Latin America.* Cambridge: Cambridge University Press, 1987.

Bethell, Leslie, ed. *Brazil: Empire and Republic, 1822–1930.* Cambridge: Cambridge University Press, 1989.

———. *Latin America: Economy and Society, 1870–1930.* Cambridge: Cambridge University Press, 1989.

Biddiss, Michael D. *Father of Racist Ideology: The Social and Political Thought of Gobineau.* London: Weidenfeld and Nicolson, 1970.

Bleier, Ruth. "Biology and Women's Policy: A View from the Biological Sciences." In *Women, Biology, and Public Policy,* ed. Virginia Sapiro, 19–40. Beverly Hills: Sage, 1985.

Boehrer, George. "The Church and the Overthrow of the Brazilian Monarchy." *Hispanic American Historical Review* 48 (1968): 380–401.

———. "The Church in the Second Reign, 1840–1889." In *Conflict and Continuity in Brazilian Society,* ed. Henry H. Keith and S. F. Edwards, 115–143. Columbia: University of South Carolina Press, 1969.

Bonner, Thomas Neville. *Becoming a Physician: Medical Education in Britain, France, Germany, and the United States, 1750–1945.* New York: Oxford University Press, 1995.

Borges, Dain Edward. "Medical Ideas, Class and Race in Brazil, 1830–1930." Paper presented to the Latin American Studies Association, Albuquerque, New Mexico, April 18–20, 1985.

———. *The Family in Bahia, Brazil, 1870–1945.* Stanford: Stanford University Press, 1992.

———. "Medical Ideas, Class, and Race in Brazil, 1830–1930" (paper presented to the Latin America Studies Association, Albuquerque, New Mexico, April 18–20, 1985).

———. " 'Puffy, Ugly, Slothful, and Inert': Degeneration in Brazilian Social Thought, 1880–1940." *Journal of Latin American Studies* 25 (1993): 235–256.

———. "The Recognition of Afro-Brazilian Symbols and Ideas, 1890–1940." *Luso-Brazilian Review* 32, 2 (1995): 59–78.

———. "Salvador's 1890s: Paternalism and Its Discontents." *Luso-Brazilian Review* 32, 2 (1995): 47–57.

Borst, Charlotte G. *Catching Babies: The Professionalization of Childbirth, 1870–1920.* Cambridge, Mass.: Harvard University Press, 1995.

Bowers, John Z., and Elizabeth F. Purcell, eds. *Aspects of the History of Medicine in Latin America.* New York: Josiah Macy Jr. Foundation, 1979.

Bowler, Peter J. *The Eclipse of Darwinism: Anti-Darwinian Evolution Theories in the Decades around 1900.* Baltimore: Johns Hopkins University Press, 1983.

Bracegirdle, Brian. "The Microscopical Tradition." In *Companion Encyclopedia of the History of Medicine,* ed. W. F. Bynum and Roy Porter, 102–119. London: Routledge, 1994.

Bradley, David J. "Tropical Medicine." In *The Oxford Companion to Medicine,* ed. John Walton, Paul B. Beeson, and Ronald Bodley Scott, 2: 1394–1397. Oxford: Oxford University Press, 1986.

Brandt, Allan M. *No Magic Bullet: A Social History of Venereal Disease in the United States since 1880.* New York: Oxford University Press, 1987.

Britto, Nara. *Oswaldo Cruz: A construção de um mito na ciência brasileira.* Rio de Janeiro: FIOCRUZ, 1995.

Britto, Nara, and Nísia Trinidade Lima. "Salud y nación: Propuesta para el sanea-
miento rural. Un estudio de la revista *Saúde* (1818–1919)." In *Salud, cultura y sociedad
en América Latina: Nuevas perspectivas históricas,* ed. Marcos Cueto, 135–158. Lima:
Instituto de Estudios Peruanos, 1966.

Bullough, Vern, and Martha Voght. "Women, Menstruation, and Nineteenth-Century
Medicine." In *Women and Health in America,* ed. Judith Walzer Leavitt, 28–37.
Madison: University of Wisconsin Press, 1984.

Burns, E. Bradford. *A History of Brazil.* 2d ed. New York: Columbia University Press,
1980.

———. *The Poverty of Progress: Latin America in the Nineteenth Century.* Berkeley: University of California Press, 1980.

Butler, Kim D. *Freedoms Given, Freedoms Won: Afro-Brazilians in Post-Abolition São
Paulo and Salvador.* New Brunswick: Rutgers University Press, 1998.

———. "Ginga Baiana: The Politics of Race, Class, Culture, and Power in Salvador,
Bahia." In *Afro-Brazilian Culture and Politics: Bahia, 1790s to 1990s,* ed. Hendrik
Kraay, 158–175. Armonk: M. E. Sharpe, 1998.

Bynum, W. F. *Science and the Practice of Medicine in the Nineteenth Century.* Cambridge:
Cambridge University Press, 1994.

Bynum, W. F., and V. Nutton, eds. *Essays in the History of Therapeutics.* Amsterdam:
Rodopi, 1991.

Cabral, Oswaldo Rodrigues. *A medicina teológica e as benzedeiras: Suas raízes na história
e sua persistência no folclore.* São Paulo: Departamento de Cultura, 1958.

Callaway, Helen. *Gender, Culture, and Empire.* London: Macmillan, 1987.

Cancian, Francesca, Louis Wolf Goodman, and Peter H. Smith, eds. "The Family in
Latin America." *Journal of Family History* 3 (1978): 314–458.

Cândido, Antônio. "The Brazilian Family." In *Brazil: Portrait of Half a Continent,* ed.
T. Lynn Smith and Alexander Merchant, 291–312. New York: Dryden, 1951.

Cannon, H. Graham. "What Lamarck Really Said." *Linnean Society Proceedings* 168
(1975): 70–85.

Carlson, Dennis G. *African Fever: A Study of British Science, Technology, and Politics in
West Africa, 1787–1864.* New York: Science History Publications, 1984.

Carlson, Eric T. "Medicine and Degeneration: Theory and Praxis." In *Degeneration:
The Dark Side of Progress,* ed. J. Edward Chamberlin and Sander L. Gilman, 121–143.
New York: Columbia University Press, 1985.

Carneiro, Edison. *Candomblés da Bahia.* Rio de Janeiro: Coquetel, n.d.

Carvalho, José Murilo de. "As forças armadas na Primeira República: O poder desestabilizador." In *O Brasil republicano,* vol. 2 of *História geral da civilização brasileira,*
ed. Boris Fausto, 183–234. São Paulo, 1971.

———. "Elite and State-Building in Imperial Brazil." Ph.D. dissertation, Stanford University, 1974.

———. *A construção da ordem: A elite política imperial.* Rio de Janeiro: Campus, 1980.

———. "Political Elites and State Building: The Case of Nineteenth-Century Brazil." *Comparative Studies in Society and History* 24 (1982): 378–399.

———. *Os bestializados: O Rio de Janeiro e a República que não foi.* São Paulo: Companhia das Letras, 1987.

Cassell, Eric J. "Ideas in Conflict: The Rise and Fall (and Rise and Fall) of New Views of Disease." *Daedalua* 115 (1986).

Castor, Josué de. *O problema da alimentação no Brasil.* São Paulo: Companhia Editora Nacional, n.d.

Castro, Dinorah D'Araújo Berbert de. "Idéias filosóficas nas teses inaugurais da Faculdade de Medicina da Bahia, 1838–1889." Master's thesis, Universidade Federal da Bahia, 1973.

Cava, Ralph dela. *Miracle at Joaseiro.* New York: Columbia University Press, 1970.

Cell, John W. "Anglo-Indian Medical Theory and the Origins of Segregation in West Africa." *American Historical Review* 91 (1986): 307–335.

Chalhoub, Sidney. "The Politics of Disease Control: Yellow Fever and Race in Nineteenth-Century Rio de Janeiro." *Journal of Latin American Studies* 25 (1993): 441–463.

———. *Cidade febril: Cortiços e epidemias na corte imperial.* São Paulo: Companhia das Letras, 1996.

Chamberlin, J. Edward, and Sander L. Gilman, eds. *Degeneration: The Dark Side of Progress.* New York: Columbia University Press, 1985.

Chandler, David L. *Health and Slavery in Colonial Colombia.* New York: Arno, 1981.

Cianfrani, Theodore. *A Short History of Obstetrics and Gynecology.* Springfield: Charles C. Thomas, 1960.

Clark, Linda. *Social Darwinism in France.* University, Ala.: University of Alabama Press, 1984.

Cobbold, Thomas Spencer. *Parasites: A Treatise on the Entozoa of Man and Animals Including Some Account of the Ectozoa.* London: J. and A. Churchill, 1879.

Codell-Carter, K. "Germ Theory, Hysteria, and Freud's Early Work in Psychopathology." *Medical History* 24 (1980): 259–274.

Codman, John. *Ten Months in Brazil.* New York: James Miller, 1972.

Coelho, Edmundo. "Físicos, sectários e charlatães: A medicina em perspectiva histórico-comparada." In *Profissões de saúde: Uma abordagem sociológica,* ed. Maria Helena Machado. Rio de Janeiro: FIOCRUZ, 1995.

Coleman, William. *Death Is a Social Disease: Public Health and Political Economy in Early Industrial France.* Madison: University of Wisconsin Press, 1982.

Collichio, Therezina Alves Ferreira. *Miranda Azevedo e darwinismo no Brasil.* Belo Horizonte: Itatiaia, 1988.

Coni, Antônio Caldas. *A Escola Tropicalista Bahiana: Paterson, Wucherer, Silva Lima.* Salvador: Progresso, 1952.

Cooper, Donald B. "Brazil's Long Fight against Epidemic Disease, 1849–1917, with

Special Emphasis on Yellow Fever." *Bulletin of the New York Academy of Medicine* 51, no. 5 (1975): 672–696.

———. "The New 'Black Death': Cholera in Brazil, 1855–56." *Social Science History* 10 (winter 1986): 467–488.

Cooper, Frederick, et al. *Confronting Historical Paradigms: Peasants, Labor, and the Capitalist World System in Africa and Latin America.* Madison: University of Wisconsin Press, 1993.

Coradini, Odaci Luiz. "Grandes famílias e elite *profissional* na medicina no Brasil." *História, Ciências, Saúde, Manguinhos,* 4, 3 (1997): 425–466.

Corrêa, Mariza. "Repensando a família patriarchal brasileira." In *Colcha de retalhos: Estudos sobre a família no Brasil,* ed. Maria Suely Kofes de Ameida et al., 13–38. São Paulo: Brasiliense 1982.

———. "As ilusões da liberdade: A Escola Nina Rodrigues e a antropologia no Brasil." Ph.D. dissertation, Universidade de São Paulo, 1982.

Costa, Emília Viotti da. *A abolição.* São Paulo: Global, 1982.

———. *Da senzala à colônia.* São Paulo: Ciências Humanas, 1982.

———. *The Brazilian Empire: Myths and Histories.* Chicago: University of Chicago Press, 1985.

———. "Brazil: The Age of Reform, 1870–1889." In *The Cambridge History of Latin America,* ed. Leslie Bethell, 5: 725–777. Cambridge: Cambridge University Press, 1986.

———. "Empire, 1870–1889." In *Brazil: Empire and Republic, 1822–1930,* ed. Leslie Bethell, 161–213. Cambridge: Cambridge University Press, 1989.

Costa, João Cruz. *A History of Ideas in Brazil.* Trans. Suzette Macedo. Berkeley: University of California Press, 1964.

Costa, Jurandir Freire. *Ordem médica e norma familiar.* 2d ed. Rio de Janeiro: Graal, 1979.

Cott, Nancy F. "Passionlessness: An Interpretation of Victorian Sexual Ideology, 1790–1850." In *Women and Health in America,* ed. Judith Walzer Leavitt, 57–69. Madison: University of Wisconsin Press, 1984.

Cournand, André. "Air and Blood." In *Circulation of the Blood: Men and Ideas,* ed. Alfred P. Fishman and Dickinson W. Richards, 48–63. New York: Oxford University Press, 1964.

Coutinho, Afrânio. *An Introduction to Literature in Brazil.* Trans. Gregory Rabassa. New York: Columbia University Press, 1969.

Crook, D. P. "Darwinism: The Political Implications." *History of European Ideas* 2 (1981): 19–34.

Cruz, Agueda María Rodríguez. *Historia de las universidades hispanoamericanas: Período Hispánico.* 2 vols. Bogotá: Instituto Caro y Cuervo, 1973.

Cueto, Marcos. "Excellence in the Periphery: Scientific Activities and Biomedical Sciences in Peru." Ph.D. dissertation, Columbia University, 1988.

_____. "The Rockefeller Foundation's Medical Policy and Scientific Research in Latin America: The Case of Physiology." *Social Studies of Science* 20 (1990): 229–254.

_____. "Sanitation from Above: Yellow Fever and Foreign Intervention in Peru, 1919–1922." *Hispanic American Historical Review* 72 (1992): 1–22.

_____. "Tropical Medicine and Bacteriology in Boston and Peru: Studies of Carrion's Disease in the Early Twentieth Century." *Medical History* 40 (1996): 344–364.

_____. "Science under Adversity: Latin American Medical Research and American Private Philanthropy, 1920–1960." *Minerva* 35 (1997): 233–245.

Cueto, Marcos, ed. *Missionaries of Science: The Rockefeller Foundation and Latin America.* Bloomington: Indiana University Press, 1994.

_____. *Salud, cultura y sociedad en América Latina: Nuevas perspectivas históricas.* Lima: Instituto de Estudios Peruanos, 1996.

Cullen, M. J. *The Statistical Movement in Early Victorian Britain: The Foundations of Empirical Social Research.* New York: Harvester, 1975.

Curpertino, Fausto. *População e saúde pública no Brasil: Povo pobre e povo doente.* Rio de Janeiro: Civilização Brasileira, 1976.

Curtin, Philip D. *The Image of Africa: British Ideas and Actions, 1780–1850.* Madison: University of Wisconsin Press, 1964.

_____. "Medical Knowledge and Urban Planning in Tropical Africa." *American Historical Review* 90 (1985): 594–613.

_____. *Death by Migration: Europe's Encounter with the Tropical World in the Nineteenth Century.* Cambridge: Cambridge University Press, 1989.

Czeresina, Dina. *Do contágio à transmissão: Ciência e cultura na gênese do conhecimento epidemiológico.* Rio de Janeiro: FIOCRUZ, 1997.

Darwin, Charles. *The Voyage of the Beagle.* New York: Dutton, 1959.

Degler, Carl. *Neither Black nor White: Slavery and Race Relations in Brazil and the United States.* Madison: University of Wisconsin Press, 1986.

del Priore, Mary, ed. *Ao sul do corpo: Condição feminina, maternidades e mentalidades no Brasil colônia.* Rio de Janeiro: José Olympio, 1993.

_____. *História das mulheres no Brasil.* São Paulo: UNESP, 1997.

Desmond, Adrian. "Artisan Resistance and Evolution in Britain, 1819–1948." *Osiris,* 2d ser., 3 (1987): 77–110.

Dias, Maria Odila Leite da Silva. *Quotidiano e poder em São Paulo no século XIX.* São Paulo: Brasiliense, 1984.

Donegan, Jane B. *Women and Men Midwives: Medicine, Morality, and Misogyny in Early America.* Westport: Greenwood, 1978.

Donghi, Tulio Halperin. " 'Dependency Theory' and Latin American Historiography." *Latin American Research Review* 17 (1982): 115–132.

_____. "The State of Latin American History." In *Changing Perspectives in Latin American Studies: Insights from Six Disciplines,* ed. Christopher Mitchell, 13–62. Stanford: Stanford University Press, 1983.

Donnison, Jean. *Midwives and Medical Men: A History of the Struggle for the Control of Childbirth*. London: Historical Publications, 1988.

Donzelot, Jacques. *The Policing of Families*. Trans. Robert Hurley. New York: Pantheon, 1979.

Drachman, Virginia G. "The Loomis Trial: Social Mores and Obstetrics in Mid-Nineteenth Century." In *Women and Health in America*, ed. Judith Walzer Leavitt, 166–174. Madison: University of Wisconsin Press, 1984.

———. "The Dilemma of Women Doctors in Late 19th-Century America." In *Sickness and Health: Readings in the History of Medicine and Public Health*, ed. Judith Walzer Leavitt and Ronald L. Numbers, 173–182. Madison: University of Wisconsin Press, 1985.

Dudley, W. S. "Institutional Sources of Officer Discontent in the Brazilian Army, 1870–1889." *Hispanic American Historical Review* 55 (1975): 44–65.

Dundas, Robert. *Sketches of Brazil; Including New Views on Tropical and European Fever*. London: John Churchill, 1852.

Eakin, Marshall C. "Race and Identity: Sílvio Romero, Science, and Social Thought in Late Nineteenth-Century Brazil. *Luso-Brazilian Review* 22, 2 (1985): 151–174.

Edelweiss, Frederico G. "A secular presença da Alemanha na Bahia." *Anais do Arquivo do Estado da Bahia* 39 (1970): 223–242.

Edler, Flávio Coelho. "As reformas do ensino médico e a profissionalização da medicina na corte do Rio de Janeiro, 1854–1884." Master's thesis, Universidade de São Paulo, 1992.

Ehrenreich, Barbara, and Deidre English. *Witches, Midwives, and Nurses: A History of Women Healers*. Old Westbury: Feminist Press, 1973.

Emerson, Elias Merhy. *A saúde pública como política, São Paulo, 1920–1948: Os movimentos sanitários, os modelos tecno-assistências e a formação das políticas governamentais*. São Paulo: Hucitec, 1992.

Ettling, John. *The Germ of Laziness: Rockefeller Philanthropy and Public Health in the South*. Cambridge, Mass.: Harvard University Press, 1981.

Evanson, Philip. "The Liberal Party and Reform in Brazil, 1860–1889." Ph.D. dissertation, University of Virginia, 1969.

Expilly, Charles. *Mulheres, costumes do Brasil*. São Paulo: Companhia Editora Nacional, 1935.

Falção, Edgard de Cerqueira. *As contribuições originais da "Escola Tropicalista Bahiana."* Centro de Estudos Bahianos, Universidade Federal da Bahia, 1976.

Faoro, Raymundo. *Os donos do poder: Formação do patronato político brasileiro*. Vols. 1 and 2. Porto Alegre: Globo, 1975.

Faria, Fernando Antônio. *Querelas brasileiras: Homeopatia e política imperial*. Rio de Janeiro: Notrya, 1994.

Farley, John. "Parasites and the Germ Theory of Disease." *Millbank Quarterly* 67 (1989): 50–68.

————. *Bilharzia: A History of Imperial Tropical Medicine.* Cambridge: Cambridge University Press, 1991.

Fausto, Boris. *Crime e cotidiano: A criminalidade em São Paulo, 1880–1924.* São Paulo: Brasiliense, 1984.

————. "Society and Politics." In *Brazil: Empire and Republic, 1822–1930,* ed. Leslie Bethell, 257–307. Cambridge: Cambridge University Press, 1989.

Fee, Elizabeth. "Since versus Science: Venereal Disease in Twentieth Century Baltimore." In *AIDS: The Burdens of History,* ed. Elizabeth Fee and Daniel M. Fox, 121–146. Berkeley: University of California Press, 1988.

Fee, Elizabeth, and Daniel M. Fox. "Introduction: AIDS, Public Policy, and Historical Inquiry." In *AIDS: The Burdens of History,* ed. Elizabeth Fee and Daniel M. Fox, 1–11. Berkeley: University of California Press, 1988.

Fernandes, Florestan. *The Negro in Brazilian Society.* New York: Columbia University Press, 1969.

Fernandes, Reginaldo. *O conselheiro Jobim e o espírito da medicina do seu tempo.* Senado Federal: Centro Gráfico, 1982.

Ferreira, Luiz Otávio. "O nascimento de uma instituição científica: Os periódicos médicos brasileiros na primeira metade do século XIX." Ph.D. dissertation, Universidade de São Paulo, 1996.

Ferreira, Luiz Otávio, Marcos Chor Maio, and Nara Azevedo. "A Sociedade de Medicina e Cirurgia do Rio de Janeiro: A gênese de uma rede institucional alternativa." *História, Ciência, Saúde, Manguinhos* 4, 3 (1997): 475–491.

Ferri, Mário Guimarães, and Shozo Motoyama, eds., *História das ciências no Brasil.* São Paulo: EPU, 1973.

Figlio, Karl. "The Historiography of Scientific Medicine: An Invitation to the Human Sciences." *Comparative Studies in Society and History* 19 (1977): 262–286.

Figlio, Karl, and Paul Weindling. "Was Social Medicine Revolutionary? Rudolf Virchow and the Revolutions of 1848." *Bulletin of the Society for the Social History of Medicine* 34 (June 1984): 10–18.

Figueiroa, Sílvia F. M. "Associativismo científico no Brasil: O Instituto Histórico e Geográfico Brasileiro como espaço institucional para as ciências naturais durante o século XIX." *Interciência* 17, 3 (1992): 141–146.

————. "A medicina no Brasil." In *História das ciências no Brasil,* ed. Mário Guimarães Ferri and Shozo Motoyama, São Paulo: EPU, 1973.

————. "Medicine in Colonial Brazil: An Overview." In *Aspects of the History of Medicine in Latin America,* ed. John Z. Bowers and Elizabeth F. Purcell, New York: Josiah Macy Jr. Foundation, 1979.

————. *História geral da medicina brasileira.* 2 vols. São Paulo: Hucitec, 1991.

Fiola, Jan. "Race Relations in Brazil: A Reassessment of the 'Racial Democracy' Thesis." Program in Latin American Studies. Occasional Paper Series No. 24. University of Massachusetts at Amherst, 1990.

Fishman, Alfred P., and Dickinson W. Richards, eds. *Circulation of the Blood: Men and Ideas.* New York: Oxford University Press, 1964.

Fletcher, James C. *Brazil and the Brazilians Portrayed in Historical and Descriptive Sketches.* Boston: Little, Brown, 1866.

Flinn, M. W., ed. *Report on the Sanitary Condition of the Labouring Population of Great Britain by Edwin Chadwick, 1842.* Edinburgh: University of Edinburgh Press, 1965.

Fontaine, Pierre-Michel, ed. *Race, Class, and Power in Brazil.* Los Angeles: Center for Afro-American Studies, University of California at Los Angeles, 1985.

Foucault, Michel. *The Birth of the Clinic.* New York: Vintage, 1975.

———. *The History of Sexuality: An Introduction.* Vol. 1. New York: Vintage, 1980.

———. *Power/Knowledge: Selected Interviews and Other Writings, 1972–77.* Ed. Colin Gordon. New York: Pantheon, 1980.

Fox, Geoffrey E. "Honor, Shame, and Women's Liberation in Cuba: Views of Working Class Emigré Men." In *Female and Male in Latin America,* ed. Ann Pescatello, 273–292. Pittsburgh: University of Pittsburgh Press, 1973.

Franco, Affonso Arinos de Mello. *Conceito de civilisação brasileira.* Vol. 70. São Paulo: Companhia Editora Nacional, 1936.

Franco, Jean. *Plotting Women: Gender and Representation in Mexico.* New York: Columbia University Press, 1989.

Fraser, Gertrude Jacinta. "Afro-American Midwives, Biomedicine, and the State: An Ethnohistorical Account of Birth and Its Transformation in Rural Virginia." Ph.D. dissertation, Johns Hopkins University, 1988.

Frederickson, George M. *The Image of the Black in the White Mind.* New York: Harper and Row, 1971.

Freitas, Octávio de. *Doenças africanas no Brasil.* São Paulo: Companhia Editora Nacional, 1935.

Freyre, Gilberto. *Perfil de Euclydes e outros perfis.* Rio de Janeiro: José Olympio, 1944.

———. *New World in the Tropics.* New York: Vintage, 1963.

———. "The Patriarchal Basis of Brazilian Society." In *Politics of Change in Latin America,* ed. Joseph Maier and Richard W. Weatherhead, 155–173. New York: Praeger, 1964.

———. *The Masters and the Slaves.* Trans. Samuel Putman. New York: Knopf, 1969.

———. *Nós e a Europa germânica: Em torno de alguns aspectos das relações do Brasil com a cultura germânica no decorrer do século XIX.* Rio de Janeiro: Grifo, 1971.

———. *Médicos, doentes e contextos sociais: Uma abordagem sociológica.* Rio de Janeiro: Globo, 1983.

———. *The Mansions and the Shanties: The Making of Modern Brazil.* Trans. Harriet de Onis. Berkeley: University of California Press, 1986.

———. *Order and Progress: Brazil from Monarchy to Republic.* Trans. Rod W. Horton. Berkeley: University of California Press, 1986.

Fundação, Carlos Chagas, ed. *Mulher brasileira: Bibliografia anotada.* Vols. 1 and 2. São Paulo: Brasiliense, 1979–81.

Furst, Lilian R. *Women Healers and Physicians: Climbing a Long Hill*. Lexington: University of Kentucky Press, 1997.

Gale, Barry G. "Darwin and the Concept of a Struggle for Existence: A Study in the Extra-Scientific Origins of Scientific Ideas." *Isis* 63 (1972): 321–344.

Gallagher, Catherine, and Thomas Laqueur. *The Making of the Modern Body: Sexuality and Society in the Nineteenth Century*. Berkeley: University of California Press, 1987.

Gelfand, M. *Tropical Victory: An Account of the Influence of Medicine on the History of Southern Rhodesia, 1890–1923*. Cape Town: Juto, 1953.

Gelfand, Toby. "Medical Nemesis, Paris, 1894: Leon Daudet's Les Morticoles." *Bulletin of the History of Medicine* 60 (1986): 155–176.

Gélis, Jacques. *History of Childbirth: Fertility, Pregnancy, and Birth in Early Modern Europe*. Boston: Northeastern University Press, 1991.

Gibson, Charles. "Latin America and the Americas." In *The Past before Us,* ed. Michael Kammen, 187–204. Ithaca: Cornell University Press, 1982.

Giffoni, O. Carneiro. *Dicionário bio-bibliográfico brasileiro de escritores médicos (1500–1899)*. São Paulo: Livraria Nobel, 1972.

Gilman, Sander L. *Difference and Pathology: Stereotypes of Sexuality, Race, and Madness*. Ithaca: Cornell University Press, 1985.

Glick, Thomas. "Science and Independence in Latin America (with Special Reference to New Granada)." *Hispanic American Historical Review* 71 (1991): 307–334.

———. "Science and Society in Twentieth-Century Latin America." In *The Cambridge History of Latin America,* ed. Leslie Bethell, 4: 463–535. Cambridge: Cambridge University Press, 1995.

Gomes, Ordival Cassiano. *Manuel Vitorino Pereira: Médico e cirurgião*. Rio de Janeiro: Agir, 1957.

Goodyear, James D. "Agents of Empire: Portuguese Doctors in Colonial Brazil and the Idea of Tropical Disease." Ph.D. dissertation, Johns Hopkins University, 1982.

Goudsblom, Johan. "Public Health and the Civilizing Process." *Milbank Quarterly* 64 (1986): 161–188.

Gould, Stephen Jay. *The Mismeasure of Man*. New York: Norton, 1981.

Graden, Dale T. " 'So Much Superstition among These People!': Candomblé and the Dilemmas of Afro-Bahian Intellectuals, 1864–1871." In *Afro-Brazilian Culture and Politics: Bahia, 1790s to 1990s,* ed. Hendrik Kraay, 57–73. Armonk: M. E. Sharpe, 1998.

Graham, Maria Dundas. *Journal of a Voyage to Brazil and Residence There During Part of the Years 1821, 1822, 1823*. New York: Praeger, 1969.

Graham, Richard. *Britain and the Onset of Modernization in Brazil, 1850–1914*. Cambridge: Cambridge University Press, 1968.

———. "State and Society in Brazil, 1822–1930." *Latin American Research Review* 22 (1987): 223–236.

———. *Patronage and Politics in Nineteenth-Century Brazil*. Stanford: Stanford University Press, 1990.

Graham, Sandra Lauderdale. *House and Street: The Domestic World of Servants and Masters in Nineteenth-Century Rio de Janeiro*. Austin: University of Texas Press, 1992.

Granshaw, Lindsay. "The Hospital." In *Companion Encyclopedia of the History of Medicine*, ed. W. F. Bynum and Roy Porter, 1180–1203. London: Routledge, 1994.

Greenfield, Gerald Michael. "The Great Drought and Elite Discourse in Imperial Brazil." *Hispanic American Historical Review* 72 (1992): 375–400.

Greenwood, Major. "Miasma and Contagion." In *Science, Medicine, and History: Essays on the Evolution of Scientific Thought and Medical Practice*, ed. E. Ashworth Underwood, 500–507. London: Oxford University Press, 1953.

Grewal, Inderpal. *Home and Harem: Nation, Gender, Empire, and the Cultures of Travel*. Durham: Duke University Press, 1996.

Guha, Ranajit, and Gayatri Chakravorty Spivak, eds. *Selected Subaltern Studies*. New York: Oxford University Press, 1988.

Guimarães, Antônio Sérgio Alfredo. "Cor, classes e status nos estudos de Pierson, Azevedo e Harris na Bahia, 1940–1960." In *Raça, ciência e sociedade*, ed. Marcos Chor Maio and Ricardo Ventura Santos, 143–158. Rio de Janeiro: FIOCRUZ, 1996.

Guimarães, Reinaldo. *Saúde e medicina no Brasil: Contribuição para um debate*. 4th ed. Rio de Janeiro: Graal, 1984.

Guy, Donna J. *Sex and Danger in Buenos Aires: Prostitution, Family, and Nation in Argentina*. Lincoln: University of Nebraska Press, 1990.

Habsburgo, Maximiliano de. *Bahia 1860: Esboços de viagem*. Rio de Janeiro: Tempo Brasileiro, 1982.

Hahner, June E. "The Brazilian Armed Forces and the Overthrow of the Monarchy: Another Perspective." *Americas* 26 (1969): 171–182.

———. *Civilian-Military Relations in Brazil, 1889–1898*. Columbia: University of South Carolina Press, 1969.

———. "Women and Work in Brazil, 1850–1920: A Preliminary Investigation." In *Essays Concerning the Socioeconomic History of Brazil and Portuguese India*, ed. Dauril Alden and Warren Dean, 87–117. Gainesville: University of Florida Press, 1977.

———. "Recent Research on Women in Brazil." *Latin American Research Review* 20 (1985): 163–179.

———. *Poverty and Politics: The Urban Poor in Brazil, 1890–1920*. Albuquerque: University of New Mexico Press, 1986.

———. *Emancipating the Female Sex: The Struggle for Women's Rights in Brazil, 1850–1940*. Durham: Duke University Press, 1990.

———. *Women through Women's Eyes: Latin American Women in Nineteenth-Century Travel Accounts*. Wilmington: SR Books, 1998.

Hale, Charles A. "Political and Social Ideas in Latin America, 1870–1930." In *The Cambridge History of Latin America*, ed. Leslie Bethell, 4: 382–414. Cambridge: Cambridge University Press, 1985.

Haller, John S. Jr. "The Physician versus the Negro: Medical and Anthropological

Concepts of Race in Late Nineteenth Century." *Bulletin of the History of Medicine* 44 (1970): 154–167.

Haller, John S. Jr., and Robin Haller. *The Physician and Sexuality in Victorian America.* Urbana: University of Illinois Press, 1974.

Hannaway, Caroline. "Environment and Miasmata." In *Companion Encyclopedia of the History of Medicine,* ed. W. F. Bynum and Roy Porter, 292–308. London: Routledge, 1994.

Hardy, Anne. "Beriberi, Vitamin B$_1$, and World Food Policy, 1925–1970." *Medical History* 39 (1995): 61–67.

Harrison, Mark. "Tropical Medicine in Nineteenth-Century India." *British Journal for the History of Science* 25 (1992): 299–318.

———. *Public Health in British India: Anglo-Indian Preventive Medicine, 1859–1914.* Cambridge: Cambridge University Press, 1994.

———. " 'The Tender Frame of Man': Disease, Climate, and Racial Difference in India and the West Indies, 1760–1860." *Bulletin of the History of Medicine* 70 (1996): 68–93.

Hasenbalg, Carlos Alfredo. *Discriminação e desigualdades raciais no Brasil.* Rio de Janeiro: Graal, 1979.

Havighurst, Robert J., and J. Roberto Moreira. *Society and Education in Brazil.* Pittsburgh: University of Pittsburgh Press, 1965.

Haynes, Douglas M. "From the Periphery to the Center: Patrick Manson and the Development of Tropical Medicine as a Medical Specialty in Britain, 1870–1900." Ph.D. dissertation, University of California at Berkeley, 1992.

Hirsch, August. *Handbook of Geographical and Historical Pathology.* Erlangen: Verlag von Ferdinand Enke, 1859–62.

Hobsbawm, E. J. *Nations and Nationalism since 1870: Programme, Myth, Reality.* Cambridge: Cambridge University Press, 1990.

Hobsbawm, E. J., and Terence Ranger. *The Invention of Tradition.* Cambridge: Cambridge University Press, 1983.

Holanda, Sérgio Buarque de, ed. *O Brasil monárquico,* Vol. 3 of *História Geral da Civilização brasileira.* São Paulo: Difusão Européia do Livro, 1969.

Holloway, Thomas H. *Immigrants on the Land: Coffee and Society in São Paulo, 1886–1934.* Chapel Hill: University of North Carolina Press, 1980.

Horner, Gustavus R. B. *Medical Topography of Brazil and Uruguay.* Philadelphia: Lindsay and Blakiston, 1845.

Hudson, Robert P. *Disease and Its Control: The Shaping of Modern Thought.* Westport: Greenwood, 1983.

Hull, Isabel V. "The Bourgeoisie and Its Discontents: Reflections on 'Nationalism and Respectability.' " *Journal of Contemporary History* 17 (1982): 247–268.

Hutchinson, Carmelita Junqueira Ayres. "Notas preliminares ao estudo da família no Brasil." In *Anais da II Reunião Brasileira de Antropologia, Bahia, Julho de 1955,* 261–274. Bahia: Universidade da Bahia, 1957.

Jones, Colin, and Roy Porter, eds. *Reassessing Foucault: Power, Medicine and the Body.* London: Routledge, 1994.

Jordanova, Ludmilla J. *Sexual Visions: Images of Gender in Science and Medicine between the Eighteenth and Twentieth Centuries.* Madison: University of Wisconsin Press, 1989.

———. "The Social Construction of Medical Knowledge." *Social History of Medicine* 7, 3 (1995): 361–381.

Karasch, Mary C. *Slave Life in Rio de Janeiro, 1808–1850.* Princeton: Princeton University Press, 1987.

Kean, B. H. et al., eds., *Tropical Medicine and Parasitology: Classic Investigations.* Vol. 1. Ithaca: Cornell University Press, 1978.

Keele, Kenneth D. "Clinical Medicine in the 1860s." In *Medicine and Science in the 1860s,* ed. F. N. L. Poynter, 1–11. London: Wellcome Institute for the History of Medicine, 1968.

Keevil, John J., et al. *Medicine and the Navy, 1200–1900.* 4 vols. Edinburgh: E. and S. Livingstone, 1957–63.

Kennedy, Dane. "The Perils of the Midday Sun: Climatic Anxieties in the Colonial Tropics." In *Imperialism and the Natural World,* ed. John M. MacKenzie. Manchester: Manchester University Press, 1990. 118–140.

Kennedy, John Norman. "Bahian Elites, 1750–1822." *Hispanic American Historical Review* 53 (1973): 415–439.

Keremitsis, Eileen. "The Early Industrial Worker in Rio de Janeiro, 1870–1930." Ph.D. dissertation, Columbia University, 1982.

Kidder, K. P., and J. C. Fletcher. *Brazil and the Brazilians, Portrayed in Historical and Descriptive Sketches.* Philadelphia: Childs and Peterson, 1857.

Kiple, Kenneth F. *The Caribbean Slave.* Cambridge: Cambridge University Press, 1984.

———. "Cholera and Race in the Caribbean." *Journal of Latin American Studies* 17 (1985): 157–177.

———. "The Nutritional Link between Slave Infant and Child Mortality in Brazil." *Hispanic American Historical Review* 69 (1989): 677–690.

Kiple, Kenneth F., ed. *The Cambridge World History of Human Disease* (Cambridge: Cambridge University Press, 1993).

Kiple, Kenneth F., and Virginia Himmelsteib King. *Another Dimension to the Black Diaspora: Diet, Disease, and Racism.* Cambridge: Cambridge University Press, 1981.

Klein, Herbert S. "Colored Freedman in Brazilian Slave Society." *Journal of Social History* 3 (1969): 30–52.

———. "The Internal Slave Trade in Nineteenth Century Brazil: A Study of Slave Importations into Rio de Janeiro in 1852." *Hispanic American Historical Review* 51 (1971): 567–585.

———. *African Slavery in Latin America and the Caribbean.* New York: Oxford University Press, 1986.

Kleinman, Arthur. "What Is Specific to Western Medicine?" In *Companion Encyclope-*

dia of the History of Medicine, ed. W. F. Bynum and Roy Porter, 15–23. London: Routledge, 1994.

Kobrin, Frances E. "The American Midwife Controversy: A Crisis of Professionalization." In *Women and Health in America,* ed. Judith Walzer Leavitt, 318–326. Madison: University of Wisconsin Press, 1984.

Koster, Henry. *Travels in Brazil.* Carbondale: Southern Illinois University Press, 1966.

Kramer, Howard D. "The Germ Theory and the Early Public Health Program in the United States." *Bulletin of the History of Medicine* 22 (1948): 233–247.

Kray, Hendrik, ed. *Afro-Brazilian Culture and Politics: Bahia, 1790s to 1990s.* Armonk: M. E. Sharpe, 1998.

Kudlick, Catherine Jean. *Cholera in Post-Revolutionary Paris: A Cultural History.* Berkeley: University of California Press, 1996.

Kupperman, Karen Ordahl. "Fear of Hot Climates in the Anglo-American Colonial Experience." *William and Mary Quarterly* 41, 2 (April 1984): 213–240.

Kuznesof, Elizabeth Anne. "An Analysis of Household Composition and Headship as Related to Changes in Mode of Production: São Paulo, 1765–1836." *Comparative Studies in Society and History* 22, no. 1 (1980): 78–108.

———. *Household Economy and Urban Development: São Paulo, 1765 to 1835.* Boulder: Westview, 1986.

———. "Sexual Politics, Race, and Bastard-Bearing in Nineteenth-Century Brazil: A Question of Culture or Power?" *Journal of Family History* 16 (1991): 241–260.

La Berge, Ann F. "The Paris Health Council, 1802–1848." *Bulletin of the History of Medicine* 49 (1975): 339–352.

———. "The Early Nineteenth-Century French Public Health Movement: The Disciplinary Development and Institutionalization of *Hygiene Publique.*" *Bulletin of the History of Medicine* 58 (1984): 363–379.

———. *Mission and Method: The Early-Nineteenth-Century French Public Health Movement.* Cambridge: Cambridge University Press, 1992.

Lambert, Royston. *Sir John Simon (1816–1904) and English Social Administration.* London: MacGibbon and Kee, 1963.

Landes, Ruth. *The City of Women.* Albuquerque: University of New Mexico Press, 1994.

Landmann, Jayme. *Evitando a saúde e promovendo a doença: O sistema de saúde no Brasil.* Rio de Janeiro: Achiame, 1981.

Laqueur, Thomas. "Orgasm, Generation, and the Politics of Reproductive Biology." In *The Making of the Modern Body: Sexuality and Society in the Nineteenth Century,* ed. Catherine Gallagher and Thomas Laqueur, 1–41. Berkeley: University of California Press, 1987.

———. *Making Sex: Body and Gender from the Greeks to Freud.* Cambridge, Mass.: Harvard University Press, 1993.

Larson, Brooke. "Shifting Views of Colonialism and Resistance." *Radical History Review* 27 (1983): 3–20.

Lavrin, Asunción, ed. *Latin American Women: Historical Perspectives.* Westport: Greenwood, 1978.

———. *Women, Feminism, and Social Change in Argentina, Chile, and Uruguay, 1890–1940.* Lincoln: University of Nebraska Press, 1995.

Leavitt, Judith Walzer. "Birthing and Anesthesia." In *Women and Health in America,* ed. Judith Walzer Leavitt, 175–184. Madison: University of Wisconsin Press, 1984.

———. "Politics and Public Health: Smallpox in Milwaukee, 1894–95." In *Sickness and Health: Readings in the History of Medicine and Public Health,* ed. Judith Walzer Leavitt and Ronald L. Numbers, 372–384. Madison: University of Wisconsin Press, 1985.

———. " 'Science' Enters the Birthing Room." In *Sickness and Health: Readings in the History of Medicine and Public Health,* ed. Judith Walzer Leavitt and Ronald L. Numbers, 81–97. Madison: University of Wisconsin Press, 1985.

———. *Brought to Bed: Childbearing in America, 1750–1950.* New York: Oxford University Press, 1986.

———. "Medicine in Context: A Review Essay on the History of Medicine." *American Historical Review* 95 (1990): 1471–1484.

Leavitt, Judith Walzer, ed. *Women and Health in America.* Madison: University of Wisconsin Press, 1984.

Leavitt, Judith Walzer, and Ronald L. Numbers, eds. *Sickness and Health: Readings in the History of Medicine and Public Health.* Madison: University of Wisconsin Press, 1985.

Leavitt, Judith Walzer, and Whitney Walton. "Down at Death's Door." In *Women and Health in America,* ed. Judith Walzer Leavitt, 155–165. Madison: University of Wisconsin Press, 1984.

Leite, Miriam Moreira. *A condição feminina no Rio de Janeiro, século XIX: Antologia de textos de viajeros estrangeiros.* São Paulo: Hucitec, 1993.

Lenoir, Timothy. *Laboratories, Medicine, and Public Life in Germany, 1830–1849: Ideological Roots of the Institutional Revolution.* Cambridge: Cambridge University Press, 1992.

L'Esperance, Jean. "Doctors and Women in Nineteenth Century Society: Sexuality and Race." In *Health Care and Popular Medicine in England,* ed. John Woodward and David Richards, 105–127. New York: Holmes and Meier, 1977.

Levi, Darrell Erville. *The Prados of São Paulo, Brazil: An Elite Family and Social Change, 1840–1930.* Athens: University of Georgia Press, 1987.

Levine, Robert M. *Vale of Tears: Revisiting the Canudos Massacre in Northeastern Brazil, 1893–1897.* Berkeley: University of California Press, 1992.

———. "The Singular Brazilian City of Salvador." *Luso-Brazilian Review* 30, 2 (1993): 59–70.

Lewin, Linda. "Some Historical Implications of Kinship Organization for Family-Based Politics in the Brazilian Northeast." *Comparative Studies in Society and History* 21 (1979): 262–292.

———. *Politics and Parentela in Paraíba: A Case Study of Family-Based Oligarchy in Brazil*. Princeton: Princeton University Press, 1987.

Lewis, Richard A. *Edwin Chadwick and the Public Health Movement, 1832–1854*. London: Longmans, Green, 1952.

Lima, Lamartine de Andrade. "Roteiro de Nina Rodrigues." *Centros de Estudos Afro-Orientais* 2 (April 1980): 1–12.

Lima, Nísia Trinidade, and Gilberto Hochman. "Descobrindo a nação, construindo o estado: O movimento pela reforma da saúde pública no Brasil da Primeira República." Paper presented at the 1995 meeting of the Latin American Studies Association, Washington, D.C., September 28–30.

———. "Condenado pela raça, absolvido pela medicina: O Brasil descoberto pelo movimento sanitarista da Primeira República." In *Raça, ciência e sociedade,* ed. Marcos Chor Maio and Ricardo Ventura Santos, 23–40. Rio de Janeiro: FIOCRUZ, 1996.

Lins, Ivan. *História do positivismo no Brasil*. 2d ed. São Paulo: Companhia Editora Nacional, 1967.

Litoff, Judy Barrett. *American Midwives, 1860 to the Present*. Westport: Greenwood, 1978.

Livingstone, David N. "Human Acclimatization: Perspectives on a Contested Field of Inquiry in Science, Medicine, and Geography." *Human Science* 25 (1987): 359–394.

Lobo, Francisco Bruno. "A primeira médica formada no Brasil." *Revista de História* 42 (April–June 1971): 483–486.

Lowy, Ilana. "Yellow Fever in Rio de Janeiro and the Pasteur Institute Mission (1901–1905): The Transfer of Science to the Periphery." *Medical History* 34 (1990): 144–163.

Loyola, Maria Andrea. "A cultura pueril da Puericultura." *Novos Estudos CEBRAP,* São Paulo, 2 (1983): 4–46.

———. *Médicos e curandeiros: Conflito social e saúde*. São Paulo: Difusão Européia do Livro, 1984.

Luchetti, Cathy. *Medicine Women: The Story of Early American Women Doctors*. New York: Crown, 1998.

Lutz, Adolpho. *A opilação ou hipoemia intertropical e sua origem ou Ankylostoma duodenale e Ankylostomíase*. Rio de Janeiro: Typ. E Lith. De Machado, 1888.

Luz, Madel T. *As instituições médicas no Brasil: Instituição e estratégia de hegemonia*. Rio de Janeiro: Graal, 1979.

———. *Medicina e ordem política brasileira: Políticas e instituições de saúde, 1850–1930*. Rio de Janeiro: Graal, 1982.

Lynch, John. *The Spanish-American Revolutions, 1808–1826*. New York: Norton, 1973.

Lyons, Maryinez. "Sleeping Sickness Epidemics and Public Health in Belgian Congo." In *Imperial Medicine and Indigenous Societies,* ed. David Arnold, 105–124. Manchester: Manchester University Press, 1987.

——. *The Colonial Disease: A Social History of Sleeping Sickness in Northern Zaire, 1900–1940.* Cambridge: Cambridge University Press, 1992.

Machado, Roberto, Angel Loureiro, Rógerio Luz, and Kátia Muricy. *Danação da norma: Medicina social e constituição da psiquiatria no Brasil.* Rio de Janeiro: Graal, 1978.

MacLeod, R., and M. Lewis, eds. *Disease, Medicine, and Empire.* London: Routledge, 1988.

Maegraith, Brian. "Tropical Medicine: What It Is Not, What It Is." *Bulletin of the New York Academy of Medicine* 48 (1972): 1210–1230.

Magali, Engel. *Meretrizes e doutores: Saber médico e prostituição no Rio de Janeiro, 1840–1890.* São Paulo: Brasiliense, 1989.

Maio, Marcos Chor. "A medicina de Nina Rodrigues: Análise de uma trajetória científica." *Cadernos de Saúde Pública* 11, 2 (1995): 226–237.

Maio, Marcos Chor, and Ricardo Ventura Santos. *Raça, ciência e sociedade.* Rio de Janeiro: FIOCRUZ, 1996.

Mallon, Florencia. "AHR Forum: The Promise and Dilemma of Subaltern Studies: Perspectives from Latin American History." *American Historical Review* 99, no. 5 (1994): 1491–1515.

——. *Peasant and Nation: The Making of Postcolonial Mexico and Peru.* Berkeley: University of California Press, 1994.

Maluf, Sônia. *Encontros nocturnos: Bruxas, bruxarias no Lago da Conceição.* Rio de Janeiro: Rosa dos Tempos, 1993.

Manchester, Alan K. *British Preeminence in Brazil: Its Rise and Decline.* Chapel Hill: University of North Carolina Press, 1933.

Manson, Patrick. *Tropical Diseases: A Manual of the Diseases of Warm Climates.* London: Cassell, 1900.

——. *Lectures on Tropical Diseases Being the Lane Lectures for 1905.* Chicago: W. T. Keener, 1905.

——. "Tropical Medicine and Hygiene." *British Medical Journal* 2 (July 1917): 103–109.

Manson-Bahr, P. E. C., and F. I. C. Apted. *Manson's Tropical Diseases* 18th ed. London: Bailliere Tindall, 1982.

Manson-Bahr, Sir Philip. *Patrick Manson: The Father of Tropical Medicine.* London: Thomas Nelson and Son, 1962.

Manson-Bahr, Philip H., and A. Alcock. *The Life and Work of Sir Patrick Manson.* London: Cassell, 1927.

Marcílio, Maria Luiza, et al. "Crescimento histórico da população brasileira até 1872." São Paulo: CEBRAP, 1973.

Marques, Eduardo César. "Da higiene à construção da cidade: O estado e o saneamento no Rio de Janeiro." *História, Ciências, Saúde, Manguinhos* 2, 2 (1995): 51–67.

Martin, Percy A. "Causes and the Collapse of the Brazilian Empire." *Hispanic American Historical Review* 4 (1921): 4–48.

Martins, Wilson. *História da inteligência brasileira, 1877–1896.* 6 vols. São Paulo: Cultrix, 1976.

Martius, C. F. Philip von. *Natureza, doenças, medicina e remédios dos índios brasileiros.* São Paulo: Companhia Editora Nacional, 1939.

Mattedi, Maria Raquel Matteo, et al. "Salvador: O processo de urbanização." In *Habitação e urbanismo em Salvador,* 341–364. Bahia: Seplantec CPE, 1979.

Mattoso, Kátia M. de Queirós. "Caminhos estatísticos na história econômica da Bahia." *Universitas,* Salvador, 8–9 (1971): 135–153.

———. *Bahia: A cidade do Salvador e seu mercado no século XIX.* São Paulo: Hucitec, 1977.

———. *Testamentos de escravos libertos na Bahia no século XIX.* Salvador: Universidade Federal da Bahia, 1979.

———. *To Be a Slave in Brazil, 1550–1888.* Trans. Arthur Goldhammer. New Brunswick: Rutgers University Press, 1986.

———. *Família e sociedade na Bahia do século XIX.* São Paulo: Corrupio, 1988.

———. "Slave, Free, and Freed Family Structures in Nineteenth-Century Salvador, Bahia." *Luso-Brazilian Review* 25, 1 (1988): 69–84.

Mattoso, Kátia M. de Queirós, and M. Johildo de Athayde. "Epidemias e flutuações de preços na Bahia no século XIX." In *Colloque international sur l'histoire quantitative du Brésil de 1800 a 1930,* ed. Frederic Mauro, 185–202. Centre Nacional de la Recherche Scientifique, no. 543. Paris: Editions du Centre National de la Recherche Scientifique, 1973.

Maulitz, Russell C. "Physician versus Bacteriologist: The Ideology of Science in Clinical Medicine." *The Therapeutic Revolution: Essays in the Social History of American Medicine,* ed. Morris J. Vogel and Charles E. Rosenberg, 91–108. Philadelphia: University of Pennsylvania Press, 1979.

McClintock, Anne. *Imperial Leather: Race, Gender, and Sexuality in the Colonial Contest.* New York: Routledge, 1995.

McGregor, Deborah Kuhn. *From Midwives to Medicine: The Birth of American Gynecology.* New Brunswick: Rutgers University Press, 1998.

McKeown, Thomas. *The Modern Rise of Population.* New York: Academic Press, 1976.

McNeill, William H. *Plagues and Peoples.* New York: Anchor, 1976.

Meade, Melinda S. "Beriberi." In *The Cambridge World History of Human Disease,* ed. Kenneth F. Kiple, 606–612. Cambridge: Cambridge University Press, 1993.

Meade, Teresa, and Mark Walker, eds. *Science, Medicine, and Cultural Imperialism.* New York: St. Martin's, 1991.

Medina, Maricela. "Tobias Barreto (1839–1889): The Intellectual Odyssey of a Nineteenth Century Brazilian." Ph.D. dissertation, University of Michigan, 1986.

Mello, Carlos Gentile de. *Saúde e assistência médica no Brasil.* São Paulo: CEBES - HUCITEC, 1977.

Mendelsohn, Everett. "The Social Construction of Scientific Knowledge." In *The Social*

Production of Scientific Knowledge, ed. Everett Mendelsohn, Peter Weingart, Richard Whitley, 1: 3–26. Dordrecht: D. Reidel, 1977.

Merchant, Carolyn. "Isis' Consciousness Raised." *Isis* 73 (1982): 398–409.

Merrick, Thomas W., and Douglas H. Graham. *Population and Economic Development in Brazil: 1800 to the Present.* Baltimore: Johns Hopkins University Press, 1979.

Metcalf, Aida C. "Searching for the Slave Family in Colonial Brazil: Reconstruction from São Paulo." *Journal of Family History* 16 (1991): 283–298.

Miller, Francesca. *Latin American Women and the Search for Social Justice.* Hanover: University Press of New England, 1991.

Miller, Rory. *Britain and Latin America in the Nineteenth and Twentieth Centuries.* London: Longman, 1993.

Mineo, Ron. "Misery and Death in the Pearl of the Pacific: Health Care in Guayaquil, Ecuador, 1870–1925." *Hispanic American Historical Review* 70 (1990): 609–637.

Miranda, Maria do Carmo Tavares de. *Educação no Brasil: Esboço de estudo histórico.* Recife: Imprensa Universitária, 1966.

Moacyr, Primitivo. *A instrução e o Império: Subsídios para a história da educação no Império, 1854–1889.* 3 vols. São Paulo: Companhia Editora Nacional, 1938.

Montero, Paula. *Da doença à desordem: A magia na umbanda.* Rio de Janeiro: Graal, 1985.

Morantz, Regina Markell. "The 'Connecting Link': The Case for the Woman Doctor in 19th-Century America." In *Sickness and Health: Readings in the History of Medicine and Public Health,* ed. Judith Walzer Leavitt and Ronald L. Numbers, 161–172. Madison: University of Wisconsin Press, 1985.

Morantz-Sanchez, Regina Markell. *Sympathy and Science: Women Physicians in American Medicine.* New York: Oxford University Press, 1985.

Morehead, C. *Clinical Researches on Disease in India.* 2 vols. London, 1856.

Morrell, Jack, and Arnold Thackray. *Gentlemen of Science: Early Years of the British Association for the Advancement of Science.* Oxford: Clarendon, 1982.

Moscucci, Ornella. *The Science of Woman: Gynaecology and Gender in England, 1800–1929.* New York: Cambridge University Press, 1990.

Mosedale, Susan Sleeth. "Science Corrupted: Victorian Biologists Consider 'The Woman Question.'" *Journal of the History of Biology* 2 (1978): 1–55.

Mosse, George L. "Nationalism and Respectability: Normal and Abnormal Sexuality in the Nineteenth Century." *Journal of Contemporary History* 17 (1982): 221–246.

Mota, Carlos Guilherme, org. *Brasil em perspectiva.* Rio de Janeiro: Difusão Européia do Livro, 1981.

Mott, Luiz R. B. *Os pecados da família na Bahia de Todos os Santos.* Salvador: Universidade Federal da Bahia, 1982.

Nascimento, Anna Amélia Vieira. "A 'cholera morbus' como fator de involução populacional da cidade de Salvador." *Anais do Arquivo do Estado da Bahia* 45 (1981): 263–289.

Navarro, Vicente, ed. *Imperialism, Health, and Medicine.* Farmingdale: Baywood, 1981.

Nazzari, Muriel. *Disappearance of the Dowry: Women, Families, and Social Change in São Paulo, Brazil, 1600–1900*. Stanford: Stanford University Press, 1991.

———. "Concubinage in Colonial Brazil: The Inequalities of Race, Class, and Gender." *Journal of Family History* 21 (1996): 107–119.

Needell, Jeffrey. *The Origins of the Carioca Belle Epoque: The Emergence of the Elite Culture and Society of Turn-of-the-Century Rio de Janeiro*. Ph.D. dissertation, Stanford University, 1982.

———. *A Tropical Belle Epoque: Elite Culture and Society in Turn-of-the-Century Rio de Janeiro*. Cambridge: Cambridge University Press, 1987.

———. "The *Revolta Contra Vacina* of 1904: The Revolt against Modernization in 'Belle Époque' Rio de Janeiro." *Hispanic American Historical Review* 67 (1987): 233–270.

———. "History, Race, and the State in the Thought of Oliveira Vianna." *Hispanic American Historical Review* 75 (1995): 1–30.

———. "Identity, Race, Gender, and Modernity in the Origins of Gilberto Freyre's Oeuvre." *American Historical Review* 100 (1995): 51–77.

Novak, Steven J. "Professionalization and Bureaucracy: English Doctors in the Victorian Public Health Administration." *Journal of Social History* 6, no. 4 (1973): 440–462.

Numbers, Ronald L., ed. *Medicine in the New World: New Spain, New France, and New England*. Knoxville: University of Tennessee Press, 1987.

Nutton, Vivian. "The Seeds of Disease: An Explanation of Contagion and Infection from the Greeks to the Renaissance." *Medical History* 27 (1983): 1–34.

———. "Humoralism." In *Companion Encyclopedia of the History of Medicine*, ed. W. F. Bynum and Roy Porter, 281–291. London: Routledge, 1994.

Nye, Robert A. *Crime, Madness, and Politics in Modern France: The Medical Concept of National Decline*. Princeton: Princeton University Press, 1984.

Obregón, Diana. *Sociedades científicas en Colombia: La invención de una tradición, 1859–1936*. Bogotá: Banco de la República, 1992.

O'Brien, Patricia. "Michel Foucault's History of Culture." In *The New Cultural History*, ed. Lynn Hunt, 25–46. Berkeley: University of California Press, 1989.

Oliveira, Carlos Roberto. "Medicina e estado: Origem e desenvolvimento da medicina social no Brasil, Bahia, 1866–1896." Master's thesis, Universidade do Estado do Rio de Janeiro, 1982.

Oliveira, Eduardo de S. *Memória histórica da Faculdade de Medicina da Bahia*. Bahia: EDUFBA, 1982.

Oliveira, Reginaldo Fernandes de. *O conselheiro Jobim e o espírito da medicina do seu tempo*. Senado Federal: Centro Gráfico, 1982.

Ott, Carlos. *A Santa Casa de Misericórdia da cidade do Salvador*. Rio de Janeiro: Diretoria do Patrimônio Histórico e Artístico Nacional, 1960.

Pang, Eul-Soo. *Bahia in the First Brazilian Republic: Coronelismo and Oligarchies, 1889–1934*. Gainesville: University of Florida Press, 1979.

Pang, Eul-Soo, and Ron L. Seckinger. "The Mandarins of Imperial Brazil." *Comparative Studies in Society and History* 14 (1972): 215–244.

Pang, Laura Jarnagin. "The State and Agricultural Clubs of Imperial Brazil, 1860–1889." Ph.D. dissertation, Vanderbilt University, 1981.

Peard, Julyan G. "Tropical Medicine in Nineteenth-Century Brazil: The Case of the 'Escola Tropicalista Bahiana,' 1860–1890." In *Warm Climates and Western Medicine: The Emergence of Tropical Medicine, 1500–1900,* ed. David Arnold, 108–132. Amsterdam: Rodopi, 1996.

———. "Tropical Disorders and the Forging of a Brazilian Medical Identity, 1860–1890." *Hispanic American Historical Review* 77 (1997): 1–44.

Pedro, Joana Maria. "Práticas abortivas e gestão do corpo feminino em Florianópolis entre 1900–1950." Paper presented at the Nineteenth LASA Congress, Washington, D.C., September 28–30, 1995.

Peixoto, Afrânio. *Crime e saúde: Introdução biogeográfica à civilização brasileira.* São Paulo: Companhia Editora Nacional, 1938. Also by A. Peixoto: *Minha terra, mi gente.* Rio de Janeiro: F. Alves, 1929.

Penna, Belisário. *O saneamento do Brasil.* Rio de Janeiro: Typ. Revista dos Tribunaes, 1918.

Pennington, T. H. "Listerism, Its Decline, and Its Persistence: The Introduction of Aseptic Surgical Techniques in Three British Teaching Hospitals, 1890–99." *Medical History* 39 (1995): 35–60.

Pereira, Antônio Pacífico. *Memória sobre a medicina na Bahia.* Salvador: Imprensa Oficial do Estado, 1923.

Pernick, Martin S. "Politics, Parties, and Pestilence: Epidemic Yellow Fever in Philadelphia and the Rise of the First Party System." In *Sickness and Health: Readings in the History of Medicine and Public Health,* ed. Judith Walzer Leavitt and Ronald L. Numbers, 356–371. Madison: University of Wisconsin Press, 1985.

Pertillar, Tammy Lynn. "Afro-Brazilian Women and Medicine: A Nineteenth-Century Social Issue, 1808–1888." Master's thesis, Howard University, 1993.

Pfeifer, Edward J. "The Genesis of American Neo-Lamarckism." *Isis* 56 (1965): 156–167.

Pick, Daniel. "The Folly of Anarchy: Lombroso and the Politics of Criminal Science in Post-Unification Italy." *History Workshop* 21 (1986): 60–86.

Pierson, Donald. *Negroes in Brazil: A Study of Race Contact in Bahia.* Carbondale: Southern Illinois University Press, 1967.

Pinero, José María López, Luis García Ballester, and Pilar Faus Seville. *Medicina y sociedad en la España del siglo XIX.* Madrid: Sociedad de Estudios y Publicaciones, 1964.

Pinho, Wanderley. *História de um Engenho do Recôncavo.* São Paulo: Companhia Editora Nacional, 1982.

———. *Salves e damas do segundo reinado.* 2d ed. São Paulo: Livraria Martins, n.d.

Poovey, Mary. " 'Scenes of an Indelicate Character': The Medical 'Treatment' of Victorian Women." In *The Making of the Modern Body: Sexuality and Society in the Nine-*

teenth Century, ed. Catherine Gallagher and Thomas Laqueur, 137–168. Berkeley: University of California Press, 1987.

Poppino, Rollie E. *Feira de Santana.* Bahia: Itapua, 1968.

Prakash, Gyan. *After Colonialism: Imperial Histories and Postcolonial Displacements.* Princeton: Princeton University Press, 1995.

———. "AHR Forum: The Promise and Dilemma of Subaltern Studies: Perspectives from Latin American History." *American Historical Review* 99, no. 5 (December 1994): 1475–1490.

Pratt, Mary Louise. *Imperial Eyes: Travel Writing and Transculturation.* London: Routledge, 1992.

Pyenson, Lewis. "'Who the Guys Were': Prosopography in the History of Science." *History of Science* 15 (1977): 155–188.

Quelle, Otto. "A atuação germânica no Estado da Bahia." *Revista do Instituto Geográfico e Histórico da Bahia* 59 (1933): 449–481.

Querino, Manoel Raimundo. *A Bahia de outrora.* Salvador: Progresso, 1955.

Quintaneiro, Tânia. *Retratos de mulher: O cotidiano feminino no Brasil sob olhar de viajeros do século XIX.* Petrópolis: Vozes, 1995.

Radcliffe, Walter. *Milestones in Midwifery.* Bristol: John Wright, 1967.

Ramos, Artur. *O negro na civilização brasileira.* Rio de Janeiro: Casa do Estudante no Brasil, 1956.

Ramos, Donald. "Marriage and Family in Colonial Vila Rica." *Hispanic American Historical Review* 55 (1975): 200–225.

———. "City and Country: The Family in Minas Gerais, 1804–1838." *Journal of Family History* 3 (1978): 361–375.

———. "Single and Married Women in Vila Rica, Brazil, 1754–1838." *Journal of Family History* 16, no. 3 (1991): 261–282.

Reis, David Onildo. "O inimigo invisível: A epidemia do cólera na Bahia, 1855–1856." Master's thesis, Universidade Federal da Bahia, 1994.

Reis, João José. *Slave Rebellion in Brazil: The African Muslim Uprising of 1835 in Bahia.* Trans. Arthur Brakel. Baltimore: Johns Hopkins University Press, 1993.

———. "'The Revolution of the *Ganhadores*': Urban Labour, Ethnicity, and the African Strike of 1857 in Bahia, Brazil." *Journal of Latin American Studies* 29 (1997): 355–393.

Reiser, Stanley Joel. *Medicine and the Reign of Technology.* Cambridge: Cambridge University Press, 1978.

Ribeiro, Leonídio. *Medicina no Brasil.* Rio de Janeiro: Imprensa Nacional, 1940.

Ribeiro, Lourival. *O Barão de Lavradio e a higiene no Rio de Janeiro imperial.* Belo Horizonte: Itatiaia, 1992.

Risse, Günter. "History of Western Medicine from Hippocrates to Germ Theory." In *The Cambridge World History of Human Disease,* ed. Kenneth F. Kiple, 11–19. Cambridge: Cambridge University Press, 1993.

———. "German Medicine and the State: Historical Perspectives." Unpublished manuscript.

Rocha, Leduar de Assis. *História da medicina em Pernambuco—século XIX*. Recife: Arquivo Público Estadual, 1962.

Rodrigues, José Honório. *Brasil e Africa: Outro horizonte*. Rio de Janeiro: Civilização Brasileira, 1961.

———. *Brazil and Africa*. Berkeley: University of California Press, 1965.

———. *The Brazilians: Their Character and Aspirations*. Trans. Ralph Edward Dimmick. Austin: University of Texas Press, 1967.

Rodrigues, Raimundo Nina. *As raças humanas e a responsabilidade penal no Brazil*. Salvador: Progresso, 1957.

———. *Memória histórica da Faculdade de Medicina e Farmácia da Bahia*. 1897.

———. *Manual de autopsia médico-legal*. Bahia: Reis, 1901.

———. *Os africanos no Brasil*. São Paulo: Companhia Editora Nacional, 1935.

———. *O animismo fetichista dos negros bahianos*. São Paulo: Companhia Editora Nacional, 1935.

Romero, Sílvio. *A filosofia no Brasil; ensaio crítico*. Porto Alegre: Typ do Deutsche Zeitung, 1878.

———. *História da literatura brasileira*. 3d ed. Vol. 1. Rio de Janeiro: José Olympio, 1949.

Rosen, George. *From Medical Police to Social Medicine: Essays on the History of Health Care*. New York: Science History Publications, 1974.

———. *The Structure of American Medical Practice, 1875–1941*. Philadelphia: University of Pennsylvania Press, 1983.

———. *A History of Public Health*. Expanded ed. Introduction by Elizabeth Fee. Baltimore: Johns Hopkins University Press, 1993.

Rosenberg, Charles E. "Cholera in Nineteenth Century Europe: A Tool for Social and Economic Analysis." *Contemporary Studies in Society and History* 8 (1966): 452–463.

———. "The Bitter Fruit: Heredity, Disease, and Social Thought." In *No Other Gods: On Science and American Social Thought*, 25–53. Baltimore: Johns Hopkins University Press, 1976.

———. "The Therapeutic Revolution: Medicine, Meaning, and Social Change in Nineteenth-Century America." In *The Therapeutic Revolution: Essays in the Social History of American Medicine*, ed. Morris J. Vogel and Charles E. Rosenberg, 3–26. Philadelphia: University of Pennsylvania Press, 1979.

———. *The Care of Strangers: The Rise of America's Hospital System*. New York: Basic, 1987.

———. *The Cholera Years: The United States in 1832, 1849, and 1866*. Chicago: University of Chicago Press, 1987.

———. "Disease and Social Order in America: Perceptions and Expectations." In *AIDS: The Burdens of History*, ed. Elizabeth Fee and Daniel M. Fox, 12–32. Berkeley: University of California Press, 1988.

————. "Disease in History: Frames and Framers." *Millbank Quarterly* 67 1 (1989): 1–15.

Rosenberg, Charles E., and Carroll Smith-Rosenberg, eds. *The Male Midwife and the Female Doctor.* New York: Arno, 1974.

Ross, Ronald. *Memories of Sir Patrick Manson.* London: Harrison and Sons, n.d.

Rothman, David J. "Social Control: The Uses and Abuses of the Concept in the History of Medicine." In *Social Control and the State: Historical and Comparative Essays,* ed. Stanley Cohen and Andrew Scull, 106–117. London: Basil Blackwell, 1983.

Russell-Wood, A. J. R. *Fidalgos and Philanthropists: The Santa Casa de Misericórdia of Bahia, 1550–1755.* Berkeley: University of California Press, 1968.

————. "Female and Family in the Economy and Society of Colonial Brazil." In *Latin American Women: Historical Perspectives,* ed. Asunción Lavrin, 60–100. Westport: Greenwood, 1978.

Russell-Wood, A. J. R., ed. *From Colony to Nation: Essays on the Independence of Brazil.* Baltimore: Johns Hopkins University Press, 1975.

Saffioti, Heleieth I. B. *Women in Class Society.* Trans. Michael Vale. New York: Monthly Review, 1978.

Sagasti, Francisco R. "Underdevelopment, Science, and Technology: The Point of View of the Underdeveloped Countries." *Science Studies* 3 (1973): 47–59.

Said, Edward. *Orientalism.* New York: Vintage, 1979.

Salles, Pedro. *História da medicina no Brasil.* Belo Horizonte: G. Holman, 1971.

Samara, Eni de Mesquita. *A família brasileira.* São Paulo: Brasiliense, 1985.

————. *As mulheres, o poder, e a família: São Paulo, século XIX.* São Paulo: Marco Zero, 1989.

Santos, Luiz Antônio de Castro. "Estado e saúde pública no Brasil (1889–1930)." *Dados* 23 (1980): 237–250.

————. "O pensamento sanitarista na Primeira República: Uma ideologia de construção da nacionalidade." *Dados* 28 (1985): 193–210.

————. "Power, Ideology, and Public Health in Brazil, 1889–1930." Ph.D. dissertation, Harvard University, 1987.

————. "A reforma sanitária pelo alto: O pionerismo paulista no início de século XX." *Dados* 36 (1993): 361–392.

Santos Filho, Lycurgo. *História da medicina no Brasil: Do século XVI ao século XIX,* 2 vols. São Paulo: Brasiliense, 1947.

Santos, Ricardo Ventura. "Da morfologia às moléculas, de raça à população: Trajetórias conceituais em antropologia física no século XX." In *Raça, ciência e sociedade,* ed. Marcos Chor Maio and Ricardo Ventura Santos, 125–142. Rio de Janeiro: FIOCRUZ, 1996.

————. "Edgar Roquette-Pinto: Os tipos antropológicos e a questão da degeneração racial no Brasil no início do século." Paper presented at the Twentieth Annual Meeting of Associação Nacional de Pós-Graduação e Pesquisa em Ciências Sociais, Caxambu, Minas Gerais, October 1996.

Savitt, Todd L. *Medicine and Slavery: The Diseases and Health Care of Blacks in Antebellum Virginia.* Urbana: University of Illinois Press, 1978.

———. "Black Health on the Plantation: Masters, Slaves, and Physicians." In *Sickness and Health: Readings in the History of Medicine and Public Health,* ed. Judith Walzer Leavitt and Ronald L. Numbers. Madison: University of Wisconsin Press, 1985.

———. "Slave Health and Southern Distinctiveness." In *Disease and Distinctiveness in the American South,* ed. Todd L. Savitt and James Harvey Young. Knoxville: University of Tennessee Press, 1988.

Scheper-Hughes, Nancy. *Death without Weeping: The Violence of Everyday Life in Brazil.* Berkeley: University of California Press, 1992.

Scholten, Catherine M. "'On the Importance of the Obstetrik Art': Changing Customs of Childbirth in America, 1760–1825." In *Women and Health in America,* ed. Judith Walzer Leavitt, 142–154. Madison: University of Wisconsin Press, 1984.

Schwarcz, Lília K. *Retrato em branco e negro: Jornais, escravos e cidadãos em São Paulo no final do século XIX.* São Paulo: Companhia das Letras, 1987.

———. *O espetáculo das raças: Cientistas, instituições a questão racial no Brasil, 1870–1930.* São Paulo: Companhia das Letras, 1993.

Schwartz, Ronald A. "The Midwife in Contemporary Latin America." *Medical Anthropology* 5, 1 (1981): 51–71.

Schwartz, Stuart B. "Somebodies and Nobodies in the Body Politic: Mentalities and Social Structures in Colonial Brazil." *Latin American Research Review* 31 (1996): 113–134.

Schwartzman, Simon. *Formação da comunidade científica no Brasil,* 60–62. São Paulo: Companhia Editora Nacional, 1979.

Scobie, James R. "The Growth of Cities." In *Latin America: Economy and Society, 1870–1930,* ed. Leslie Bethell, 149–182. Cambridge: Cambridge University Press, 1989.

Scott, H. Harold. *A History of Tropical Medicine.* 2 vols. Baltimore: Williams and Wilkins, 1939.

Scott, Joan Wallach. "History in Crisis? The Others' Side of the Story." *American Historical Review* 94 (1989): 680–692.

Scott, Rebecca J., et al. *The Abolition of Slavery and the Aftermath of Emancipation in Brazil.* Durham: Duke University Press, 1988.

Seed, Patricia. "Colonial and Postcolonial Discourse." *Latin American Research Review* 26 (1991): 181–200.

Shapiro, Martin F. "Medicine in the Service of Colonialism: Medical Care in Portuguese Africa, 1885–1914." Ph.D. dissertation, University of California at Los Angeles, 1983.

Sheridan, Richard B. *Doctors and Slaves: A Medical and Demographic History of Slavery in the British West Indies, 1680–1834.* Cambridge: Cambridge University Press, 1985.

Shorter, Edward. *A History of Women's Bodies.* New York: Basic, 1982.

———. *Bedside Manners: The Troubled History of Doctors and Patients.* New York: Simon and Schuster, 1985.

Shyrock, Richard. *The Development of Modern Medicine: An Interpretation of the Social and Scientific Factors Involved.* New York: Knopf, 1947.

———. *Medicine and Society in America, 1660–1860.* Ithaca: Cornell University Press, 1960.

Sigaud, Joseph-F.-X. *Du climat et des maladies du Bresil; ou statistique medicale de cet empire.* Paris: Fortin, Masson, 1844.

Silva, Alberto. *A primeira médica do Brasil.* Rio de Janeiro: Pongetti, 1954.

Silva, Maria Beatriz Nizza da. *Sistema de casamento no Brasil colonial.* Ed. T. A. Queiroz. São Paulo: Universidade de São Paulo, 1984.

———. "O pensamento científico no Brasil na segunda metade do século XVIII." *Ciência e Cultura* 40, 9 (1988): 859–868.

Singer, Charles, and E. Ashworth Underwood. *A Short History of Medicine.* 2d ed. New York: Oxford University Press, 1962.

Singer, Paul, Oswaldo Campos, and Elizabeth Nachado de Oliveira. *Prevenir e curar: O controle social através dos serviços de saúde.* Rio de Janeiro: Forense-Universitária, 1978.

Skidmore, Thomas E. *Black into White: Race and Nationality in Brazilian Thought.* New York: Oxford University Press, 1974.

———. "Racial Ideas and Social Policy in Brazil, 1870–1940." In *The Idea of Race in Latin America, 1870–1940,* ed. Richard Graham, 7–36. Austin: University of Texas Press, 1990.

———. "Studying the History of Latin America: A Case of Hemispheric Convergence." *Latin American Research Review* 33 (1998): 105–127.

Smith, Hilda. "Gynecology and Ideology in Seventeenth Century England." In *Liberating Women's History: Theoretical and Critical Essays,* ed. Berenice A. Carroll, 97–114. Urbana: University of Illinois Press, 1976.

Smith-Rosenberg, Carroll. *Disorderly Conduct: Visions of Gender in Victorian America.* New York: Knopf, 1985.

———. "Puberty to Menopause: The Cycle of Femininity in Nineteenth-Century America." In *Disorderly Conduct: Visions of Gender in Victorian America,* ed. Carroll Smith-Rosenberg, 186–196. New York: Knopf, 1985.

Smith-Rosenberg, Carroll, and Charles Rosenberg. "The Female Animal: Medical and Biological Views of Woman and Her Role in Nineteenth Century America." In *Women and Health in America,* ed. Judith Walzer Leavitt, 12–27. Madison: University of Wisconsin Press, 1984.

Soares, Luís Carlos. "Da necessidade do bordel higienizado: Tentativas de controle da prostituição carioca no século XIX." In *História e sexualidade no Brasil,* ed. Ronaldo Vainfas, 143–168. Rio de Janeiro: Graal, 1986.

Socolow, Susan M. "Acceptable Partners: Marriage Choice in Colonial Argentina, 1778–1810." In *Sexuality and Marriage in Colonial Latin America,* ed. Asunción Lavrin, 209–251. Lincoln: University of Nebraska Press, 1989.

Sodré, Antônio Augusto de Azevedo. "Considerações históricas sobre o beriberi." *Brasil Médico* 75, 1–2 (January–July 1961): 51–56.

Solorzano, Armando. "The Rockefeller Foundation in Mexico: Nationalism, Public Health, and Yellow Fever (1911–1924)." Ph.D. dissertation, University of Wisconsin, 1990.

Sontag, Susan. "AIDS and Its Metaphors." *New York Review of Books,* 27 October 1988, 89–98.

Souza, Antônio Cândido de Melo e. *Formação de literatura brasileira.* São Paulo: Martins, 1959.

Spivak, Gayatri Chakravorty. *In Other Worlds: Essays in Cultural Politics.* New York: Methuen, 1987.

Stanton, William Ragan. *The Leopard's Spots: Scientific Attitudes towards Race in America, 1815–1859.* Chicago: University of Chicago Press, 1960.

Starr, Paul. *The Social Transformation of American Medicine.* New York: Basic, 1982.

Stebbins, Robert E. "France." In *The Comparative Reception of Darwinism,* ed. Thomas F. Glick, 117–163. Chicago: University of Chicago Press, 1988.

Stein, Stanley J. *Vassouras, A Brazilian Coffee County, 1850–1900: The Roles of Planter and Slave in a Plantation Society.* Princeton: Princeton University Press, 1985.

Stepan, Nancy Leys. "Initiation and Survival of Medical Research in a Developing Country: The Oswaldo Cruz Institute of Brazil, 1900–1920." *Journal of the History of Medicine and Allied Sciences* 30 (1975): 303–325.

———. "The Interplay between Socio-Economic Factors and Medical Science: Yellow Fever Research, Cuba, and the United States." *Social Studies of Science* 8 (1978): 397–423.

———. *Beginnings of Brazilian Science: Oswaldo Cruz, Medical Research, and Policy, 1890–1920.* New York: Science History Publications, 1981.

———. *The Idea of Race in Science: Great Britain, 1800–1960.* London: Macmillan, 1982.

———. "Biological Degeneration: Races and Proper Places." In *Degeneration: The Dark Side of Progress,* ed. J. Edward Chamberlin and Sander L. Gilman, 97–120. New York: Columbia University Press, 1984.

———. "Eugensia, genética y salud pública: El movimiento eugenésico brasileño y mundial." *Quipu* 2 (1985): 351–384.

———. "Race and Gender: The Role of Analogy in Science." *Isis* 77 (1986): 261–277.

———. "Race, Gender and Science: Strategies of Resistance." Talk given at the Institute of Women and Gender, Columbia University, February 4, 1988.

———. *"The Hour of Eugenics": Race, Gender, and Nation in Latin America.* Ithaca: Cornell University Press, 1991.

———. "Tropical Medicine and Public Health in Latin America." *Medical History* 42 (1998): 104–112.

Stern, Steve J. "Feudalism, Capitalism, and the World System in the Perspective of Latin America and the Caribbean." *American Historical Review* 93 (1988): 829–872.

Stocking, George W. "Lamarckism in American Social Sciences: 1890–1915." *Journal of the History of Ideas* 27, 2 (1962): 239–256.

———. "The Persistence of Polygenist Thought in Post-Darwinian Anthropology." In *Race, Culture, and Evolution: Essays in the History of Anthropology,* ed. George W. Stocking, 42–68. New York: Free Press, 1968.

Stoler, Ann L. "Making Empire Respectable: The Politics of Race and Sexual Morality in 20th-Century Colonial Cultures." *American Ethnologist* 16, 2 (1989): 634–659.

Sussmann, Hector J. "Culture, Ideology, and Science." In *From Military Rule to Liberal Democracy in Argentina,* ed. Monica Peralta-Ramos and Carlos H. Wasiman, 147–158. Boulder: Westview, 1987.

Swanson, Maynard W. "The Sanitation Syndrome: Bubonic Plague and Urnad Policy in the Cape Colony, 1900–1909." *Journal of African History* 13, 3 (1977): 387–410.

Tannenbaum, Frank. *Slave and Citizen.* Boston: Beacon, 1992.

Taussig, Michael. *Shamanism, Colonialism, and the Wild Man: A Study in Terror and Healing.* Chicago: University of Chicago Press, 1987.

Tavares, Luís Henrique Dias. *História da Bahia.* São Paulo: Ática, 1973.

———. *A independência do Brasil na Bahia.* Salvador: Civilização Brasileira, 1982.

Taylor, William. "Between Global Process and Local Knowledge: An Inquiry into Early Latin American Social History, 1500–1900." In *Reliving the Past: The Worlds of Social History,* ed. Oliver Zunz, 115–190. Chapel Hill: University of North Carolina Press, 1985.

Teixeira, Luiz Antônio. "Da raça à doença em *Casa-grande e senzala.*" *História, Ciências, Saúde, Manguinhos* 4, 2 (1997).

Temkin, Oswei. "A Historical Analysis of the Concept of Infection." In *The Double Face of Janus,* 456–471. Baltimore: Johns Hopkins University Press, 1977.

Thackray, Arnold. "Natural Knowledge in Cultural Context: The Manchester Model." *American Historical Review* 79 (1974): 672–709.

Tomes, Nancy. "The Private Side of Health: Sanitary Science, Domestic Hygiene, and the Germ Theory, 1870–1900." *Bulletin of the History of Medicine* 64 (1990): 503–539.

Toplin, Robert B. *The Abolition of Slavery in Brazil.* New York: Atheneum, 1975.

Torres, Octávio. *Esboço histórico dos acontecimentos mais importantes da vida da Faculdade de Medicina da Bahia, 1808–1946.* Salvador: Vitória, 1952.

Towler, Jean, and Joan Bramall. *Midwives in History and Society.* London: Croom Helm, 1986.

Treichler, Paula A. "Feminism, Medicine, and the Meaning of Childbirth." In *Body Politics: Women and the Discourses of Science,* ed. Mary Jacobus, Evelyn Fox Keller, and Sally Shuttleworth, 113–138. New York: Routledge, 1990.

Tuchman, Arleen Marcia. *Science, Medicine, and the State in Germany: The Case of Baden, 1815–1871.* New York: Oxford University Press, 1993.

Uricoechea, Fernando. *O minotauro imperial: A burocratização do estado patrimonial brasileiro no século XIX.* Rio de Janeiro: Difusão Européia do Livro, 1978.

Vainfas, Ronaldo. *História e sexualidade no Brasil*. Rio de Janeiro: Graal, 1986.

Valle, José Ribeiro do. "A farmacologia no Brasil." *História das ciências no Brasil,* ed. Mário Guimarães Ferri and Shozo Motoyama, 175–190. São Paulo: EPU, 1973.

Varnahagen, Francisco Adolfo de. *História da independência do Brasil*. Rio de Janeiro: Imprensa Nacional, 1940.

Ventura, Roberto. *Escritores, escravos e mestiços em um país tropical: Literatura, historiografia e ensaísmo no Brasil*. Nürnberg: Wilhelm Fink Verlag München, 1987.

———. *Estilo tropical: História cultural e polêmicas literárias no Brasil, 1870-1914*. São Paulo: Companhia das Letras, 1991.

Verger, Pierre. *Notícias da Bahia—1850*. Salvador: Corrupio, 1981.

Vianna, Ataliba. *Gente sem raça*. Vol. 234. São Paulo: Companhia Editora Nacional, 1944.

Vilhena, Luis dos Santos. *A Bahia no século XVIII*. Vols. 1–3. Bahia: Itapua, 1969.

Voeks, Robert A. *Sacred Leaves of Candomblé: African Magic, Medicine and Religion in Brazil*. Austin: University of Texas Press, 1997.

Vogel, Morris J., and Charles E. Rosenberg, eds. *The Therapeutic Revolution: Essays in the Social History of American Medicine*. Philadelphia: University of Pennsylvania Press, 1979.

Von Spix, John Baptiste, and C. F. Philip von Martius. *Travels in Brazil in the Years 1877-1820*. London: Longman, Hurst, Rees, Orme, Brown and Green, 1824.

Waddell, D. A. G. "International Politics and Latin American Independence." In *The Independence of Latin America,* ed. Leslie Bethell, 195–226. Cambridge: Cambridge University Press, 1987.

Wade, Peter. *Race and Ethnicity in Latin America*. London: Pluto, 1997.

Wagley, Charles. *Race and Class in Rural Brazil*. New York: UNESCO, 1963.

———. "Luso-Brazilian Kinship Patterns: The Persistence of a Cultural Tradition." In *Politics of Change in Latin America,* ed. Joseph Maier and Richard W. Weatherhead, 174–189. New York: Praeger, 1964.

Walsh, Mary Roth. *"Doctors Wanted: No Women Need Apply": Sexual Barriers in the Medical Profession, 1835-1875*. New Haven: Yale University Press, 1977.

Warner, John H. *The Therapeutic Perspective: Medical Practice, Knowledge, and Identity in America, 1820-1885*. Cambridge, Mass.: Harvard University Press, 1986.

Warren, Donald. "A medicina espiritualizada: A homeopatia no Brasil do século XIX." *Religião e Sociedade* 13 (1986): 88–107.

———. "A terapia espírita no Rio de Janeiro por volta de 1900." *Religião e Sociedade* (1984): 56–83.

Watts, Sheldon. *Epidemics and History: Disease, Power, and Imperialism*. London: Yale University Press, 1997.

Willems, Emilio. "Structure of the Brazilian Family." *Social Forces* 31 (1953): 339–345.

Williams, Robert R. *Toward the Conquest of Beriberi*. Cambridge: Harvard University Press, 1961.

Williams, Steven. "Nationalism and Public Health: The Convergence of Rockefeller

Foundation Techniques and Brazilian Federal Authority during the Time of Yellow Fever, 1925–1930." In *Missionaries of Science: The Rockefeller Foundation and Latin America,* ed. Marcos Cueto, 23–51. Bloomington: Indiana University Press, 1994.

———. "A River of Tears: Corporate Interests and Public Consequences during Rio de Janeiro's First Yellow Fever Outbreak, 1849–1850." Paper presented at the 1995 meeting of the Latin American Studies Association, Washington, D.C., September 28–30.

Wilson, Adrian. *The Making of Man-Midwifery: Childbirth in England, 1660–1770.* London: University of California Press, 1995.

Winant, Howard. *Racial Conditions: Politics, Theory, Comparisons.* Minneapolis: University of Minnesota Press, 1994.

Winslow, Charles-Edward Amory. *The Conquest of Epidemic Disease: A Chapter in the History of Ideas.* Madison: University of Wisconsin Press, 1980.

"Women in Latin America." *Signs* 5 (1979): 1–204.

Wood, Charles H., and José Alberto Magno de Carvalho. *The Demography of Inequality in Brazil.* Cambridge: Cambridge University Press, 1988.

Worboys, Michael. "The Emergence of Tropical Medicine: A Study of the Establishment of a Scientific Specialty." In *Perspectives on the Emergence of Scientific Disciplines,* ed. G. Lemaine et al., 75–98. The Hague: Mouton, 1976.

———. "Science and British Colonial Imperialism, 1895–1940." Ph.D. dissertation, University of London, 1979.

———. "The Emergence and Early Development of Parasitology." In *Parasitology: A Global Perspective,* ed. Kenneth S. Warren and John Z. Bowers, 1–18. New York: Springer-Verlag, 1983.

———. "Tropical Diseases." In *Companion Encyclopedia of the History of Medicine,* ed. W. F. Bynum and Roy Porter, 512–536. London: Routledge, 1994.

Wright, Winthrop R. *Café con Leche: Race, Class, and National Image in Venezuela.* Austin: University of Texas Press, 1993.

Yoeli, M. "The Evolution of Tropical Medicine: A Historical Perspective." *Bulletin of the New York Academy of Medicine* 48 (1972): 1231–1246.

Young, Robert J. C. *Colonial Desire: Hybridity in Theory, Culture, and Race.* London: Routledge, 1995.

Zeldin, Theodore. *France 1848–1945.* Oxford: Clarenson, 1973.

INDEX

Abolition, 7, 44, 66–67, 87–88, 134, 144. *See also* Politics; Slavery

Abortion, 118, 126

Acclimatization: Europeans in the tropics, 99

Africa: influences in Brazil, 105–6; as subject of colonial history, 106

Agassiz, Louis, 85

Agriculture: production in Brazil, 87–89, 165; women's participation in, 131. *See also* Women

Ainhum, 89, 99, 237 n.92. *See also* Diseases

Allopathic medicine, 179

Alvares dos Santos, Luís: in debate over positivism, 144–50

A Mulher, 134

Anais Brasilenses de Medicina, 42, 45, 77, 164, 203–4 n.98

Anais de Medicina do Rio de Janeiro, 18

Anajatuba: leper colony, 102

Andrade e Silva, José Bonifácio de: on Brazilian university system, 155

Andrews, George Reid, 106

Anesthesia: development of, 32, 34; used in childbirth, 118, 122–24. *See also* Drugs; Women's health

Anoxemia: as cause of beriberi, 59–60; as explanation of Brazilian degeneracy, 95–97. *See also* Degeneracy; Diseases; Pereira, Antônio Pacífico

Anthropology: criminal, 166 (*see also* Criminality; Legal medicine); in development of scientific racism, 102, 104, 166 (*see also* Race; Scientific racism); in historical writing, 6 (*see also* Historiography)

Anticlericalism, 147. *See also* Catholic Church; Politics; Religion

Antisepsis: application of method in Brazil, 31–34; development of, 25; in female disorders, 116, 119, 123–24. *See also* Lister, Joseph; Women's health

Aparadeiras. See Midwifery

Araroba, 37, 153. *See also* Brazilian pharmacopoeia

Atavism: atavistic inheritance, 103

Australia: research of Joseph Bancroft, 73–75. *See also* Bancroft, Joseph

Austria: influence on Brazilian medicine, 153. *See also* Germany

Autopsy, 31, 47, 58, 64, 133, 153

Azevedo, Fernando de, 155

Bacteriology, 1, 4, 48; in childbirth, 119; in explanation of berberi, 51–63; new

Julyan Peard is Associate Professor with the Department
of History at San Francisco State University.

Library of Congress Cataloging-in-Publication Data
Peard, Julyan G.
Race, place, and medicine : the idea of the tropics in
nineteenth-century Brazilian medicine / Julyan G. Peard.
p.   cm.
Includes bibliographical references and index.
ISBN 0-8223-2376-1 (alk. paper). —
ISBN 0-8223-2397-4 (pbk. : alk. paper)
1. Escola Tropicalista Bahiana—History—19th century.   2. Tropical
medicine—Brazil—Bahia (State)—History—19th century.   3. Medicine—
Brazil—Bahia (State)—History—19th century.   I. Title.
RC962.B6P43   1999
616.9′883′098109034—dc21   99-34867   CIP